DOUBT IS THEIR PRODUCT

DOUBT

HOW INDUSTRY'S ASSAULT ON SCIENCE

IS THEIR

THREATENS YOUR HEALTH

PRODUCT

DAVID MICHAELS

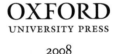

OXFORD
UNIVERSITY PRESS
2008

OXFORD

UNIVERSITY PRESS

Oxford University Press, Inc., publishes works that further
Oxford University's objective of excellence
in research, scholarship, and education.

Oxford   New York
Auckland   Cape Town   Dar es Salaam   Hong Kong   Karachi
Kuala Lumpur   Madrid   Melbourne   Mexico City   Nairobi
New Delhi   Shanghai   Taipei   Toronto

With offices in
Argentina   Austria   Brazil   Chile   Czech Republic   France   Greece
Guatemala   Hungary   Italy   Japan   Poland   Portugal   Singapore
South Korea   Switzerland   Thailand   Turkey   Ukraine   Vietnam

Copyright © 2008 by Oxford University Press, Inc.

Published by Oxford University Press, Inc.
198 Madison Avenue, New York, New York 10016

www.oup.com

Oxford is a registered trademark of Oxford University Press

Library of Congress Cataloging-in-Publication Data
Michaels, David, 1954–
Doubt is their product : how industry's assault on science
threatens your health / by David Michaels.
p. ; cm.
Includes bibliographical references.
ISBN 978-0-19-530067-3
1. Industrial toxicology—United States.   2. Environmental health—United States.
3. Science and industry—United States.   4. Lobbying—United States.
5. Health risk assessment—United States.
[DNLM: 1. Environmental Pollution—adverse effects—United States.
2. Carcinogens—toxicity—United States.   3. Industry—standards—United States.
4. Liability, Legal—United States.   5. Lobbying—United States.
6. Public Policy—United States. WA 670 M621d 2007] I. Title.
RA1229.M53 2007
615.9'02—dc22   2007010959

1 3 5 7 9 8 6 4 2

Printed in the United States of America
on acid-free paper

For Gail,
Joel, and Lila

Contents

Introduction: "Sound Science" or "Sounds Like Science"?

Since 1986 every bottle of aspirin sold in the United States has included a label advising parents that consumption by children with viral illnesses greatly increases their risk of developing Reye's syndrome, a serious illness that often involves sudden damage to the brain or liver. Before that mandatory warning was required by the Food and Drug Administration (FDA), the toll from this disease was substantial: In one year—1980—555 cases were reported, and many others quite likely occurred but went unreported because the syndrome is easily misdiagnosed. One in three diagnosed children died.[1]

Today, less than a handful of Reye's syndrome cases are reported each year—a public health triumph, surely, but a bittersweet one because an untold number of children died or were disabled while the aspirin manufacturers delayed the FDA's regulation by arguing that the science establishing the aspirin link was incomplete, uncertain, and unclear. The industry raised seventeen specific "flaws" in the studies and insisted that more reliable ones were needed.[2] The *medical community* knew of the danger, thanks to an alert issued by the Centers for Disease Control (CDC), but *parents* were kept in the dark. Despite a federal advisory committee's concurrence with the CDC's conclusions about the link with aspirin, the industry even issued a public service announcement claiming "We *do* know that *no* medication has been *proven* to cause Reyes" (emphasis in the original).[3] This campaign and the dilatory procedures of the White House's Office of Management and Budget delayed a public education program for two years and mandatory labels for two more.[4] Only litigation by Public Citizen's Health Research Group forced the recalcitrant Reagan Administration to act. Thousands of lives have now been saved—but only after hundreds had been lost.

Of course, the aspirin manufacturers did not invent the strategy of preventing or postponing the regulation of hazardous products by questioning the science that reveals the hazards in the first place. I call this strategy "manufacturing uncertainty"; individual companies—and entire industries—have been practicing it for decades. Without a doubt, Big Tobacco has manufactured more uncertainty over a longer period and more effectively than any other industry. The title of this book comes from a phrase unwisely committed to paper by a cigarette executive: "*Doubt is our product* since it is the best means of competing with the 'body of fact' that exists in the minds of the general public. It is also the means of establishing a controversy" (emphasis added).[5]

There you have it: the proverbial smoking gun. Big Tobacco, left now without a stitch of credibility or public esteem, has finally abandoned its strategy, but it showed the way. The practices it perfected are alive and well and ubiquitous today. We see this growing trend that disingenuously demands *proof* over precaution in the realm of public health. In field after field, year after year, conclusions that might support regulation are always disputed. Animal data are deemed not relevant, human data not representative, and exposure data not reliable. Whatever the story—global warming, sugar and obesity, secondhand smoke—scientists in what I call the "product defense industry" prepare for the release of unfavorable studies even before the studies are published. Public relations experts feed these for-hire scientists contrarian sound bites that play well with reporters, who are mired in the trap of believing there must be two sides to every story. Maybe there are two sides—and maybe one has been bought and paid for.

* * *

As it happens, I have had the opportunity to witness what is going on at close range. In the Clinton administration, I served as Assistant Secretary for Environment, Safety, and Health in the Department of Energy (DOE), the chief safety officer for the nation's nuclear weapons facilities. I ran the process through which we issued a strong new rule to prevent chronic beryllium disease, a debilitating and sometimes fatal lung disease prevalent among nuclear weapons workers. The industry's hired guns acknowledged that the current exposure standard for beryllium is not protective for employees. Nevertheless, they claimed, it should not be lowered by *any* amount until we know with certainty what the exact final number should be.

As a worker, how would you like to be on the receiving end of this logic?

Christie Todd Whitman, the first head of the Environmental Protection Agency under the second President Bush, once said, "The absence of certainty is not an excuse to do nothing."[6] But it is. Quite simply, the regulatory agencies in Washington, D.C., are intimidated and outgunned—and quiescent. While it is true that industry's uncertainty campaigns exert their influence regardless of the party in power in the nation's capital, I believe it is fair to say that, in the administration of President George W. Bush, corporate interests successfully infiltrated the federal government from top to bottom and shaped government science policies to their desires as never before. In October 2002 I was the first author of an editorial in *Science* that alerted the scientific community to the replacement of national experts in pediatric lead poisoning with lead industry consultants on the pertinent advisory committee.[7] Other such attempts to stack advisory panels with individuals chosen for their commitment to a cause—rather than for their expertise—abound.

Industry has learned that debating the *science* is much easier and more effective than debating the *policy*. Take global warming, for example. The vast majority of climate scientists believe there is adequate evidence of global warming to justify immediate intervention to reduce the human contribution. They understand that waiting for absolute certainty is far riskier—and potentially far more expensive—than acting responsibly now to control the causes of climate change. Opponents of action, led by the fossil fuels industry, delayed this policy debate by challenging the science with a classic uncertainty campaign. I need cite only a cynical memo that Republican political consultant Frank Luntz delivered to his clients in early 2003. In "Winning the Global Warming Debate," Luntz wrote the following: "Voters believe that there is *no consensus* about global warming within the scientific community. Should the public come to believe that the scientific issues are settled, their views about global warming will change accordingly. Therefore, *you need to continue to make the lack of scientific certainty a primary issue in the debate. . . . The scientific debate is closing [against us] but not yet closed. There is still a window of opportunity to challenge the science*" (emphasis in original).[8]

Sound familiar? In reality, there is a great deal of consensus among climate scientists about climate change, but Luntz understood that his clients can oppose (and delay) regulation without being branded as antienvironmental by simply manufacturing uncertainty.

* * *

Polluters and manufacturers of dangerous products tout "sound science," but what they are promoting just *sounds like science* but isn't. Only the truly naïve (if there are any of these folks left) will be surprised to learn that the sound science movement was the brainchild of Big Tobacco, as we shall see. While these corporations and trade associations are always on the side of sound science, everyone else in the public health field, according to this construct, favors "junk science." Posthumously, George Orwell has given us a word for such rhetoric. The vilification of any research that might threaten corporate interests as "junk science" and the sanctification of its own bought-and-paid-for research as "sound science" is indeed Orwellian—and nothing less than standard operating procedure today. But to give credit where credit is due, the sound science/junk science dichotomy has worked wonders as a public relations gimmick and has gained widespread acceptance in the current debate over the use of scientific evidence in public policy.[9]

We are at a crossroads, I believe. The scientific enterprise is at a crossroads. We need to understand what is going on in the name of "sound science" and what the consequences may be—and have already been—for public health. At its heart, this book documents the way in which product defense consultants have shaped and skewed the scientific literature, manufactured and magnified scientific uncertainty, and influenced policy decisions to the advantage of polluters and the manufacturers of dangerous products.

During my service at the Department of Energy, I was the chief architect of the historic initiative to compensate nuclear weapons workers who developed cancer and other diseases as a result of their work protecting America's security. In addition, my research has contributed to the scientific literature on the health effects of exposure to asbestos and lead. I have been in the middle of the national debates over the regulation of beryllium, chromium, and diacetyl (the chemical in artificial butter flavor that is destroying workers' lungs) and a leader in the science community's response to the Bush administration's attempts to stack scientific advisory committees and weaken federal regulatory agencies. All are the subject of this book. I have reluctantly omitted many other sagas equally damning but in which I have had no involvement.

Throughout, I have included what may be an overabundance of references, but I make some strong claims and raise questions about the motives of some scientists and corporations along the way. I have been very careful to document these claims. I have posted many important unpublished documents, including the "smoking guns" that support these assertions, at www. DefendingScience.org, the website of the George Washington University School of Public Health and Health Services' Project on Scientific Knowledge and Public Policy. These documents provide much additional and damning detail. I wish I could promise that the documents will be available on this website in perpetuity, but that is not the way the web or the world works. Regardless, you can rest assured that every story and every outrage presented in this book is absolutely true.

DOUBT IS THEIR PRODUCT

1

The Manufacture of Doubt

What did Big Tobacco know, and when did it know it? Lengthy books have been written to answer this question, but the short answer is "enough—and early." For decades, cigarette manufacturers have known that their product is hazardous to our health, did not care, and took whatever measures were necessary to protect their profits. The industry's scientists were not surprised in the least by the U.S. Surgeon General's famous report in 1964,[1] which made crystal clear to the public the compelling conclusions of the scientific community. In fact, Big Tobacco knew the facts about smoking better than anyone. In their public statements, however, tobacco executives and their public relations coconspirators fudged, weaved, bobbed, and roped-a-dope almost to perfection.

In the 1970s, a decade after the famous report, researchers were hard at work trying to create the "safe" cigarette.[2] Safe from what? From the health hazards that were "not a statement of fact but *merely an hypothesis*" [emphasis in original], in the words of a Brown and Williamson Tobacco Corporation (B&W) public relations statement.[3] In the eighties, the industry's PR firms created the "sound science" movement as just one aspect of the all-out war declared on the regulation of secondhand smoke. In the nineties Big Tobacco beat down the FDA, the EPA, and OSHA. In 1994 Thomas Sandefur, the chairman and CEO of Brown and Williamson, sat before a committee of the U.S. House of Representatives and said with a straight face, "I do not believe that nicotine is addictive. . . . Nicotine is a very important constituent in the cigarette smoke for taste."[4] (For Jeffrey Wigand,

3

a former B&W scientist, this testimony was the final straw. He later approached *60 Minutes* with his inside knowledge of the industry deceit. Wigand's story first became a magazine article in *Vanity Fair*[5] and then a movie, *The Insider*, with Russell Crowe as Wigand and Al Pacino as Lowell Bergman, the *60 Minutes* producer who saw his story about Wigand quashed by executives of Westinghouse, CBS's corporate parent.)

For almost half a century, the tobacco companies hired consultants and scientists—swarms of them, in times of greatest peril—initially to deny (sometimes under oath) that smokers were at greater risk of dying of lung cancer and heart disease, then to refute the evidence that secondhand smoke increases disease risk in *nonsmokers*. The industry and its scientists manufactured uncertainty by questioning every study, dissecting every method, and disputing every conclusion. What they could not question was the enormous, obvious casualty count—the thousands of smokers who die every day from a disease directly related to their habit—but no matter. Despite the overwhelming scientific evidence, the tobacco industry was able to wage a campaign that successfully delayed regulation and victim compensation for decades—and it is still doing so.[6–9]

Tobacco wins the prize—hands down. No industry has employed the strategy of promoting doubt and uncertainty more effectively, for a longer period, and with more serious consequences. That last qualifier about consequences is what sets the tobacco story apart from, say, asbestos, or chromium, or beryllium. As a later Surgeon General's report concluded, "Smoking is responsible for more than one of every six deaths in the United States. Smoking remains the single most important preventable cause of death in our society."[10]

The number is still correct; the superlative is still the case.[11] Let's see how Big Tobacco accomplished this feat.

* * *

Practically from the moment people began smoking "certain dried leaves," as Columbus referred to one gift received from the indigenous residents of the New World (and unwittingly discarded), it became apparent that long-term smokers could pay a price for whatever benefits they received in return. By the eighteenth century, doctors were writing about the oral tumors of the mouth and throat that seemed to afflict smokers, although many therapeutic effects were attributed to smoking at the time. The much lower life spans of that era, along with a lower incidence of smoking, somewhat concealed the mortality risk itself, but by the twentieth century, alert observers were beginning to wonder about that as well. In 1938 a study by a Johns Hopkins University scientist suggested a strongly negative correlation between smoking and lifespan.[12] The Associated Press wire service picked up this story, but it was generally ignored—or actively suppressed, in the view of George

Seldes, foreign correspondent in the 1920s who turned muckraking press critic in the thirties. Seldes accused the press of caving in to the tobacco companies, all of whom bought reams of evocative advertising featuring happy smokers, similar to claims that producers of patent medicines made at the turn of the century. Incensed, Seldes started a newsletter in 1941, in which he published dozens of stories over the following decade linking tobacco to disease and premature death.[13]

In 1950 the scientific picture changed dramatically: Five studies in which smoking was powerfully implicated in the causation of lung cancer were published that year.[14–18] Among these was Richard Doll and Austin Bradford Hill's now classic paper "Smoking and Carcinoma of the Lung," which appeared in the *British Medical Journal.* Doll and Hill reported that heavy smokers were fifty times as likely as nonsmokers to contract lung cancer.[14] In 1952, researchers demonstrated that cigarette smoke "tar" painted on the backs of mice produced tumors, and the industry soon responded by introducing new, filtered cigarettes. By the following year, thirteen alarming case-control studies comparing smoking rates among smokers and non-smokers were circulating through the scientific community (and therefore the tobacco industry). Because association is not necessarily *causation,* however, there were many questions, What was the mechanism by which the tobacco smoke caused cancer? Were there other factors associated with both lung cancer and tobacco that might be responsible? Was there something in one's constitution (which today we would explain as genetic) that increased both lung cancer risk and the propensity to smoke? If so, then smoking would not cause lung cancer; a third factor would cause them both. Smoking apparently increased risk not just of lung cancer but of a host of other diseases as well. To some researchers steeped in infectious disease epidemiology, it seemed implausible that many different diseases could be associated with a single cause.[19]

At the time, tobacco growers and cigarette manufacturers did not have even a trade association, primarily because they feared running afoul of antitrust legislation.[20] Wake up! cried John Hill of the public relations firm Hill and Knowlton (H&K). Get organized! In December 1953 he warned tobacco industry officials of big trouble looming just over the horizon. (Two years earlier, the chemical industry had hired Hill and Knowlton to handle the response to a well-publicized investigation by Representative James Delaney (D-NY) into carcinogens in the nation's food supply, a probe prompted by public concern about additives that had proven carcinogenic in animals.[21,22])

In 1953, with his success holding off Congressional action on food contamination, John Hill and his colleagues were well positioned to design a new campaign to convince the world that cigarette smoking is not dangerous.

For starters, Hill warned the cigarette companies that they needed to embrace the principle that "public health is paramount to all else." They should issue a statement to that effect. He shrewdly suggested that the word "research" be included in the name of a new committee, and indeed the Tobacco Industry Research Committee (TIRC; later renamed the Council for Tobacco Research, or CTR) was soon up and running.[8,20]

"Will the companies agree to sponsor new research which will provide definite answers to the charges?" Hill asked. On this question, a "clear-cut answer" was "deferred for the time being," he wrote, because the industry was confident it could supply "comprehensive and authoritative scientific material which completely refutes the health charges." Nevertheless, Hill had his doubts—and wisely so. Where was this research? He told the companies to get busy with a PR campaign that would be "pro-cigarette" and not merely defensive.[20] The only way they could fight science was *with* science. This prescient judgment was surely correct—but there was one catch. Could the industry come up with better science that independent observers would recognize as such?

Just six months later, the prospects did not look good. On June 21, 1954, E. Cuyler Hammond and Daniel Horn of the American Cancer Society (ACS) presented to the American Medical Association (AMA) the findings of the largest and most rigorous study to date on tobacco and health.[23] The conclusions from the study of the causes of death among 187,766 white men ages fifty to sixty-nine, who had been previously interviewed by twenty-two thousand ACS volunteers around the country, were so dramatic and so incendiary that the survey had actually been halted so the news could be published. Cigarette smokers had 52 percent more deaths (3,000 instead of 1,980). The heavier the smoking, the heavier the consequences. The Hammond-Horn report, published later that year in the *Journal of the American Medical Association (JAMA)*, made headlines around the country, and that should have been the end of the debate about whether smoking is dangerous.[24] Then and there, in 1954, every scientist and every executive should have said, "Yes, more research is needed, but until we find out that these results are incorrect, let's assume that cigarettes are killers and treat them accordingly."

At the AMA convention, Dr. Charles S. Cameron, medical and scientific director of the American Cancer Society, downplayed the call for action that was implicit within the study, which he had previously lauded. "Personally," Cameron said, "I believe that a life of outward productiveness and inward serenity is more important than how long a life is, and therefore I could not try to convert anyone from what he believes contributes to his productivity and his happiness."[23] With complicated statistics, he minimized the significance of the risks from smoking, while the public would have been better served if he had put the issue this way: A lifetime of smoking decreases a man's lifespan by six to eight years on average. Perhaps that might have gotten the attention of Joe Two-Pack.

Or maybe not—because Big Tobacco was on the case now. The Tobacco Industry Research Committee responded cautiously to the Hammond-Horn report. Shortly before the AMA convention bombshell, Dr. Clarence Cook Little, former ACS director, was named scientific director for the industry's committee.[25] (Little had been forced out of his ACS position a decade earlier by Mary Lasker, who led the effort to turn ACS into a powerful volunteer health organization. Lasker went on to become one of the leading figures in the philanthropic support of medical research; ironically, her fortune derived from the work of her husband, the advertising executive who transformed Lucky Strikes into the nation's leading brand of cigarettes.[9])

In responding to Hammond-Horn on behalf of the tobacco industry, Dr. Little called for "greatly extended, amplified and diversified basic research on the relation of various habits of the different types of human beings to their health and well-being throughout their life cycle." The greatest need was for "further experimentation wisely conceived, patiently executed, and fearlessly and impartially interpreted in our search for truth."[23]

How about some honest research on *cigarettes?* That was not part of the agenda, however. Nor was any aspect of the industry's uncertainty campaign ever guided by the glowing principles set forth in Dr. Little's statement. If they had been, imagine the positive impact of Dr. Cameron's blunt statement that the Hammond-Horn results "appear to be of first importance in consideration of the changing death rates of the past 25 years. If further validated, they point the way to the means of still further lengthening man's life span."[23]

Indeed they did, but instead of industry research wisely conceived, patiently executed, and fearlessly and impartially interpreted in our search for truth—truth that might have saved hundreds of thousands of lives—the public and the scientific community got something else instead. Here I would like to cite some headlines from "Reports on Tobacco and Health Research," a rather short-lived journal published under the auspices of the Tobacco Institute. The primary audience was doctors and scientists, but also the news media; many of the articles reported information taken from published papers or unpublished presentations delivered at scientific meetings.[26] Remember that these headlines and the studies they describe date from 1961 to 1964, years after Dr. Little's clarion promise of cooperation in the search for truth:

- "Cancer Personality Pattern Is Reported to Begin in Childhood" (the report of a Scottish psychologist)[27]
- "Lung Specialist Cites 28 Reasons for Doubting Cigarette-Cancer Link"[27]
- "Test Results: Smoking Fails to Raise Cholesterol Levels"[27]
- "Inhalation Tests Fail to Cause Lung Cancer; Virus Suggested"[28]
- "Scientists Report Lung Cancer Rise Linked to Decline in TB"[29]
- "Marital Data Show 'Fallacy' of Using Correlations to Find Disease Causes"[30]
- "Psychological, Familial Factors May Have Roles in Lung Cancer"[31]
- "Measles Virus Proposed as Cause of Emphysema" (this from a New York internist)[27]
- "Smokers, Non-Smokers Differ in Weight, Size" (this from a Harvard anthropologist)[32]
- "March Birth, Lung Cancer Linked" (a Dutch study)[32]

The list goes on and on:

- "Heart Rate Deaths Reported Levelling [*sic*]; Elderly Smokers' Health Studied"[32]
- "Miners' Lung Cancers Triple Average"[32]
- "Smoke 'Tars' Give Negative Results"[32]
- "Do British Doctors Smoke More or Less Than Other Graduates?" (This study refuted the idea that doctors smoke less because of their "special knowledge" of the alleged health hazards.)[32]
- "Rare Fungus Infection Mimics Lung Cancer" (Two Toronto physicians studied three cases.)[32]
- "Follow-up Study Sheds New Light on Smoking and Infant Survival" (This study from a University of California biostatistician showed that small babies of smoking mothers were much *less* likely to die than those born to nonsmokers.)[33]
- "Lung Cancer Rare in Bald Men" (Two New Orleans physicians conducted this research.)[33]
- "Massive German Study Points to Occupational Hazards in Lung Cancer"[33]
- "Nicotine Effect Is Like Exercise"[33]
- "Scientist Links Amount of Smoking with Degree of Extroversion/ Personality Types, Cancer Also Found Associated"[34]
- "Reverse Smokers Are Free of Cancer" (The head of Harvard's Forsyth Dental Center conducted this study of Caribbean smokers who inhale from the lighted end.)[34]
- "English Surgeon Links Urbanization to Lung Cancer"[34]

- "In 4,012 Cancer Autopsies…Find 26% Metastasize to Lung"[34]
- "Finds Occupational Tie in Lung, Gastric Cancer"[35]
- "Nearly Half of 1,000 Lung Cancer Cases Found to Be Non-Smokers"[35]

Some of these studies sound reasonably plausible, whereas some sound ludicrous, but all of them were motivated by the same principle: Find other causes for disease, find smokers who do not have disease, find new associations of whatever sort, find this, find that, find *anything*—but the truth. Also and always contest the methods that epidemiologists used. Argue that "expectation-led" interviewers bias results.[36,37] And because everyone knows our memories are faulty, emphasize "recall bias."[38] Industry documents argued that this bias was the Achilles' heel of epidemiology, and that "failure to consider how the peculiarities of memory affect the studies underlying the policy decisions may fatally flaw the policies themselves." As Hill and Knowlton promised, the headlines "strongly call out the point—Controversy! Contradiction! Other Factors! Unknowns!"[26]

The industry understood that the public is in no position to distinguish good science from bad. Create doubt, uncertainty, and confusion. Throw mud at the "antismoking" research under the assumption that some of it is bound to stick. And buy time, lots of time, in the bargain.

All that said, one means by which science moves toward the real truth is by challenging and disproving supposed truth and received wisdom. It is certainly legitimate for scientists to work to prove one hypothesis in the cause of disproving another. Nor was the industry alone in its search for other causes of lung cancer that might work in tandem with smoking or even be the actual cause of the disease among smokers—"confounders" is the technical term. Moreover, because the question was important, academic researchers were also busily searching for confounders. So couldn't the industry's research of half a century be seen in this light—as a legitimate effort to disprove the correlation of smoking and disease? The answer is a no. The millions of pages of Big Tobacco's internal documents and studies that have come to light as a result of lawsuits demonstrate that the industry worked tirelessly for decades to promote only the studies that would support their preordained conclusions and suppress any findings that suggested otherwise.

A full decade passed between the landmark Hammond-Horn report and the even more important U.S. Surgeon General's report of 1964, generally regarded as a turning point in the whole tobacco saga, the moment when the public, including smokers, had no choice but to see the light. A scientific consensus was reached. Forgotten is the fact that the report was actually a fairly moderate document, perhaps not surprisingly, as Big Tobacco was given the right to veto the appointments of the scientists on the report-writing committee. The report made the blunt statement that smoking was associated with a 70 percent increase in the age-specific death rates of males, but it corroborated the link between smoking and lung cancer for men only, as if women's lungs might somehow be different.[1]

Former Surgeon General C. Everett Koop, in his foreword to the important book *The Cigarette Papers,* deplored the "sleazy behavior of the tobacco industry in its attempts to discredit legitimate science as part of its overall effort to create controversy and doubt." He plausibly suggested that the public health of the United States would have been much better if the industry had simply shared with the 1964 Surgeon General's committee the scientific studies that it—and it alone—knew to be the best work available at the time.[39] Among the hundreds of secret industry documents cited in *The Cigarette Papers,* he might have been thinking of those in which executives of Brown and Williamson did consider passing along to the Surgeon General the results of its own "safe cigarette" research, commissioned from a laboratory in Geneva. The basic idea in Switzerland was to find a carcinogen-free nicotine-delivery system. The study, titled "A Tentative Hypothesis on Nicotine Addiction," lays out the probable biochemical pathways that would explain the addictive properties of nicotine.[40] The addiction itself was never questioned. After judicious consideration, the company forwarded the incriminating study to the Tobacco Institute Research Committee and other industry bodies—but *not* to the Surgeon General of the United States.[8]

The following year, 1965, Congress passed legislation that required warning labels on all cigarette packages in the United States, another watershed and the first time any such label had been ordered for any retail product in the nation. However, this was no public health triumph; in fact, it was the opposite. The tobacco industry understood that warnings would have little effect on smokers. It used its powerful voice in Washington to craft legislation that ensured that cigarette marketing would continue unabated. In the same bill that required warning labels, Congress prohibited the Federal Trade Commission from regulating tobacco advertising and barred state and local governments from taking any action on cigarette labeling or advertising.[41,42] Given the warnings now printed on every pack, smokers could hardly argue that they had been deceived by the cigarette makers. Many subsequent tobacco lawsuits turned on whether the disease predated the 1966 warning labels.

The industry would use the label for legal purposes while simultaneously denying the charges and muddying the waters at every opportunity. Perhaps my favorite of the many, many self-incriminating documents uncovered in the forty million pages now in the public domain (mostly as a result of discovery during litigation; I have not read all of them, I admit) is the 1969 memo in which an executive gloated, "Doubt is our product since it is the best means of competing with the 'body of fact' that exists in the minds of the general public. It is also the means of establishing a controversy."[43]

Another personal favorite is a letter dated 1972, in which a staffer for the Tobacco Institute wrote to a colleague that the strategy of the past twenty years or so—"litigation, politics, and public opinion"—had been "brilliantly conceived and executed" but was not "a vehicle for victory." It was only a holding action, one based on "creating doubt about the health charge without actually denying it; advocating the public's right to smoke, without actually urging them to take up the practice; encouraging objective scientific research as the only way to resolve the question of health hazard."[44]

There you have it: *creating doubt about the health charge without actually denying it.*

2

Workplace Cancer before OSHA

WAITING FOR THE BODY COUNT

Although not quite as infamous as the tobacco scandal, the asbestos cover-up of the past seventy years or so has been just as tragic in terms of lives diminished and lost. The "magic mineral" is a natural insulator against heat and flame. Currently it is also responsible for one hundred thousand deaths a year worldwide, according to the World Health Organization.[1] Paul Brodeur,[2-4] Barry Castleman,[5] and numerous others[6-10] have documented in damning detail the industry's denigration of the risks associated with asbestos exposure and its efforts over the decades to keep vital information out of the scientific literature and the popular press. No one—not even those subject to litigation today—defends the attitudes and actions of the original asbestos corporations. (Well, almost no one. Former Senate minority leader William Frist, a medical doctor, described the Johns-Manville Corporation and W. R. Grace and Company as "large, reputable companies that have gone bankrupt because of this crisis with the associated job losses" rather than as large, reputable companies that knowingly produced and sold a product that killed thousands of Americans.[11]) As with the tobacco story, I will not retell the whole tragedy. I intend to focus on those aspects that involved the manipulation of science, as well as the absence of responsible corporate behavior in the period before the development of our regulatory system.

Asbestos is a bizarre mineral. It can be crushed into fibers and woven into cloth that is remarkably resistant to heat and fire. From ancient times, its uses were manifest—but so were its hazards. As Roman historian Pliny reports, the earliest producers understood that mining and working with asbestos fibers were deleterious to healthy breathing. With the coming of the industrial era, the uses of asbestos were even more manifest and more numerous—hundreds, perhaps thousands, of products contained and in some cases still contain asbestos—but this popularity only served to amplify the dangers. Perhaps the first authoritative acknowledgment of this down-side in the industrial age was the Annual Report of Her Majesty's Lady Inspectors. This British initiative, dated 1898, described in no uncertain terms the "evil" that asbestos dust posed: "The worker falls into ill-health and sinks away out of sight in no sudden or sensational manner."[12] Asbestos workers did not drop dead on the factory floor. Laboring to breathe, they just faded away—out of sight, out of mind—until a group of dedicated re-searchers and proselytizers brought this outrage to the world's attention.

The sad—outrageous—fact is that the epidemiological research that proved the hazards of working with asbestos fibers had reached critical mass decades *before* virtually every major U.S. manufacturer entered bankruptcy, due mainly to large awards for damages made to asbestos disease victims and their families. There is little question that this enormous human and eco-nomic toll is the direct result of the industry's obdurate, short-sighted program to deny the risks associated with exposure, to delay whenever pos-sible protective regulation of workers, and to denigrate those who stepped forward to speak the truth. They played fast and loose with the science with a vengeance, and they reaped what they sowed, but only after thousands of workers had died.

One of the most famous documents cited by every chronicler of this story is the following admission by the chief actuary of the Prudential Life In-surance Company: "In the practice of American and Canadian life insurance companies asbestos workers are generally declined on account of the assumed health-injurious conditions of the industry."[13] The year was 1918. That early in the saga, the truth was officially out. Anyone in the industry who wanted to know about asbestos-related disease could have known, should have known—and almost certainly did know. By the thirties, the evidence was simply overwhelming. Why then didn't the industry do something? The usual reason: It did not have to. Workers' compensation for occupational "dust diseases" (silicosis and asbestosis) was a rising concern for U.S. em-ployers.[5] Early on, therefore, executives must have decided that they had no choice but to keep plugging the holes in the dam because if it ever broke . . .

One famous smoking gun in the asbestos story comprises the 1934 letters from Vandiver Brown, attorney for Johns-Manville, then one of the world's largest producers of asbestos products, to Dr. Anthony Lanza, the Metropolitan Life Insurance Company's assistant medical director, who had conducted an industry-funded study about both asbestosis and silico-sis, a separate lung disease caused by exposure to silica dust. At that time silicosis was perceived to be an even greater problem for the industry world-wide than was asbestosis. In the infamous Gauley Bridge tunnel episode early in the decade, hundreds of workers had been felled by silicosis—workers who would not have died had they used a "wet drilling" method to hold down the dust levels. Alas, that process slowed down the job, so the construction company used it only when inspectors were present.[6,14] Following the Gauley Bridge episode, states began moving toward classifying silicosis as a compensable disease under their workers' compensation programs. Therefore, the asbestos industry desperately wanted to distance its own asbestos problem from silicosis, and Brown asked Dr. Lanza to include in his published report the assertion that asbestosis was a much milder disease than silicosis.[5] Early in his research Lanza had believed this was the case. By 1934 he knew that the opposite was more likely, as it has turned out to be.[6]

Writing to Lanza about suggested changes for the published report, Brown said, "I am sure that you understand that no one in our organization is suggesting that you alter by one jot or tittle any scientific facts or inevitable conclusions revealed or justified by your preliminary survey. All we ask is that all of the favorable aspects of the survey be included and that none of the unfavorable be intentionally pictured in darker tones than the circumstances justify. I feel confident that we can depend on you . . . to give us this 'break.'"[6]

Vandiver Brown was also in the middle of a dispute regarding the industry's control over the animal studies it was funding at the Saranac Laboratory in upstate New York, the research facility of the Trudeau Sanatorium, the renowned tuberculosis treatment facility directed by the great-grandfather, grandfather, and then father of Garry Trudeau, the muckraking cartoonist who created "Doonesbury."[15] In 1936 Brown wrote Dr. Leroy Gardner, the director of the laboratory, "It is our further understanding that the results obtained will be considered the property of those who are advancing the required funds, who will determine whether, to what extent and in what manner they shall be made public."[5]

* * *

In 1938 Waldemar Dreessen led a team of U.S. Public Health Service (PHS) and state investigators in an epidemiological study of three asbestos textile plants in North Carolina. At the time, the PHS was a quiescent body that was unequipped in every way to face off with the companies.[6] Unfortunately, the study was somewhat compromised by the fact that about 150 workers—more than one-quarter of the workforce—had been fired before the investigators showed up. Nor had these men and women been chosen for termination at random. They were the workers with the longest tenure in the plant and working in the most "exposed" jobs, therefore most likely to have asbestosis. Alerted to the deceit, the PHS was able to track down 69 of the fired employees. Forty-three had asbestosis. Hobbled as they were by the management's scorched-earth employment policy, the investigators were still able to determine that of the workers who had been exposed to a total of 5–10 million particles per cubic foot (mppcf) for more than ten years, 68 percent had asbestosis. In many of the areas the PHS surveyed, the exposure levels often rose to 5 or 10 or occasionally even 100 mppcf. No cases of asbestosis were seen among the few workers (5 in all) who were exposed to less than 5 mppcf for more than ten years.[16]

Dreessen recognized that the percentage of workers with asbestosis "increases greatly with increasing length of employment" and that virtually no one employed at these factories had been there more than 15 years. But averaging 5 mppcf per year, their careers would be short: perhaps 20 or 30 years. At some point in this time frame, they were likely to develop asbestosis.[16]

Yet Dreessen "tentatively" recommended a standard (then called a "threshold value") of 5.0. Why? He concluded that the industry could meet the 5.0 standard with the current technology, and since exposure above that level yielded indisputable disease, the government scientists could perhaps sell that number to the industry.[6] (This was three decades before the creation of the Occupational Safety and Health Administration [OSHA]). The Public Health Service had no enforcement power whatsoever. In fact, it could not even enter the plants without permission. Considering that many jobs in the industry exposed workers to levels many times higher than 5 mppcf, reasonable compliance with even that level would have been a public health triumph, relatively speaking. Nevertheless, it did not happen. No one bothers to argue that the 5.0 standard was effectively enforced or even monitored. What happened is that the American Conference of Governmental Industrial Hygienists, despite its name a private organization that made recommendations for voluntary exposure limits, adopted Dreessen's insufficient "tentative" standard in 1946, and it remained the only one, official or otherwise, enforced or unenforced, for more than twenty years. By then it was too late. An exposure limit that was far too lenient in the first place, combined with lax observance and enforcement, yielded the epidemic in asbestos disease with which we are dealing to this day.

In 1947 the Industrial Hygiene Foundation (a research group that worked for various employer trade associations) conducted a far-reaching study under the leadership of W. C. L. Hemeon, with the results intended for use only by its sponsor, the manufacturers who composed the Asbestos Textile Institute. Hemeon did not tell the ATI members what they wished to hear. He said the 5.0 exposure level was insufficiently researched and "*does not* permit complete assurance" of worker safety (emphasis in original).[17]

Indeed it did not. In one of the factories surveyed, where the average exposure level was only 2.0 mppcf—less than half the operative standard—Hemeon found that 20 percent of the workers had asbestosis. Hemeon told the asbestos companies that "a new yardstick of accomplishment" needed to be found "[because] the elimination of future asbestosis depends on the degree of control effected now."[17]

Vandiver Brown, the in-house counsel for Johns-Manville, saw the results differently. He saw a golden opportunity to manufacture uncertainty. In a truly classic example of double-talking, he said in a speech at a Saranac Laboratory symposium, "So far as I have ever been able to ascertain, no one can state with certainty what is the maximum allowable limit for asbestos dust. I am certain no study has been made specifically directed toward ascertaining this figure and I question whether there exists sufficient data correlating the disease to the degree of exposure to warrant any determination that will even approximate accuracy."[18]

Follow the slippery logic here: Because the industry did not want to be held to any standard at all, it simply never conducted the studies that would have ascertained the proper standard. It would then use this *self-imposed* lack of "certainty" to defend itself against regulation and liability. (We will later see exactly the same ploy in other industries.)

* * *

The asbestos industry wanted nothing to do with cancer, which is exactly what the Saranac researchers and others started to find in the 1930s. Director Gardner was "startled" to discover that of eleven white mice inhaling asbestos dust for two years, nine developed pulmonary cancer.[5] But the human evidence started appearing about the same time. Dr. Wilhelm Hueper, a German immigrant toxicologist who became a world-renowned expert in environmental carcinogenesis, identified the correlation between asbestosis and lung cancer in his classic text of 1942, *Occupational Tumors and Allied Disease.*[19] By 1949 both the *Journal of the American Medical Association* and *Scientific American* had cited the evidence that asbestos is a carcinogen.[20,21] Recognition of this relationship progressed faster in Europe; in fact, the wartime Nazi government made asbestos-induced lung cancer a compensable disease.[22]

Following World War II, Johns-Manville pressured Saranac Laboratory to produce a report on the industry-funded research, which included the study with the white mice. The resulting report said not one word about cancer, while including a gratuitous—and utterly false—statement about the nonprogressive character of asbestosis.[23]

In like fashion, the authors of a 1957 study on lung cancer among asbestos miners in Canada removed, at the request of the Quebec Asbestos Mining Association (QAMA), all reference to high rates of lung cancer found in workers with asbestosis. The authors of the study had suggested that one reason for the relatively high rate of cancers might have been the general *underdiagnosis* of asbestosis: the industry did not like the high cancer incidence, but it also did not like the underreporting hypothesis. Ultimately it failed to pursue either possibility.[8]

Apprised of the editorial decision to quash the cancer issue, Dr. Kenneth W. Smith, Johns-Manville's medical director, filed this prescient (but obvious) caveat: "It must be recognized . . . that this report will be subjected to criticism when published because all other authors today correlate lung cancer and cases of asbestosis."[5] Wilhelm Hueper, chief of the National Cancer Institute's Environmental Cancer Section, was the most prominent such voice. He derided the study's "statistical acrobatics."[5] That Canadian study was cited by an oversight committee of the Asbestos Textile Institute as the reason for not funding its own comprehensive study. For one thing, they would receive the results from Canada. For another, as the committee stated in its minutes, "There is a feeling among certain members that such an investigation would stir up a hornet's nest and put the whole industry under suspicion." Finally, "We do not believe there is enough evidence of cancer or asbestosis, or cancer and asbestosis, in this industry to warrant this survey."[24]

A fascinating statement because this was not a document intended for the public; it was the "eyes only" minutes of a meeting. So these were *people deceiving themselves.* In 1957 no insider could have plausibly believed that last statement. Yet here it is. I believe that these asbestos executives needed to believe they were producing a safe product, so they pulled out all of the stops to convince not just the public *but also themselves* that this was the case. Comfortable within this self-delusion, they felt no hesitation to do whatever they could to defeat those people who were threatening their profits. Personal experience and observation also play a key role in these situations. Everyone knew asbestos-exposed workers who did *not* have asbestos-related disease, even after decades of exposure. It is just like cigarettes: "My grandfather smoked till he was eighty, and he was as strong as a bull, so it can't be that harmful." Epidemiological evidence involving statistics is harder to grasp. That is one reason there is always work for epidemiologists. However, the asbestos executives also ignored the obvious when it interfered with their worldview. I suspect this is how William Cooling, treasurer of Canada's Asbestos Corporation, Ltd., viewed the world before dying at age sixty-three of mesothelioma, the almost always fatal cancer of the lining of the chest cavity or of the abdomen and whose only known occupational cause is asbestos exposure.[25]

By consensus, 1964 was the year in which the asbestos industry's decades-long cover-up fell apart. (This was also the year of the landmark

Surgeon General's report on smoking.[26]) It did so almost overnight, at the historic Conference on the Biological Effects of Asbestos, organized for the New York Academy of Sciences by Dr. Irving Selikoff, of Mount Sinai Hospital.[27] Selikoff is the most prominent figure in the entire asbestos saga (perhaps in tandem with Paul Brodeur, whose lengthy article four years later in the *New Yorker* brought Dr. Selikoff and the asbestos scandal and crisis to national attention[28] and whose subsequent 1985 book, *Outrageous Misconduct,* is one of the seminal works in the field[4]).

Almost predictably, the industry tried to silence Dr. Selikoff. Immediately after the conference, industry lawyers wrote to him and urged caution in public discussion of the relationship between asbestos and mesothelioma. The letter discussed the "possibly damaging and misleading news stories" that might be derived from the doctor's statements about asbestos and mesothelioma.[29]

In 1967 Johns-Manville retained the public relations and consulting firm Hill and Knowlton, which, thanks to its experience in defending tobacco, had much to offer the asbestos industry. The firm set up the Asbestos Information Association (AIA). Matt Swetonic, a Johns-Manville public relations staffer who would later become director of H&K's Division of Scientific, Technical, and Environmental Affairs and do extensive work for the tobacco industry, served as the AIA's first full-time executive secretary.[30,31] Years later, when H&K was promoting its product defense expertise to industries facing regulatory challenges, the public relations firm summarized the approach it had developed for the asbestos companies. They advised the industry "to admit to the hazards of asbestos *where they are demonstrable*" (emphasis added).[32] One wonders what advice they would give about any hazard about which there was even a small amount of uncertainty.

In this period, the industry emphasized a new defense of its business: The voluminous body of epidemiologic literature demonstrating asbestos's harmful effects does not pertain to asbestos *products*. Yes, the magic mineral does cause illness among workers processing the raw fiber, but retail products containing these fibers are perfectly safe. In 1968, for example, QAMA, the Canadian trade association, asserted that "Arising from recent press publicity, sometimes ill informed and exaggerated, widespread concern has been expressed, suggesting that the use of certain asbestos products might result in hazards to public health, such as lung cancer. These implications are naturally of great concern to the asbestos industry and it would seem somewhat premature, to say the least, to accept theories of this sort, when not corroborated by unequivocal scientific evidence."[33]

Whatever traction this argument might have had would be convincingly undermined by Dr. Selikoff's 1968 study of workers who installed asbestos insulation, whose lung cancer rate was seven times the expected number.

This was also the study that established conclusively the powerfully syn-ergistic impact of asbestos exposure combined with smoking. Asbestos workers with high exposures who also smoke have *ninety times* as many lung cancers as the nonsmoking population.[34] Both industries looked the other way—except when necessary in the courtroom, where, as we will see later in this chronicle, they might blame each other.

* * *

In the summer of 1979 I ran the program at the Montefiore Medical Center/Albert Einstein College of Medicine in the Bronx that introduced medical students to occupational medicine. As part of that curriculum, we placed the first-year students with the International Chemical Workers Union, which represented workers at the old Calco Chemicals (later called Amer-ican Cyanamid and now Wyeth) plant in Bound Brook, New Jersey. The workers at the factory manufactured, along with many other products, commercial dyes. The students' assignment was to investigate the hazards the workers faced and to design and implement an educational program to reduce these dangers.

Never allowed into the factory, we would meet with the workers in diners and parking lots. The union members told us that the Raritan River down-stream from the factory would run red some days, blue others, and green others, depending on the work product at the time. They also told us about the bladder cancers that were afflicting several of their coworkers and about their lawsuit against DuPont, which produced the chemicals then used in the manufacture of the dyes. These chemicals are known generically as ar-omatic amines (not that they are particularly fragrant, but aromatic is what chemists call molecular structures that are based on the benzene ring). The workers' lawsuits had ended abruptly some years earlier, when DuPont's lawyers produced a letter dated 1947 from a medical director for the com-pany warning the medical director of Calco of the hazards of beta-Naph-thylamine (BNA), one of the chemicals in question. The workers' attorney told them DuPont would have been legally liable only if it had known or should have known of the risk posed by BNA and then failed to tell its cus-tomers. Since it had warned Calco of the dangers, their attorneys explained, DuPont was off the legal hook, and under workers' compensation laws, workers are barred from suing their employer. The men with bladder cancer would have to settle for workers' compensation payments, which would cover their medical bills and only a portion of their lost wages, with no pay-ments for pain and suffering.

One of the workers gave us a copy of the DuPont letter, which contains information that, to my knowledge, had never been made public. The second paragraph begins this way: "The question of health control of em-ployees in the manufacture of Beta Naphthylamine is indeed a grave one.

As you know, we have manufactured Beta Naphthylamine for many years. Of the original group, who began the production of this product, approximately 100% have developed tumors of the bladder."[35]

Now *that* is a smoking gun. Reading the letter for the first time, I stared in disbelief. I knew that the link between the aromatic amines and bladder cancer was well established, but I had never heard of any chemical that caused cancer in every one of a group of exposed workers. Could "100%" have been a typo? Should the number have been 10 percent, bad enough in itself? Either way, the admission by a medical director at DuPont demanded an investigation, and the more I learned, the more appalled I became. The number was not a mistake. The aromatic amines are killers, and the manufacturers knew this and did little until it was too late. In the annals of callous indifference to the health of industrial workers, this story is just as unseemly as the asbestos story, if less well known and affecting fewer people.

* * *

The saga begins in 1856, when William Henry Perkin, an eighteen-year-old British chemistry student, was attempting to synthesize quinine, a drug used throughout the British Empire to prevent malaria, from the coal tar that formerly had been a useless by-product of the distillation of coal to produce gas for lighting. Instead of quinine, however, Perkin came up with a delicate purple solution, which he named mauveine, which the French would shorten to mauve. His discovery became the first commercially feasible synthetic dye and the first of a series of scientific and industrial advances relating to dyes achieved in Europe in the second half of the nineteenth century, thereby creating an important new industry that provided the growing textile industry with bright and inexpensive colors.[36]

Armed with the first patents, the English chemical industry dominated the global dye market—but not for long, as Germany rushed to catch up. Seeing an opportunity for sustained industrial development, the German government built formidable university laboratories to train scientists and provide the basic research the organic chemical industry needed—perhaps the earliest example of a large-scale "industrial policy." With the private sector matching the government's efforts, German scientists soon obtained hundreds of patents. Their nation quickly surpassed the British and dominated the market for decades.[36,37]

The early dye industry was large and profitable, but its importance in economic history stems primarily from its relationship to the development of the synthetic organic chemical industry; aspirin, sulfa drugs, and phenolic resins were all derived from coal tar. The patents and production processes for the new dyes became the basis for the global expansion of organic chemical production, a vast and incalculably important contributor to modern industry and modern life.[38]

However, a darker downside also existed: bladder cancer. The first cases among dye workers were diagnosed in 1895 by Ludwig Rehn, a surgeon in Frankfurt-am-Main, a center of the German chemical industry.[39] Rehn reported that three of the forty-five workers employed in the production of fuchsine, another early purple dye, developed bladder cancer, an exceedingly rare disease at the time. Ten years later he had identified thirty-eight workers with bladder cancer, and other physicians in Germany and Switzerland soon reported dozens of additional cases among dye workers.[40] In those initial reports, the chemical or chemicals responsible for the cancer were the subject of speculation. Published reports consisted primarily of a listing of cases, accompanied by the names of the chemicals to which each worker was known to have been exposed. Over the course of several decades a consensus developed, as reported in the 1921 International Labour Organization (ILO) monograph *Cancer of the Bladder among Workers in Aniline Factories*. Examining the accumulated evidence, the ILO asserted that the chemicals most likely responsible for the cancer cases were benzidine and beta-naphthylamine. It urged "the most rigorous application of hygienic precautions" to prevent further cases from developing.[41]

On this side of the Atlantic, the United States also had a synthetic dye industry in the late 1800s, but these small-scale operators were dominated by the European chemical colossus, primarily because German and Swiss producers controlled virtually all of the important patents in the field. Then came the climactic months of World War I, when U.S. government officials accompanied the conquering U.S. Army into German manufacturing plants, seized their formulas and patents, and then distributed them at low cost to U.S. chemical companies. The recipients of these spoils of war, E. I. du Pont de Nemours and Company, Calco Chemicals, and Allied Chemical and Dye Corporation (later Allied-Signal and now Honeywell) became the three largest synthetic dye producers in the United States, worthy rivals to their European competitors.[42]

DuPont constructed its first organic chemicals factory in Deepwater, New Jersey, across the Delaware River from Wilmington, the center of its booming industrial empire.[43,44] The plant would become known as the Chambers Works, after Arthur Chambers, the chemist who led DuPont's expansion into the dye industry.[44] Among the first chemicals produced there with the newly procured patents were benzidine and BNA. An internal DuPont document describes the workplace in 1919: "[BNA] was cast in open pans, broken with a pick, and transferred by hand into barrels, ground in an open mill, and shoveled by hand into operating equipment. There was no ventilation provided. Gross exposures occurred."[45-47]

DuPont's physicians recognized the first bladder cancers among workers at the Chambers Works in 1932.[45] The cancers may have started appearing some years earlier,[48] but even if they did not, the date is irrelevant. The physicians and executives of all of the U.S. chemical companies were in regular, direct contact with the dye producers of Central Europe and England. It was *their job* to know about the cancer cases in those countries. By 1932 the etiology, treatment, and prevention of the disease had already been discussed at length in numerous epidemiologic studies and review articles published in the medical journals of Britain, Germany, Switzerland, and Austria.[36,40,49] Germany and Switzerland had even made bladder cancer among dye workers a compensable occupational disease in 1925.[40] Most important, the International Labour Organization had published its monograph on occupational bladder cancer in 1921, only a few years after DuPont began dye production at the Chambers Works. The explicit purpose of this report was to inform dye manufacturers around the world about the dangers posed by the production processes.[41]

Despite the wealth of information and warnings, DuPont allowed "gross exposures" to known carcinogens to go unabated for more than a decade at the Chambers Works. The company ultimately made some improvements to its operations in 1934, a few years after the beginning of a cancer epidemic, but significant levels of exposure were nevertheless allowed.[45] Recognizing that the chemicals it produced were extremely dangerous, that same year DuPont also established the Haskell Laboratory for Toxicology and Industrial Medicine, named after Harry Haskell, a DuPont executive who had started the firm's medical division. The Haskell Laboratory remains one of the leading industrial toxicology laboratories in the world. It has supported a series of well-known researchers, the first of whom was Dr. Wilhelm Hueper.[44,47]

Hueper joined DuPont in 1934, more than a year after writing an unsolicited memorandum to Irénée du Pont, great-grandson of E. I. du Pont, suggesting that employees at the Deepwater plant were being exposed to known bladder carcinogens and were likely to develop cancer.[50] Early in his tenure as a DuPont toxicologist, he requested permission to visit the Chambers Works. In his unpublished memoirs he recorded his shocked reaction at some length:

> When the betanaphthylamine [BNA] experiment had been well under way for several months, I requested that I should be shown the incriminated operation in the Chambers Works, so that I could form an enlightened judgment of the occupational hazard. Several associates and I crossed the river a short time later to fulfill this task. The manager and some of his associates brought us first to the building housing this operation, which was located in a part of a much larger building. It was separated from other operations in the building by a

large sliding-door allowing the ready spread of vapors, fumes and dust from the betanaphthylamine operation into the adjacent workrooms. Being impressed during this visit by the surprising cleanliness of the naphthylamine operation, which at that occasion was not actively working, I dropped back in the procession of visitors, until I caught up with the foreman at its end. When I told him 'Your place is surprisingly clean,' he looked at me and commented, 'Doctor, you should have seen it last night; we worked all night to clean it up for you.' The purpose of my visit was thereby almost completely destroyed. What I had been shown was a well-staged performance. I, therefore, approached the manager with the request to see the benzidine operation. After telling him what I just had been told, his initial reluctance to grant my request vanished and we were led a short distance up the road where the benzidine operation was housed in a separate small building. With one look at the place, it became immediately obvious how the workers became exposed. There was the white powdery benzidine on the road, the loading platform, the window sills, on the floor, etc. This revelation ended the visit. After coming back to Wilmington, I wrote a brief memorandum to Mr. Irenee Du Pont describing to him my experience and my disappointment with the attempted deception. There was no answer but I was never allowed again to visit the two operations.[51]

Hueper and his Haskell lab colleagues were soon able to perfect the first experimental animal "model" for chemically induced bladder cancer.[52] Meanwhile, the number of bladder cancers continued to grow, and by 1936 at least eighty-three cases had been diagnosed.[53] But despite the mounting evidence about the culpability of the DuPont operation—or perhaps *because of* the mounting evidence—Hueper's disagreements with the company intensified, and he was not allowed to publish or present data on his work.[47,54]

It is quite likely that the rapid evolution—perhaps "devolution" is a more accurate description—of DuPont's policy on the role of scientific research in its chemical operations was influenced by an earlier episode of occupational disease at the Chambers Works, unrelated to dye production. In the early 1920s DuPont and General Motors, which at the time DuPont partly owned, had agreed to manufacture and distribute leaded gasoline, a product designed to reduce automobile engine knock. DuPont chose the Chambers Works for its production facility. The neurological effects of exposure to the organic lead were so severe and widespread—hallucinations were a common symptom—that workers labeled the plant the "House of Butterflies." The *New York Times* reported that more than three hundred workers had been poisoned, eight of them fatally, during the first two years of production.[55,56]

This may seem like ancient history, but to those workers still employed at Chambers, where they manufactured deadly organic lead for gasoline into the 1980s, it is not. While the most severe lead exposures were eventually controlled at the Chambers Works, the union representing the plant's employees hired me in 1990 to represent them on a management-labor committee that was overseeing a new study of neurological effects among the lead-exposed workers. In that study, researchers from Johns Hopkins documented these effects among workers who were employed *sixty years* after the initial poisonings.[57,58]

The national notoriety of the "House of Butterflies" scandal may have convinced DuPont that occupational disease epidemics would have to be handled differently in the future. Perhaps cover-up and denial would be better for the company, if not for the workers. In any event, the company fired Hueper in 1937, just three years after hiring him to do exactly what he did so splendidly: investigate the relationship between the aromatic amines and bladder cancer.[51,54]

In 1940 the industrial giant considered additional improvements to reduce exposure to aromatic amines but decided to delay any changes, citing World War II as its excuse. No further improvements in the BNA production process were implemented until 1948. Total enclosure of the production line was finally completed in 1951, twenty years after the epidemic was recognized and thirty-plus years after production of the carcinogenic chemicals was begun with full knowledge of the dangers involved.[45,59] The human toll was substantial: at least 450 Chambers Works employees have developed work-related bladder cancer.[60]

After his dismissal, Dr. Hueper incorporated the DuPont research in his 1942 text *Occupational Tumors and Allied Diseases*, the most thorough review of world literature on occupational cancer to date.[19] Outraged by the bladder cancer epidemic at the Chambers Works, Dr. Hueper initially wanted the dedication of the book to read "To the victims of cancer who made things for better living through chemistry"—a caustic allusion to DuPont's well-known advertising slogan, "Better things for better living through chemistry."[50] Perhaps fearful of the company's retribution, in the end he dedicated the book "[t]o the memory of those of our fellow men who have died from occupational disease contracted while making better things for an improved living for others."[47]

Hueper wrote later, with great bitterness, that he believed DuPont had attempted to undermine his scientific credibility and his ability to earn a living by denouncing him first as a Nazi and later as a Communist sympathizer.[51] Any such attempt failed. Hueper served as chief of the National Cancer Institute's Environmental Cancer Section from 1948 until 1964.

His refusal to separate his scientific work from his crusade for a noncarcinogenic environment made him a lightning rod for controversy, but in addition to his groundbreaking work on occupational bladder cancer, he made important contributions in the study of air and water pollution, synthetic hydrocarbons, and food additives. His work provided much of the scientific basis for the "Delaney Clause," as it is known, a 1958 amendment to the Food, Drug, and Cosmetic Act of 1938, which banned any food additive known to cause cancer in animals, no matter how small the exposure.[61]

* * *

While Wilhelm Hueper invented the laboratory method to investigate the carcinogenic properties of aromatic amines, one of England's pioneer epidemiologists, Robert A. M. Case, produced the most important epidemiologic study linking these chemicals with bladder cancer in humans. As Dr. Case recounts the history, by 1938 the British government and the British chemical industry were "totally convinced" that both BNA and benzidine were bladder carcinogens.[62] Hueper's animal studies in the United States were conclusive regarding BNA. No one could deny that link. Still—and no surprise—the industry desired additional data on humans before it would publicly acknowledge that the chemicals caused cancer. (Animal studies are important, but manufacturers often hold out for epidemiological evidence with humans before accepting any label that a substance is a carcinogen. Alternatively, they will hold out for animal studies if the only existing evidence comes from epidemiologic studies.) The looming world war interrupted research in this area, but a gentleman's agreement between the British government and the Association of British Chemical Manufacturers (ABCM) went into effect on January 1, 1939, and provided the equivalent of workers' compensation payments to men who developed occupational bladder cancer. The industry agreed to reduce exposure as much as possible, but it would not halt production or sales.[36,62,63]

After the war Dr. Case received a research fellowship from the British manufacturers' group, with which he designed and conducted one of the first occupational cohort mortality studies, pioneering an approach that has attained widespread usage in occupational epidemiology.[64] He tracked down lists of workers who had been employed years earlier and followed them through time, identifying who had died by the end of the study period. He compared the risk of a worker dying from bladder cancer (and other causes) with the likelihood of a person of the same sex and age, from the general population of England and Wales, dying of these diseases. The results of the study, published in 1954, quantified the excess risk of bladder cancer for the chemical workers exposed to BNA and benzidine and exonerated the chemical aniline as a cause of the disease. As we have seen, previous reports had documented the risk, but none had measured the tremendous excesses.[65]

While examining bladder cancer rates in the general British population, Case focused on Birmingham, England, because it was a large industrial city *without* a significant dye industry. To his surprise, he found twenty-two cases of bladder cancer among the rubber workers in Birmingham. Too many. Only four would have been expected. What was the source problem in these factories? The workers were exposed to antioxidants, chemicals used to slow the oxidation or decay of the rubber. The antioxidants were made from BNA. Almost accidentally, Case had identified an entirely new industry in which aromatic amines were causing bladder cancer among the line workers. The British rubber industry elected not to sponsor a comprehensive cancer study comparable to the one the chemical industry had commissioned, but it acknowledged the problem and eliminated the use of BNA.[66] Unfortunately, it continued to rely on *other* aromatic amines as antioxidants, several of which were later determined to be bladder carcinogens, and rubber workers paid for this practice with increased risk of bladder cancer for years.[66,67]

While Hueper's early animal studies confirmed that BNA was a carcinogen, the early animal studies on benzidine, another dye chemical, were negative.[36] DuPont's toxicologists were also unable to induce bladder cancer with benzidine in a small study involving four dogs,[68] and the epidemiological evidence on the carcinogenicity in humans was strong but not definitive, primarily because few workers were exposed to benzidine *alone;* most (if not all) of them were exposed to BNA as well. Dye manufacturers therefore had the "scientific" cover they needed to exempt benzidine from classification as a human carcinogen and to permit almost unfettered exposure to the chemical.

Hueper believed that the evidence against benzidine was sufficiently strong to mandate action, but Dr. George Gehrmann, DuPont's medical director, declared otherwise at a 1948 international industrial medicine conference: "We feel that it cannot be concluded that Benzidine is a cause of bladder tumours until conclusive proof that Benzidine workers who have developed tumours have never been exposed even in the slightest degree to Beta Naphthylamine (even an old Beta contaminated building constitutes exposure) and that the incidence of bladder tumours in workers exposed to Benzidine is greater than the incidence of idiopathic bladder tumours in such a group."[68]

This is a remarkably disingenuous statement because fifteen years earlier, after a visit to Germany, Dr. Gehrmann had recommended to his employer that it should consider benzidine, along with BNA and aniline, as "the causative materials and take immediate steps to construct all operations so that there shall be absolutely no dust, no fumes nor any skin contacts."[69] What had caused his change of heart? Corporate policy, plain and simple. In an especially unguarded moment in the backseat of a car, the good doctor admitted to two visiting British researchers (one of them, Dr. Case, was pretending to be asleep[69]), "We here know very well that benzidine is causing bladder cancer, but it is company policy to incriminate only the one substance, Beta-naphthylamine."[70]

Soon enough—in 1950—DuPont and the other manufacturers lost their only remaining cover on benzidine when animal studies supported by Allied Chemical provided indisputable evidence that the chemical caused cancer.[71] Allied had been producing both BNA and benzidine for many decades, had known about the risks for many decades, and had done little to protect its employees from several of them. Even now, the managers did not fully modernize and enclose the production line for half a dozen years, and production continued for nearly two decades. As a result, more than one hundred men at Allied's Buffalo facility developed bladder cancer.[47,72,73]

In 1951 the medical officer of Clayton Aniline Company Ltd., the British subsidiary of Ciba Chemicals, the Swiss conglomerate that is now called Novartis, reported that sixty-six workers, including twenty-three who were exposed only to benzidine, had developed bladder cancer.[74] This was perhaps the most powerful epidemiological evidence yet, but the Swiss conglomerate ignored that evidence from the factory they operated in Cincinnati, Ohio. They failed to apply the protective measures in effect in *the conglomerate's own European factories.* Laborers at the Cincinnati plant shoveled benzidine by hand, with no controls provided.[75]

Did the Cincinnati managers feel safe from repercussions because this particular facility was in the United States, not in Europe? It is difficult to avoid this conclusion. When the first cases of bladder cancer were recognized at this facility in 1958, management claimed surprise and subsequently contracted with a group of scientists from the University of Cincinnati to undertake a screening program. (Among this group was Dr. Eula Bingham, who went on to become the head of OSHA during the Carter administration.) Of the twenty-five men who were screened, all but two of whom were working on the benzidine line, thirteen eventually developed bladder cancer.[76] Such radically excessive rates were also detected at a second benzidine manufacturing plant in Ohio owned by the Swiss group.[77] (This work was done by Dr. Thomas Mancuso, a colleague of Hueper and another pioneer in occupational epidemiology.)

Still, change was coming, even at DuPont. The 1954 edition of the textbook *Modern Occupational Medicine,* written and edited by DuPont staff, admitted that BNA caused cancer but maintained that benzidine was only a "suspected cause of tumors."[78] The following year, the company threw in the towel with BNA and terminated production, only four years after introducing new production methods. However, it was not until 1967—seventeen years after the publication of Allied Chemical's indisputable animal studies—that DuPont shut down its production line for benzidine. Even then, it continued to use supplies purchased from other manufacturers for five more years.[79]

This history underscores the limitation of voluntary compliance with workplace health regulation. The aromatic amines were also responsible for bladder cancer outbreaks involving hundreds of cases in Germany, Switzerland, England, France, Italy, Austria, and the former Soviet Union.[40,80] In each country the chronology of events is similar to that in the United States. The carcinogens were regulated or banned only after the epidemics had occurred. But the Europeans were certainly first. Acknowledging that BNA could not be manufactured safely, Switzerland banned its production in 1938, and Great Britain followed suit in 1952.[40]

In the absence of regulation in the United States, DuPont did not stop producing this carcinogen until 1955, and Allied continued to manufacture BNA-containing chemicals through 1955 and to purchase them until 1962.[73] In the absence of regulation in the United States, the Swiss-owned factory in Cincinnati produced benzidine with an operation that neither the government nor management would have tolerated in Switzerland or any other Western European nation.[76] Smaller companies maintained production, often with virtually no protection for their workers, until federal intervention finally began a decade later.[73,81]

3

America Demands Protection

From the beginning, and most famously with Henry David Thoreau's *Walden,* published in 1854, American literature featured evocative testimonies to the awesome beauty of the North American landscape and the intricacy of its ecology. In the twentieth century, however, writers began to sound warning notes, and then in 1962 Rachel Carson hit a national nerve with *Silent Spring.*[1] Almost overnight, the perfect, potent title and Carson's devastating revelations about pesticide blight (DDT, specifically) gave unofficial birth to the environmental movement. The trade-off between economic development on the one hand and the natural world and public health on the other was now front and center for mainstream America, and it has stayed there for more than forty years.

Less than a year following the publication of *Silent Spring,* President John F. Kennedy directed the Presidential Science Advisory Committee to study and make recommendations on the use of pesticides; the group called for more research and a gradual phaseout of all "persistent toxic pesticides."[2] In 1964 the Surgeon General issued his incendiary report on smoking,[3] and the asbestos industry's decades-long cover-up fell apart at the historic conference organized by Dr. Irving Selikoff of Mount Sinai Hospital.[4] As the 1960s progressed, the environmental movement took off. Industry lost its exclusive control of the agenda on environmental and public health issues. In those authority-doubting times, industry's credibility became suspect on every front. Its every action was subjected to much closer scrutiny—and not just by activists and policy wonks. Now members of the news media were watching closely—and the political world was therefore forced to pay attention.

In June 1969 the Cuyahoga River outside Cleveland, Ohio, caught fire. In its prominent coverage of the story, *Time Magazine* described the Cuyahoga as the river that "oozes rather than flows."[5] In fact, it had gone up in flames before, but the times had changed, and now the Cuyahoga became a potent symbol and yet another call to arms. (A couple of years later Randy Newman immortalized the event in a song with the memorable refrain "Burn on, big river, burn on.")

For decades, government at all levels had taken a pass on many far-reaching public health issues. For one thing, there was no real means of enforcement. (For the most part, it was civil litigation that eventually brought the tobacco and asbestos industries to account.) Now the nation's environmental problems could no longer be ignored. *A river on fire?* No political leader could defend or ignore that national embarrassment, which was symbolic of our rapidly deteriorating environment, and the nation took action—and on a bipartisan basis. President Richard Nixon created the Environmental Protection Agency (EPA) and supported the congressional legislation that created the Occupational Safety and Health Administration (OSHA). With the broad support of Democrats and Republicans (who could, after all, read the national opinion polls), the federal government quickly set up the modern regulatory state. Gradually the EPA, OSHA, and a host of agencies known by their acronyms (e.g., MSHA, the Mine Safety and Health Administration; NHTSA, the National Highway Traffic Safety Administration; CPSC, the Consumer Product Safety Commission) were created with the goal of acting *preemptively* to protect the environment and the public's health and safety. The public demanded action in the 1970s and by and large still supports such protection today.

The EPA, the biggest of these new agencies, was given a set of laws to work with, most prominently the Clean Air Act, the Safe Drinking Water Act, the Toxic Substances Control Act, and the Clean Water Act. These laws were not just window dressing, either. Rather, they provided the enforcement agency with real teeth. The Clean Air Act decreed that the EPA should consider only one factor—public health—as it developed its regulations. Any compliance cost to industry was explicitly *not* to be a consideration. The agency banned DDT in 1972,[6] aerosol fluorocarbons in 1978,[7] and PCBs in 1979.[8] That year it also ordered the clean-up of the infamous Love Canal toxic cesspool, on which a housing development had been built in Niagara Falls, New York—a worldwide symbol of industrial indifference.[9,10]

All in all, the seventies were a decade of tremendous improvement in public health and environmental protection. The movement to clean up

America enjoyed strong support from the public and its leaders, and it reversed the deterioration of the nation's air and water. The Clean Air Act charged the EPA with reducing the emissions of six principle air pollutants: nitrogen dioxide, ozone, sulfur dioxide, particulate matter, carbon monoxide, and lead. From 1970 (the year the act was passed) to 2002, total emissions of these six pollutants dropped almost 50 percent.[11] Our rivers and waterways are much cleaner, and the Cuyahoga has not caught fire in years.

The federal system of public health and environmental protection is now under fierce attack, orchestrated by corporate polluters and manufacturers of dangerous products. Given what is going on in the regulatory world today, it is important to remember that the groundwork for these early results was laid by the *Republican* administrations of Presidents Nixon and Ford. President Nixon's initial embrace of the regulatory state was an important component of his strategy to peel components of the labor and environmental movements away from the Democratic Party. Although the key pieces of legislation were enacted by the Democrat-controlled Congress, which monitored the agencies' progress through strong oversight, bipartisan support existed for the entire regulatory endeavor.

The federal rule-making procedure that produced these results was not draconian, however. Out-of-control regulators did not bludgeon industry into submission. Congress charged the agencies with bringing the best possible science to bear on the issues. Even when Congress instructed the EPA to consider only the public's health, the affected parties had (and still have) manifold means of challenging any regulation during the rule-making process and then again in the courts before any rule actually went into effect. Our system of governance does not make regulation easy, nor should it. If anything, the checks and balances built into the system *favor* those affected by regulation.

For OSHA, these were also the halcyon years. Under the trailblazing leadership of Dr. Eula Bingham, the University of Cincinnati toxicologist appointed by President Carter to run the agency, OSHA issued standards for many well-known hazards, including benzene, lead, and cotton dust. When new hazards were identified, OSHA was on the case quickly and proactively. A telling but not widely known example was the identification of an agricultural pesticide known as DBCP (its chemical name is 1,2-dibromo-3-chloropropane) as a potent cause of sterility. I learned the details of the story from a young filmmaker, Josh Hanig, a close friend who died of pancreatic cancer a few years ago. At that time, Josh was making a documentary about occupational health titled *Song of the Canary*.[12] Like miners' canaries, workers in the chemical industry are often the first line of exposure to environmental toxins. Several of the workers at an Occidental

Chemical factory in the San Francisco Bay area revealed to Josh what they had never been comfortable talking about with their friends—that they had been unable to father a baby. Struck by the "coincidence," Josh paid for sperm tests for this informal cohort and found that all seven of the men tested had sperm counts of virtually zero. Josh told me the workers had never been informed of the study by Dow Chemical's toxicologist Theodore Torkelson, who sixteen years earlier had found "testicular atrophy" in lab rats after exposure to DBCP.[13] In September 1977, less than two months after the sperm tests, OSHA issued an emergency temporary standard of 10 parts per billion (ppb).[14]

From the start, however, OSHA recognized that centralized standard setting and top-down enforcement of regulations would never be sufficient. In a world with thousands of toxic chemicals, the agency could never set workplace regulations for all of them, nor could it ever have enough inspectors to visit every workplace on any sort of regular basis. (Right now it has enough inspectors to visit every workplace under its jurisdiction once every 133 years.[15]) Labor unions and local Committees for Occupational Safety and Health (COSHs) demanded "the right to know," asserting that workers could not be protected if they did not know the names and properties of the hazards to which they were exposed, and their employers had no legal obligation to inform them. (In the 1970s these committees, which were union health activist organizations, sprung up in cities with a strong labor presence.) In 1977, therefore, OSHA first proposed a requirement that chemicals be identified and labeled. When Reagan-appointed Labor Department officials shelved the proposal, states and cities around the country started enacting their own right-to-know laws. The chemical industry, recognizing the problems associated with meeting numerous different locality-specific laws, pushed OSHA to issue a national hazard communications standard. This rule, finalized in 1983, requires that employers provide their employees with access to material safety data sheets, which distill into plain English the information workers need in order to protect themselves from toxic exposures.[16]

In 1977 Dr. Bingham also proposed a generic carcinogen standard; simply stated, if a chemical were found to cause cancer in one human study or in two animal studies, it would be declared a human carcinogen and regulated as such until science proved the initial designation wrong.[17] This prudent initiative was derailed by the Supreme Court, however, which ruled in 1980 that OSHA must demonstrate a significant risk associated with each chemical and that the proposed standard would reduce that risk.[18]

This ruling, known as the "benzene decision," in fact handcuffed the agency because establishing each new standard would now take years and thousands of staff-hours to produce. In 1989 OSHA tried to adopt industry's own consensus voluntary (and therefore unenforceable) recommendations as its official and enforceable standards. This initiative was killed by a follow-up judicial ruling that decreed that the agency must indeed conduct a new risk analysis for each individual chemical.[19]

In that era, Congress also addressed the health and safety of the nation's miners, spurred in large measure by an early-morning explosion at Consolidation Coal Company's number nine mine near Farmington, West Virginia. The date was November 20, 1968. Working the midnight shift, 78 miners were entombed beyond any rescue. The mine was sealed several days later. More than 170 other miners lost their lives in less-publicized accidents in the following months.[20] Following these accidents and a series of wildcat strikes in the Appalachian coal fields, Congress passed the Federal Coal Mine Health and Safety Act of 1969, which required at least four inspections of every underground coal mine each year. The act also established a compensation program for miners with pneumoconiosis, more commonly known as black lung.[21]

Again, this initiative of the new Nixon administration was thoroughly bipartisan, closely marking legislation proposed by President Johnson in the last months of his administration. Submitting the proposal to Congress, President Nixon said, "Death in the mines can be as sudden as an explosion or a collapse of a roof and ribs, or it comes insidiously from pneumoconiosis or black lung disease. When a miner leaves his home for work, he and his family must live with the unspoken but always present fear that before the working day is over, he may be crushed or burned to death or suffocated. This acceptance of the possibility of death in the mines has become almost as much a part of the job as the tools and the tunnels. The time has come to replace this fatalism with hope by substituting action for words. Catastrophes in the coal mines are not inevitable. They can be prevented, and they must be prevented."[22]

On May 2, 1972, ninety-one miners died in a tragic fire at the Sunshine silver mine near Kellogg, Idaho. This tragedy highlighted one glaring inadequacy in the 1969 legislation: It provided little protection for workers in the other sorts of mines. This would be remedied with legislation in 1977 that created the Mine Safety and Health Administration, which replaced the Mining Enforcement and Safety Administration and gave real enforcement powers to the regulators.[23] Notably, MSHA inspectors are not required to have a search warrant to enter a workplace. Other employers may require one from an OSHA inspector, however.

* * *

The movie *The Graduate* was released in 1967, just before the beginning of the environmental movement and the regulatory era. In a memorable scene, the not-yet cuckolded Mr. Robinson (Murray Hamilton) gave new college graduate Benjamin Braddock (Dustin Hoffman) one word of advice: "Plastics." That cinematic moment became an iconic joke that invited a generation of rebellious, draft-dodging youths to laugh at such a mundane career choice. A few years later the joke acquired an extra kick when the plastics industry and an infant regulatory agency found themselves embroiled in a crisis with major national repercussions.

Corporate stakeholders, the new agencies, unions, public health officials, environmentalists, and politicians all had a stake in the fight. Is this chemistry as toxic as it is valuable? Because plastics were *new*—the wave of the future for the culture and the economy—the answer was profoundly important. For its part, the manipulation of science by the plastic industry was at least as flagrant and self-serving as the behavior of any other industry I have cited. The industry also claimed that the level of regulation clearly required to protect workers would be financially devastating and might even put companies out of business, with catastrophic results for the entire economy.

What happened? As we shall see, strict environmental controls for vinyl chloride were imposed, and the economy seemed not to notice. Vinyl chloride was regulated, and two years later the headline in the September 1976 issue of *Chemical Week* read: "PVC Rolls out of Jeopardy, into Jubilation."[24] The cost of doing the right thing did not cripple the industry after all. Ben Braddock could have had a good career in plastics. The lesson from this story is that industry itself, to say nothing of its employees and the public, is often well served by a strong regulatory regime. This is a lesson that must be too frequently relearned, as the shareholders of Merck and Company experienced in the years after Vioxx was found to cause heart attacks.

* * *

In October 1961, eight months before *Silent Spring* was serialized in the *New Yorker*, scientists employed by Dow Chemical's Biochemical Research Laboratory published the results of a series of experiments in which laboratory animals (rats and rabbits) were exposed to different levels of vinyl chloride for up to six months. (Vinyl chloride is converted into a resin called polyvinyl chloride, or PVC, which can be extruded [i.e., shaped] into the plastic products sometimes known simply as "vinyl." Vinyl chloride, not PVC, is the primary hazard for employees in the industry.) Chief investigator Theodore Torkelson (the same toxicologist who reported "testicular atrophy" in the rats exposed to DBCP, the chemical that caused low sperm counts in the pesticide workers) detected liver changes in the animals at exposure levels as low as 100 parts per million (ppm); no effects were detected at 50 ppm. In those pre-regulatory years, the industry's recommended (but voluntary) limit for worker exposure was 500 ppm averaged over eight hours. On the basis of the new findings, Dr. Torkelson recommended that the workplace exposure level be lowered to 50 ppm, or one-half the level at which liver changes had been found, but his suggestion was never implemented.[25]

In 1964 Dr. John Creech, who conducted physicals at the B. F. Goodrich polyvinyl chloride plant in Louisville, Kentucky, discovered four cases of acroosteolysis, a rare disease in which some fingers of the victims become progressively shorter as their bones disappear, among workers from the same department. In 1969 a study conducted at the University of Michigan, paid for by the industry, recommended that the exposure threshold for vinyl chloride be lowered to 50 ppm, the same level the Dow researchers had recommended eight years earlier. However, when the study was published in the *Archives of Environmental Health*,[26] the recommendation had mysteriously disappeared.[27]

Confronted with unfriendly science, the industry had simply censored it. It refused to fund more research into the causes of acroosteolysis and disbanded its health advisory committee. The registry that had been created at the University of Michigan was allowed to die. And this was just the beginning. As Gerald Markowitz and David Rosner chronicle in *Deceit and Denial: The Deadly Politics of Industrial Pollution*, their excellent book on the scandalous behavior of the lead and plastics industries, "The reactions of the industry to the link between vinyl chloride and acroosteolysis were a mere preview to how the industry would react when faced with . . . the link between vinyl chloride and cancer. . . . When cancer became an issue . . . the industry moved from denial and obfuscation to outright deception."[27]

None of this research had much impact on workplace exposures, however. When OSHA was created in 1971, for the most part it simply adopted industry's voluntary standards, including 500 ppm for vinyl chloride.

The cancer issues came front and center in 1970, shortly before OSHA's birth. That year, Dr. Pierluigi Viola, an Italian toxicologist, presented a paper at an international cancer research meeting in Houston,[28] reporting that when he and his colleagues exposed rats to 30,000 ppm of vinyl chloride monomer for twelve months, "almost all the animals developed tumors of the skin and lungs."[29] European manufacturers immediately hired Dr. Cesare Maltoni, also an Italian toxicologist, for follow-up experiments. His results were even more alarming. By early 1973 Dr. Maltoni told his sponsors that his group had found tumors, including angiosarcomas of the liver, in experimental animals exposed to levels of vinyl chloride as low as 250 ppm, after eighty-one weeks of observation.[30] This level was half the exposure limit that OSHA permitted at the time. The Europeans conveyed this information to their U.S. counterparts but insisted that the U.S. manufacturers sign an agreement in October 1972 not to release the information without the Europeans' permission.[31,32]

The U.S. vinyl chloride manufacturers were soon in a terrible quandary concerning the still-secret, still-damning animal studies in Italy. In January 1973 the newly formed National Institute for Occupational Safety and Health (an agency created by the OSHA legislation signed by President Nixon) made a formal request for information on the health hazards associated with vinyl chloride. The Europeans still required secrecy, so the industry officials who met with NIOSH came up with this plan: They would reveal the Italian animal studies *only if* they were asked about them.[33,34] Officials from several U.S. chemical companies and the industry's trade association requested a meeting with the director of NIOSH, Dr. Marcus Key. The conference took place on July 11, 1973. The industry plan was a success: The manufacturers were not required to tell Dr. Key about the European studies. One company's representative at the meeting subsequently reported that their "presentation was very well received and the chances of precipitous action by NIOSH on vinyl chloride were materially lessened."[35]

The picture changed dramatically in January 1974, however, when Goodrich informed NIOSH that Dr. John Creech, the physician who had discovered the earlier cases of acroosteolysis at the Goodrich plant in Louisville, had found four cases of angiosarcoma of the liver.[36] This type of cancer is exceedingly rare in humans. It is also one of the cancers that Maltoni had found when he exposed rats to vinyl chloride.[37]

The following month OSHA convened an emergency hearing.[38] Joining forces to demand that the government set an exposure standard for vinyl chloride were Irving Selikoff, the iconic figure most responsible for exposing the asbestos tragedy and scandal ten years earlier, and Thomas Mancuso, another giant in these pages who contributed groundbreaking studies of workers exposed to asbestos, beryllium, chromium, dyes, radiation, rayon, and a host of other toxins while making important contributions to the development of the methodology used in the field. At the emergency hearing Mancuso stated bluntly, "Invariably, whenever a new occupational cancer is discovered, it is played down for fear of alarming the workers and the general public. . . . Nevertheless, from past experience, what happens is that as further [scientific] work is undertaken and information obtained, the problem gets broader and broader with more implications."[39]

Subsequently, OSHA proposed a permanent standard of "no detectable level."[40] Given the instrumentation available at the time, this meant 1 ppm, the equivalent of an ounce of vermouth in eighty thousand gallons of gin. Public hearings on the proposal were scheduled for June 1974. The industry hired Hill and Knowlton to set its strategy, a job not made any easier when NIOSH's Dr. Key realized that the industry had deceived him the previous year by withholding the results of the Italian studies.[41] Thus did the plastics industry find itself in the same straits as many others before it: another corporate emperor with no clothes.

The manufacturers decided to circle the wagons in the way that Hill and Knowlton had perfected for tobacco—by mounting an uncertainty campaign. The industry opposed the 1 ppm proposed standard. It was true that both animal and epidemiological studies confirmed cancer, but none corroborated cancer risk at the lowest exposure levels. (An internal Hill and Knowlton memo to the public affairs committee of the Society of the Plastics Industry [SPI] Vinyl Chloride Committee indicates that this last point might seem to be the clincher, but "it should be remembered that the corollary to this statement is that it has not been scientifically demonstrated that the SPI recommended levels are truly safe."[42]) Industry could live with a 10 ppm standard. Anything lower would be ruinous. Tens of thousands of jobs would be lost: an economic tailspin—another Great Depression. The sky might even fall. Not coincidentally, *Fortune* weighed in with a story titled "On the Horns of the Vinyl Chloride Dilemma," in which the author put the choice before the nation in these harsh terms: "If government allows workers to be exposed to the gas, some of them may die. If it eliminates all exposure a valuable industry may disappear.... [M]edical and economic considerations collide head-on."[43]

Ultimately OSHA gave the industry a small break by setting the exposure level at 1.0 (rather than no detectable level) for vinyl chloride monomer. The agency also required that warning labels be affixed to vinyl chloride containers to alert workers of the cancer hazard.[44] The industry took OSHA to court—the Court of Appeals for the Second Circuit—where it was rebuffed in an opinion written by retired Supreme Court justice Tom Clark, who summarized the saga pretty much as I have here and in equally critical language.[45] The Supreme Court declined to hear industry's appeal, and the new standard went into effect on April 1, 1975.[46]

Industry's predictions of $1 billion in upgrading costs turned out to be greatly exaggerated. A 1995 report on OSHA's "analytic approach" by Congress's Office of Technology Assessment stated, "As events turned out, costs did increase and production capacity was eroded, but only modestly. Furthermore, there was little evidence that the financial status or ability to respond to customer needs in the affected industries had been strained."[47] Perhaps this assessment was even giving a slight benefit of the doubt to the manufacturers. Remember that headline in the September 1976 issue of *Chemical Week:* "PVC Rolls out of Jeopardy, into Jubilation." In this case, the new regulatory system had worked.

4

Why Our Children Are Smarter Than We Are

In *Deceit and Denial: The Deadly Politics of Industrial Pollution*, Gerald Markowitz and David Rosner anoint lead as "the mother of all industrial poisons."[1] It's a tough call, but I agree. The metal is that nasty, and, in the not so recent past, it was that ubiquitous. Lead was in the sky above and the mud below and the waters, too. But not now. Here we have one of the great public health triumphs of the twentieth century. The business with the aromatic amines was frustrating and unnecessary, asbestos a needless tragedy that killed hundreds of thousands around the world, and Big Tobacco the ultimate outrage, but with the health hazards posed by lead the newly empowered regulatory system actually worked—haltingly and over the bitter opposition of the industry. In the end, the science could no longer be denied or distorted. While children are still being exposed to lead, those born in the 1990s have higher IQ scores than those born twenty years earlier because the regulatory system forced the lead out of gasoline.[2,3]

We want as little lead as possible in our bodies. The metal is a potent toxin that affects the brain, the kidney, blood, bones, sperm, everything, and it is especially toxic in rapidly growing bodies—that is, infants and young children.

By the early part of the twentieth century it was both widely utilized and widely known as hazardous to our health. Lead-based paints were acknowledged as a particular problem because paint chips could be eaten by children. Children can also ingest lead from contaminated dirt, but peeling paint and contaminated household dust were (and remain) the most easily identifiable lead hazard. Blood lead levels greater than 70 μg/dl (or micro-grams per deciliter of blood), generally from eating paint chips, can cause seizure, coma, and death in children. Lead exposure also affects behavior and learning abilities, but often without overt symptoms. By the 1920s, all this was well known.

But so what? By the 1930s, several European countries, including France, Belgium, and Austria, had banned or severely restricted the use of white lead (the main culprit) as an ingredient in interior paint, but when the Metropolitan Life Insurance Company wrote openly about the hazards, the U.S. industry successfully pressured the company to shut up. When articles in the *JAMA* and the *American Journal of Disease in Children* gained wide attention, the industry rejected the claims, challenged the proof of causa-tion, defended their products, and even tried to blame the poisoned chil-dren, who were "sub-normal to start with," and irresponsible parents who would allow their children to eat the paint peeling from the walls of poorly maintained homes.[1]

What was the visual emphasis of many of the ads in the all-out PR campaign? Children, of course. As Markowitz and Rosner write, for fifty years the National Lead Company had "linked lead, whiteness, healthiness, prosperity, and purity with its 'pure white lead' paint."[1]

By the 1940s, the paint manufacturers were phasing out lead, but not for health reasons. Lead paint required thorough mixing, so some manufac-turers began marketing ready-to-use paints with zinc and especially tita-nium pigments, which are still widely used today. In 1971 President Nixon signed the Lead-Based Paint Poisoning Prevention Act, which severely restricted the lead content in paint used in housing built with federal money. This legislation also provided funds for the states to establish lead abatement programs.[4]

On the run but still fighting, the industry's public relations flacks—Hill and Knowlton—prepared a report on childhood lead poisoning. Now all they needed, as we learn from the minutes of a committee meeting at the Lead Industries Association, was a recognized scientist who would act as the author. However, someone pointed out that the report would be part of a package to be distributed to science writers at a series of seminars around the country the following month, so there would not be enough time to set up the authorship charade.[1]

The game was up. Amendments to the original legislation in 1973 and 1975 placed further restrictions on lead paint, and one of the new agencies, the Consumer Product Safety Commission (created in 1972), would ef-fectively ban the product in 1976—all in all, landmark legislation and regulation in the cause of sane public health policies in this country.[5] Of course, legislation and regulation have their limits: They cannot require the removal of crumbling lead paint from thousands of houses painted before the legislation was enacted. States and municipalities across the country are now suing the lead industry for the cost of lead abatement; a Providence jury ruled that three paint companies must pay to remove the lead paint from more than three hundred thousand Rhode Island homes.[6]

* * *

The control of leaded paints was a public health triumph, and the second aspect of the lead story, while not quite so simple, also demonstrates that the regulatory system *has worked* in the not-too-recent past. The product in question now is tetraethyl lead, more commonly known as "Ethyl," an additive that raised the octane level of gasoline, thereby affording two benefits to the combustion of those early engines: more power and less knock. Gasoline with the highest dose of Ethyl soon became known simply as "premium," and the highest-performing engines in the most expensive cars required premium. But was adding lead to gasoline really such a good idea? Even the president of the National Lead Company had acknowledged in a letter of 1921 to the dean of the Harvard Medical School that "lead is a poison when it enters the stomach of man." The hazards of lead were well known. Even the GM researcher who developed Ethyl soon took a leave of absence to recover from lead poisoning![1,7]

Of course leaded gasoline was a good idea. In order to substantiate this assertion, General Motors, the first of the car makers to introduce the big machines that required premium gas, and DuPont, a major supplier of ethyl, asked the Bureau of Mines to conduct a study. Clearly, GM and DuPont trusted the Bureau to proceed in the proper spirit of cooperation. The Bureau repaid that trust by agreeing to put a gag order on its own scientists until the work was complete and avoiding the word "lead" even in its internal communications ("ethyl" was used instead). When GM demanded that "all manuscripts, before publication, will be submitted to the company for comment and criticism," the Bureau acquiesced. Two months later, when a new GM edict arrived with the word "approval" added to the list of demands, the Bureau genuflected one more time.[1]

That was in 1922. In 1924 the Ethyl producers' problems were exacerbated by a series of poisoning cases and fatalities in the processing refineries. In addition to the publicity generated by the poisonings at DuPont's "House of Butterflies" Chambers Works[8] (the same site where 100 percent of the men manufacturing dye chemicals would develop bladder cancer), an incident at Standard Oil's plant in Elizabeth, New Jersey, prompted this headline in the *New York Times:* "Odd Gas Kills One, Makes Four Insane."[9] The "insane" workers soon died. Something of a media riot followed, and the public did not seem overly interested in the distinction between the organic lead the workers were dealing with—the raw product—and the inorganic lead to which everyone would be exposed by way of car exhaust. New York City, Philadelphia, and other jurisdictions banned the sale of leaded gasoline.[1]

Conveniently enough, the preliminary results from the Bureau of Mines study could not have been clearer: There is no proof of lead poisoning from car exhaust; the only problem is worker exposure. Less than a year later, a committee rushed into service by the Surgeon General gave Ethyl a clean bill of health, but with an asterisk that called for regulation and further study. The committee based its pronouncement on a rudimentary study of garage and gas station employees and chauffeurs, 252 people in all, divided into cohorts exposed to leaded and unleaded gas.[1] "There you go!" the industries declared. "Lead-exposed workers who did not show any adverse health effects"—that is to say, no overt signs of poisoning.

Indeed, neither the Surgeon General's study nor any other had offered specific "proof" of the lead in car exhaust. There was only the proof of lead, period. Nevertheless, as automobile usage grew, so did lead consumption. By 1959, fifteen percent of the nation's consumption of the heavy metal was added to gasoline in the form of tetraethyl lead and burned in automobile combustion engines. Thousands of tons of lead were inevitably deposited in the nation's air, soil, and water.[7]

Then, in the 1960s a geochemist named Clair Patterson and a colleague, using core drillings of the ice in Greenland, documented a correlation between the industrial use of lead and its presence in the polar ice cap, an isolated environment far from the nearest sources of emissions. The deeper (and therefore older) the ice, the less the lead.[7] This was news. The industry's lobby had always denied that lead in the atmosphere posed any environmental threat at all and had contended that, since lead had always been in the air, it was somehow natural and therefore not dangerous. The American Petroleum Institute reacted to the Patterson research by arguing that "all 'accepted medical evidence . . . proves conclusively' that lead in the environment presents no threat to public health."[10]

(Fast-forwarding to the early twenty-first century, we see virtually the same line of argument now with mercury, another metallic neurotoxin that can produce adverse neurological, cognitive, and behavioral effects, especially in infants and children. In 2004 the EPA and the Food and Drug Administration issued a joint advisory [years in the making, including a comprehensive review of the scientific evidence by the National Academy of Sciences[11]] that recommended that pregnant women, nursing mothers, and young children avoid certain fish and shellfish known to contain elevated levels of methylmercury.[12] Strong opposition to the advisory came not just from the fishing industry, which had much to lose if consumers stopped eating its catch, but also from the electrical utilities that operated coal-fired power plants, which were responsible for emitting the mercury in the first place. Like the lead industry, these firms readily agreed that high-level poisoning is dangerous but argued through public relations campaigns and captive think tanks that the scientific evidence linking low-level exposure to adverse health effects is scant. In December 2003 the Bush administration proposed federal regulation of mercury emissions and announced that power plants would have fifteen years to reduce mercury exposures by 70 percent, although the EPA's own models suggest that the proposed system will actually take far longer to reach that goal. Shortly after the proposal was made, it came out that sizable hunks of the EPA's proposal were taken verbatim from memoranda sent to the EPA by power industry lawyers.[13,14] At least one more generation of children—and possibly several—will be born before significant reductions in exposure occur. The cost to society may turn out to be enormous.[15] Mercury, it appears, has become the twenty-first-century's lead.)

In his work, Clair Patterson did not stop with his documentation of the lead build-up in the environment. He estimated that the average blood lead level of U.S. citizens was 20 μg/dl, about one hundred times higher than the "natural" level. Patterson also helped focus national attention on the evidence that lower levels of lead exposure might lead to subclinical chronic conditions.[16] Until that time, the industry had effectively defended the self-serving argument that the only allowable "evidence" of ill effects from lead was full-blown intoxication and poisoning—the "House of Butterflies" effect. Christian Warren, in *Brush with Death: A Social History of Lead Poisoning,* reports that Patterson's work upended that contention. Describing a U.S. Public Health Service symposium in 1965, Warren writes that "Patterson, half a world away in Antarctica, still stole the show."[7]

The following year, an aroused U.S. Senate held hearings. Hill and Knowlton orchestrated the defense, but the firm could do little more than emphasize that the only people who needed regulatory protection were lead employees and that the standard in effect at the time, 80 μg/dl, was sufficient.[1]

In 1967 an industry poll showed that more than 40 percent of respondents identified lead as harmful to human health. In fact, it was the second most frequently identified substance. (Carbon monoxide was first.) That was the bad news for the industry, but the good news was that the public did not seem to know which products contained lead, and the really good news was that the public was "*not now aware* of use of lead in gasoline or emission of lead from auto exhaust" (emphasis in original).[17] (Remember, forty years had passed since the headlines of the 1920s. "Premium" gas was as American as apple pie.) However, the internal report on the poll continues: "this should not lead to complacency that [the public] will not be made increasingly aware of leaded gasoline, as the official and mass media publicity campaigns on air pollution intensify."[17]

Or put it this way: We cannot rest assured that the public will remain in the dark forever. Just in case the poll numbers should start moving in the wrong direction, the industry's strategy called for vigorous challenges to any suggestion that leaded gasoline was responsible for environmental pollution. In a 1968 pamphlet titled "Facts about Lead in the Atmosphere," the lead lobby outlined its plan "to refute the many claims made in the technical journals and the lay press that lead in the ambient air is reaching dangerous levels." The policy would "keep attention focused on old, leaded paint [as the source of pollution] and make clear that other sources of lead are not significantly involved."[1]

With the coming of the environmental movement, the credibility of industry as a whole in those tempestuous times was under a cloud of suspicion. In any event, two years after the comforting poll of 1968, Congress passed and President Nixon signed the Clean Air Act, with the Environmental Protection Agency empowered—mandated—to clean up the nation's fouled air.

Now lead paint had company: Leaded gasoline was also on its way out. The EPA gave notice in 1972.[18] The industry sued, but the courts upheld the EPA's action as reasonable.[19] Another key factor working against lead this time was the fact that tetraethyl lead fouled the catalytic converters that new cars needed to meet the EPA-mandated reductions in engine emissions. Automobile manufacturers needed catalytic converters more than leaded gasoline, so the lead industry was now on its own—and losing. Within a decade, sales of leaded gasoline had decreased by 50 percent. Not coincidentally, the Centers for Disease Control and Prevention (CDC) found a 37 percent decline in blood lead levels.[20]

In 1984 the U.S. Senate considered a bill to ban the use of lead in gasoline.[21] The bill's chief sponsor, Senator Dave Durenberger, Republican from Minnesota, hoped it would "build some momentum [to] ban lead at the earliest possible date." He noted that "the principle source of lead in our environment is the family car. Automobiles are, in effect, high-speed aerosol cans of lead poisoning that clog up our city streets . . . and the ironic thing is that automobiles don't need leaded gasoline."[22] Testifying in favor of the ban was Dr. Herbert Needleman, pediatrician at the University of Pittsburgh.[23] His work with lead over the years had been incendiary because it found a correlation between lead exposure and lower IQ in children with no signs of acute poisoning and blood levels *below 40 µg/dl.*[24] As we will see later in this saga, scientists using more powerful methods have recently found environmental lead exposure among children with blood levels below 10 µg/dl.[2,3]

Vernon Houk, director of the CDC's Center for Environmental Health, reported to the committee that "if no lead had been allowed in gasoline since 1977, there would have been approximately 80 percent fewer children identified with lead toxicity. . . . In spite of some other views which you may hear this morning—and I predict you will hear other views—evidence is overwhelming that the gasoline lead is a major controllable source of lead exposure."[20]

Houk's prediction about "other views" was correct. The proverbial parade of witnesses and in-house scientists from the lead industry testified that leaded gasoline was not a major contributor to lead poisoning. Jerome Cole, testifying on behalf of the Lead Industries Association, stated that "Lead has been used in gasoline for over 60 years. Over that time, despite extensive research efforts . . . there is simply no evidence that anyone in the general public has ever been harmed by this usage."[25] He disputed the Needleman studies on the adverse neurobehavioral effects in children from low-level exposure to lead. (The industry would also conduct an extended vendetta against Needleman by questioning not just his work's accuracy but even his personal honesty.[26] Dr. Needleman's work withstood the challenge, and his conclusions that low-level lead exposure have deleterious effects on the development of brain function in children are now widely accepted.)

Soon after the Durenberger hearing, the EPA proposed to ban the use of leaded gasoline. The industry challenged the move, however. Taking no chances that the regulations would be delayed by regulatory maneuverings or legal challenges, Congress passed the Clean Air Act Amendments of 1990, which outlawed leaded gas in this country as of December 31, 1995.[27]

And so it was. Between 1976 and 1991 lead essentially disappeared from gasoline in this country. This is why our children and especially our grandchildren will be smarter than we are. As a *direct* result, the average blood lead level of children between the ages of one and five years declined by more than 80 percent, a change directly attributable to the elimination of leaded gasoline. Preschool-aged children in the United States in the late 1990s had IQs that were, on average, 2.2–4.7 points higher than the comparable group two decades earlier. In terms of productivity and higher income, the effects are huge: Government researchers estimate that the economic value of this increased intelligence is between $100 and $300 billion dollars for each age cohort (i.e., all of the kids born in the United States in a single year).[28]

5

The Enronization of Science

Lead...Hill and Knowlton. Vinyl chloride...Hill and Knowlton. Asbestos...Hill and Knowlton. Tobacco...Hill and Knowlton. Are we beginning to see a pattern here? Given where we are today, it is hard to believe that the cigarette manufacturers did not even have a trade association until 1953, when public relations guru John Hill warned the industry to get organized before it was too late and offered his firm's services for that dubious purpose. In 1966 Hill and Knowlton set up its Division of Scientific, Technical, and Environmental Affairs, which in later years would brag in solicitation brochures that this founding was "years before the first 'Earth Day' or the establishment of the Environmental Protection Agency."[1] Regarding the vinyl chloride story, the firm boasted that it assisted the producers of this carcinogen "to help fight and finally bring under control one of the most violent media and government regulatory firestorms ever experienced by a single industry," with the result that the final OSHA standards "were significantly less onerous than had been originally proposed."[2] When three scientists linked chlorofluorocarbon gas—Freon—to the destruction of the ozone layer[3] and users of the chemicals began to look for alternatives, Hill and Knowlton went into action. On behalf of the Freon manufacturers, the firm attacked the science as uncertain and later boasted that its work helped DuPont gain "two or three years before the government took action to ban fluorocarbons."[4] In fact, the science was of the highest quality: The three researchers subsequently won a Nobel Prize.

While Hill and Knowlton continues to provide public relations services to polluters, since the 1970s the sophistication of the "product defense industry" has grown apace with the federal regulatory apparatus established by Congress. For thirty years, therefore, it has been pretty much smooth sailing—that is, lots of lucrative work—for the key players in the new industry who specialize in helping corporations fight regulation. Ironically, more work is assured them with every advance in our ability to identify the deleterious health effects of toxic exposures. Only in the last few decades have we perfected the techniques that allow us to recognize and measure the illness and premature death toll associated with specific components of air pollution. New laboratory techniques have enabled scientists to examine the endocrine-disrupting properties of chemicals at almost unthinkably low levels of concentration. As a general rule, the more we know, the more regulation is required. Industry and free-market ideologues despise this logic, but what is the alternative? *Ignore* the health impact of these toxins? Yes, or better yet, let's debate the impact!

As the product defense work has gotten more and more specialized, the makeup of the business has changed; generic public relations operations like Hill and Knowlton have been eclipsed by product defense firms, specialty boutiques run by scientists. Having cut their teeth manufacturing uncertainty for Big Tobacco, scientists at ChemRisk, the Weinberg Group, Exponent, Inc., and other consulting firms now battle the regulatory agencies on behalf of the manufacturers of benzene, beryllium, chromium, MTBE (methyl tertiary-butyl ether), perchlorates, phthalates, and virtually every other toxic chemical in the news today. Their business model is straightforward. They profit by helping corporations minimize public health and environmental protection and fight claims of injury and illness. In field after field, year after year, this same handful of individuals and companies comes up again and again.

The range of their work is impressive. They have on their payrolls (or can bring in on a moment's notice) toxicologists, epidemiologists, biostatisticians, risk assessors, and any other professionally trained, media-savvy experts deemed necessary. They and the larger, wealthier industries for which they work go through the motions we expect of the scientific enterprise, salting the literature with their questionable reports and studies. Nevertheless, it is all a charade. The work has one overriding motivation: advocacy for the sponsor's position in civil court, the court of public opinion, and the regulatory arena. Often tailored to address issues that arise in litigation, they are more like legal pleadings than scientific papers. In the regulatory arena, the studies are useful not because they are good work that the regulatory agencies have to take seriously but because they clog the machinery and slow down the process.

Public health interests are beside the point. Follow the science wherever it leads? Not quite. This is science for hire, period, and it is extremely lucrative. Court records show that the big three U.S. auto companies paid product defense scientists $23 million between 2001 and 2006 to help defend them against disease claims by mechanics and other workers exposed to asbestos contained in automobile brakes.[5]

The coterie of consulting firms that specialize in product defense have done a great job—so great that manufacturing uncertainty has become a big business in itself. The scientific studies these firms do for their clients are like the accounting work that some Arthur Andersen Company accountants did for Enron (until both companies went bankrupt): They appear to play by the rules of the discipline, but their objective is to help corporations frustrate regulators and prevail in product liability litigation.

* * *

Should the public lose all interest in its health, these product defense firms would be out of luck. Exponent, Inc., one of the premier firms in the product defense business, acknowledges as much in this filing with the Securities and Exchange Commission:

> Public concern over health, safety and preservation of the environment has resulted in the enactment of a broad range of environmental and/or other laws and regulations by local, state and federal lawmakers and agencies. These laws and the implementing regulations affect nearly every industry, as well as the agencies of federal, state and local governments charged with their enforcement. To the extent changes in such laws, regulations and enforcement or other factors significantly reduce the exposures of manufacturers, owners, service providers and others to liability, the demand for our services may be significantly reduced.[6]

Exponent, Inc., began its existence as an engineering firm, calling itself Failure Analysis Associates and specializing in assisting the auto industry in defending itself in lawsuits involving crashes.[7] "Failure analysis" is a standard methodology for investigating the breakdown of a system or machine, but the firm must have realized that "Failure" in its name might not work well outside the engineering world and switched to the more palatable Exponent, Inc., when it went public in 1998.[8]

Exponent's scientists are prolific writers of scientific reports and papers. While some may exist, I have yet to see an Exponent study that does not support the conclusion needed by the corporation or trade association that is paying the bill. Here are brief sketches of a few recent Exponent projects:

- The taste and smell of the gasoline additive MTBE are so foul that a tiny amount makes water undrinkable. This is bad because MTBE has contaminated drinking water sources across the country. (Moreover, it causes cancer in animals and may do so in people also, but this will be difficult to determine because the exposure levels are very low, exactly the sort of situation that epidemiology has the most difficulty addressing. The state of California has categorized MTBE as a possible human carcinogen.[9]) Communities across the country have sued the major oil companies and the MTBE manufacturers for the costs of cleaning up their water supplies. In response, a firm that provides the methanol used for making MTBE hired Exponent to produce a series of studies that concluded, not surprisingly, that MTBE is unlikely to pose a public health hazard and has not significantly impacted California's drinking water.[10] When the defendants in certain lawsuits tried to convince Congress to end the litigation by fiat and bail out the polluters, Exponent's economists produced a report for the American Petroleum Institute that concluded that the cost of the cleanup would be relatively low, which would make the proposed taxpayer bailout of the industry more acceptable to fiscal watchdogs.[11]

- An article in the *Annals of Emergency Medicine* suggested that the new generation of amusement park rides exposed thrill seekers to g-forces (a measure of acceleration) that exceed those experienced by astronauts and recommended that emergency physicians consider these rides as "a possible cause of unexplained neurologic events in healthy patients."[12] Six Flags Theme Parks, Inc., immediately commissioned Exponent to produce an "Investigation of Amusement Park Roller Coaster Injury Likelihood and Severity."[13] The press release on the report was headlined "Roller Coasters, Theme Parks Extraordinarily Safe."[14]

- Given the skyrocketing obesity rates among teenagers, many school systems and even some states have considered banning soda machines from high schools in order to discourage teenagers from consuming the empty calories. In 2005 an Exponent scientist conducted a study on behalf of the American Beverage Association that concluded that the number of beverages consumed from school vending machines "does not appear to be excessive."[15,16] In this case, however, the public just could not be convinced. The soft drink industry jettisoned these findings and in 2006 agreed to stop selling soda in schools.[17]

- Defense giant Lockheed Martin turned to Exponent when faced with the huge potential cost of cleaning up underground water sources contaminated with perchlorate, a rocket fuel component that according to the National Academy of Sciences causes thyroid disease in infants.[18] Exponent's studies minimized the risk associated with perchlorate exposure.[19,20]

- When a study by consulting epidemiologists discovered a high rate of prostate cancer cases at a Syngenta plant that produced the pesticide atrazine,[21] Exponent's scientists produced a study that found no relationship between the chemical and the disease.[22]
- After numerous studies that linked pesticide exposure and Parkinson's disease appeared in prestigious scientific journals, Exponent's scientists produced a literature review for CropLife America, the trade association of pesticide producers, whose conclusion maintained that "the animal and epidemiologic data reviewed do not provide sufficient evidence to support a causal association between pesticide exposure and Parkinson's disease."[23]
- Exponent specializes in literature reviews that draw negative conclusions. The company's scientists have produced several reviews of the asbestos literature for use in litigation, all of which conclude that certain types of asbestos and certain types of asbestos exposure are far less dangerous than previously believed.[24–26]

Another major player is the Weinberg Group, which was founded in 1983 by Dr. Myron Weinberg, formerly of Booz, Allen, and Hamilton. "Asbestos, Tobacco, Pharmaceuticals—We're All Next!" shouts the PowerPoint presentation of one Weinberg executive. Here is his bottom line: "Without the science you cannot win, but having it carries no guarantee."[27] In one promotional brochure the firm touts its work for a company that was confronted with a Superfund problem. On behalf of this client Weinberg's scientists "analyzed existing studies to find any design flaws to support legal defense.... [B]y reanalyzing the raw data from this study, a biostatistician from THE WEINBERG GROUP helped to demonstrate the study's numerous design and analysis flaws."[28]

In 2003 DuPont hired the Weinberg Group to address "the threat of expanded litigation and additional regulation by the EPA" of perfluorooctanoic acid (PFOA),[29] a chemical used in the production of Teflon. (The majority of members on an EPA scientific advisory board have labeled PFOA a "likely" carcinogen.[30]) Paul Thacker, a reporter, uncovered a letter from Terry Gaffney, Weinberg's vice president for Product Defense, to a DuPont vice president, explaining that "DUPONT MUST SHAPE THE DEBATE AT ALL LEVELS." (This firm appears to favor uppercase exhortations.) Gaffney lays out a comprehensive strategy, including "analyzing existing data, and/or constructing a study to establish not only that

PFOA is safe...but that it offers real health benefits."[29,31] At the time, Gaffney was also running the campaign of a major manufacturer of ephedra-based dietary supplements to stop the FDA from banning ephedra, a product that the agency had already linked to 164 deaths.[32]

In my work on beryllium, I first came across the work of Dr. H. Daniel Roth. This was a reanalysis by Dr. Roth and Dr. Paul Levy on behalf of the beryllium industry, and it yielded the usual result: By changing some of the parameters, the researchers had managed to demonstrate that the statistically significant elevation of lung cancer risk was no longer statistically significant.[33] Such reanalyses are a specialty of some of the product defense firms, whereby one epidemiologist reanalyzes another's raw data in ways that almost always exonerate the chemical, toxin, or product in question. The studies are carefully designed to do just this. Statistically significant differences disappear; estimates of risk are reduced. Such alchemy is rather easily accomplished, whereas the opposite—turning insignificance into significance—is extremely difficult.

Intrigued by the work of Levy and Roth on behalf of the beryllium industry, I wanted to see whether the two had bestowed similar benefits on other industries, so I Googled them. Among the many exhibits I found were a number of tobacco documents showing how both men had worked for this industry. Dr. Levy was hired by R. J. Reynolds (RJR) to conduct a reanalysis of a study examining the link between lung cancer and workplace exposure to secondhand smoke; in 1998 he presented his findings to a National Toxicology Program panel that was considering whether to designate environmental tobacco smoke (ETS) as a carcinogen. No link existed, he concluded.[34] Dr. Roth's work with tobacco was more extensive. In 1985 he was one of the experts hired by Philip Morris to assist with its litigation, especially to develop ways to attribute lung cancer among smoking asbestos workers to asbestos rather than to smoking.[35] In 1987 he applied for the position of executive director of the Center for Indoor Air Research (CIAR), a creation of the Tobacco Institute. The evaluation of Dr. Roth by CIAR's executive search firm was very positive. "Simply put," it concluded, he "believes in the mission of the Center and in his ability to achieve its objectives."[36] The tobacco documents do not reveal whether he was offered the job, but it is clear he later played a key role in Big Tobacco's efforts to stop OSHA's proposed indoor air quality standard in 1994.[37]

The tobacco relationship did not surprise me, but the coal connection did. For the past thirty years Dr. Roth has worked for producers and users of coal, turning out reanalysis after reanalysis refuting studies of the health effects of airborne pollutants from coal-burning power plants. On behalf of the North Dakota Lignite Research Council, which represents companies that produce coal with a high mercury content, he reviewed the literature on the effects of human exposure to mercury and, taking a page from the tobacco playbook, told the coal producers that most of the studies were "highly questionable" and that the overall picture was inconclusive. Even so, he recommended that "it would be valuable to reanalyze the raw data."[38]

In 1977 Dr. Roth produced a report for the electrical power industry that attacked the EPA's research on the relationship between exposure to fine particles in the air and the risk of asthma attacks. This reanalysis was required, he wrote, because the acceptance by the public and policy makers of the original EPA study was "making it most difficult to generate wise policy decisions on such matters as the rapid expansion of the use of coal."[39] Interestingly, both of Dr. Roth's coauthors on this study went on to become key scientists in Big Tobacco's campaign to manufacture uncertainty about the health effects of secondhand smoke. One of them, Dr. Anthony Colucci, was appointed director of RJR's Scientific Litigation Support Division.[40]

A jack of all trades within the product defense business, Dr. Roth also turned up in a book, *The Expert Witness Scam,* written by Leon Robertson, a retired professor of epidemiology from Yale and one of the two or three leading injury epidemiologists of the twentieth century. Dr. Robertson was appalled that for at least a decade Dr. Roth had been presented as an expert in vehicle rollovers although, according to Robertson, Roth had never published a research paper on any aspect of motor vehicle injuries.[7]

Dr. Roth also collaborated with Dr. Levy in refuting the risks associated with liquor; the Distilled Spirits Council of the United States hired them to critique the studies on alcohol consumption and breast cancer.[41,42]

Yet another major product defense consultant is ChemRisk, founded in the 1980s by Dennis Paustenbach, perhaps the leading figure in the field. Dr. Paustenbach has an unassailable scientific background. He is the author of two textbooks on risk assessment and hundreds of scientific articles and book chapters. At first, ChemRisk was part of a larger consulting firm, McLaren/Hart Environmental Engineering Corporation, of which Dr. Paustenbach eventually became president and chief executive officer. In 1998, when McLaren/Hart was facing bankruptcy, Dr. Paustenbach and several ChemRisk colleagues moved to Exponent, Inc.

In 2003 Dr. Paustenbach left Exponent and revived the name ChemRisk for his firm, which has prospered, quickly opening six offices around the country. He and his colleagues are important players in this book and are featured in upcoming discussions of benzene, beryllium, and chromium. In each case they have developed arguments that could have the effect of delaying or weakening public health regulation of a powerful toxin. Paustenbach is a veteran of the Love Canal and Times Beach, Missouri, catastrophes, and has been a key participant in the attempted rehabilitation of dioxin.[43] He has worked for the initiative funded by the auto industry that attempts to show that asbestos liberated from automobile brakes does not cause disease,[44,45] and he was also among the scientists used by the tobacco industry to question the EPA's risk assessment of secondhand tobacco smoke.[46]

According to a report in the *Wall Street Journal,* Dr. Paustenbach and his colleagues at ChemRisk pulled off a particularly audacious stunt on behalf of Pacific Gas and Electric (PG&E).[47] The California utility was fighting several lawsuits, including the one portrayed in the movie *Erin Brockovich,* in which chromium-contaminated groundwater was alleged to have caused a range of illnesses. In mounting its defense, PG&E turned to ChemRisk, which had already been working for the chromium industry in New Jersey (trying to convince that state's regulators that the metal was not so dangerous as to require cleaning up a massive toxic waste dump.[48]) According to a report in the *Wall Street Journal,* ChemRisk's product defense experts, through an affiliate in Shanghai, obtained the raw data of a 1987 study that had implicated chromium-polluted water in high cancer rates.[49] This study was a major problem for the defendants. The *Wall Street Journal* reported that ChemRisk paid Dr. Zhang JianDong, the lead author, two thousand dollars, reanalyzed his data, and obtained different results that appeared to exonerate chromium. The renalysis was then published under the names of Dr. Zhang and a Chinese colleague, without any mention or acknowledgement of ChemRisk's role.[47,50,51]

This initiative was remarkably successful; for almost a decade, the fabricated study was promoted in courts and regulatory proceedings. Fortunately, the questionable history of the article is now public knowledge. After much uproar, the editor of the journal in which the paper was published withdrew the work,[52] and a California state epidemiologist has reexamined the original data and determined that Dr. Zhang's first analysis was the accurate one: Drinking chromium in your water increases your risk of stomach cancer.[53] (Paustenbach has said that his involvement in the paper was relatively minor and has defended the "underlying science." ChemRisk has also claimed that its scientists "wanted to be co-authors on the paper."[54] A year after the *Wall Street Journal* reported the story, the Chinese paper's second author claimed that the newspaper's coverage was inaccurate.[55] But the *Wall Street Journal* has not corrected or retracted its story.)

This episode was outrageous but not all that out of line with the standards of the industry. When product defense specialists cannot get the raw data required for a reanalysis, they have even been known to make them up. I learned this when I came across an abstract that described the reanalysis of the data of a study of older adults that had found reduced performance on neuropsychological tests associated with polychlorinated biphenyl (PCB) levels. The reanalysts did not have access to the raw data, so they came up with a simulated data set based on the overall distribution of subjects in the original study. Not surprisingly, their results called into doubt the validity of the original findings.[56] My curiosity piqued, I called the author of the original study, toxicologist Susan Schantz of the University of Illinois. Dr. Schantz had never heard of the reanalysis. She had never been asked to provide her raw data, and when I read her the abstract, she laughed. Dr. Shantz told me the new work was simply wrong, as she could have explained to the reanalysts if they had asked her. (One of those reanalysts was the same scientist who would later defend the cause of selling soda in schools for the American Beverage Association.)

* * *

Peer review is a complex issue, one that is widely misunderstood by the public and by some individuals in the regulatory and legal systems. Even rigorous peer review by honest scientists does *not* guarantee a study's accuracy or quality. Peer review is just one component of a larger quality control process through which scientific knowledge is developed and tested—a process that never ends. Nevertheless, it has been granted an important role in both the regulatory and legal systems. Some agencies, including the International Agency for Research on Cancer (IARC), will not consider using a paper in its deliberations if it has not undergone peer review.[57] Articles that have been published in peer-review journals are assumed, often mistakenly, to be of high quality. This is not necessarily so.

The credibility given peer-reviewed studies encourages product defense firms to manipulate and distort the process. They play the peer-review card beautifully. They understand that their studies and reanalyses need this imprimatur, but how do they get this seal of approval? Easy. They establish vanity journals that present themselves to the unwary as independent sources of information and science, but the peer reviewers are carefully chosen, like-minded corporate consultants sitting in friendly judgment on studies that are exquisitely structured to influence a regulatory proceeding or court case.

There is now a slew of these "captured" journals. The tobacco industry, for example, secretly financed the journal *Indoor and Built Environment* to promote (and position for legal purposes) the idea that indoor air pollution was a problem caused not by secondhand smoke but by inadequate ventilation.[58] The best-known of these publications is *Regulatory Toxicology and Pharmacology*, the official mouthpiece of the International Society for Regulatory Toxicology and Pharmacology (ISRTP)—an impressive name, but really just an association dominated by scientists who work for industry trade groups and consulting firms.[59] The sponsors of the ISRTP include many of the major tobacco, chemical, and drug manufacturing companies. Its leadership consists of corporate and product defense scientists and attorneys, along with a small number of government scientists who have apparently bought in or who do not know better. The immediate past president was Terry Quill, an attorney who became senior vice president for product defense of the Weinberg Group.[60] Quill also has roots in the tobacco wars but not as a scientific expert. Rather, he served as outside counsel to Philip Morris in the secondhand-smoke litigation.[61]

The editor of *Regulatory Toxicology and Pharmacology* is Gio Gori, well known in the public health community as one of the tobacco industry's most prominent and long-standing defenders—after serving from 1968 to 1980 as director of the National Cancer Institute's highly regarded Smoking and Health Program. Then he changed sides and embarked on a lucrative career defending Big Tobacco on the secondhand smoke issue.[62]

Does the peer-review process at these journals play a role in improving the published papers or do studies of questionable validity move to publication unchallenged? Here is a recent story that speaks volumes. One well-known epidemiologist and corporate consultant recently conducted what is called a meta-analysis, in which several studies on the same exposure were combined into a single large study, theoretically at least more powerful than several smaller ones. The study, which was paid for by PG&E for use in the chromium-contaminated drinking water suits, concluded that, contrary to fifty years of epidemiologic studies, chromium was "only weakly carcinogenic for the lungs."[63]

Published in *Regulatory Toxicology and Pharmacology*, the study makes the most basic (and fatal) mistake of combining all types of exposure and cancer rates and treating them as comparable. Heavy exposures to airborne chromium among the workers in pigment factories were combined with light exposures among residents of towns with contaminated water. Of course, there was no increased lung cancer risk among the community residents—they were not *breathing* chromium. However, since there were several times more community residents than workers, they were weighted more heavily in the analysis, thereby diluting the effects seen in the worker study and making it appear that chromium was "only weakly carcinogenic for the lungs." That is an elementary error. The peer reviewers evidently did not mind, though, since the study achieved its product defense purpose for the industry.

Another story also illustrates how polluters use these journals-for-hire to impede public health measures. The International Agency for Research on Cancer is the branch of the World Health Organization devoted to cancer prevention. In February 2006 an IARC advisory panel met to consider whether carbon black, an important industrial chemical that is the foundation for many new "nanoproducts," should be categorized as a carcinogen. One of the papers that the panel planned to consider was a study that had found that workers who had been exposed to carbon black had twice the expected risk of lung cancer.[64] The weekend before IARC's meeting was to start, a scientist who was working for the International Carbon Black Association (ICBA) breathlessly delivered to the IARC panel three manuscripts[65–67] that reanalyzed data from that first study. All three of these papers had been first presented at a conference sponsored by the ICBA and held less than *one month* before the IARC meeting.[68] The three new reanalyses had been put into a fast-track (two week) peer review and accepted for publication in the *Journal of Occupational and Environmental Medicine (JOEM)*, whose work appears all too frequently in these pages. I should explain that peer review in a scientific journal generally takes at least several months, sometimes more than a year, and that authors generally revise articles based on reviewers' feedback. As we would surmise, the fast-track papers disputed the causal relationship between carbon black and lung cancer.

The IARC advisory panel voted that carbon black was "possibly carcinogenic" and concluded that, although sufficient evidence for carcinogenicity in animal studies existed, the human evidence was inadequate.[69] Did the three new reanalyses help shape the panel's conclusion? It is hard to say, but it is clear that most of the negative evidence from human studies was provided by the industry. No new independent studies have been undertaken, let alone fast-track peer-reviewed.

Skewed studies produced for the most mercenary of purposes are now accepted as part of the game. I saw this at the Department of Energy. Regarding the beryllium industry's advocacy briefs masquerading as scientific papers (they had been published in peer-review journals, after all), my career colleagues in the department shrugged. "It's all part of the game," they said. "We know what these papers are worth." The lack of outrage by honest scientists and regulators is distressing. The late senator Daniel Patrick Moynihan had a phase for it—he called it "defining deviancy down."[70] Conduct that was once considered unacceptable and that *should* be considered unacceptable is no longer stigmatized or even acknowledged as being corrupt. Moreover, some scientists and certainly most nonscientists (including reporters, judges, juries, and members of Congress) do *not* know what those papers are worth. They are often fooled—which is the whole idea.

* * *

Polluters and manufacturers of dangerous products also fund think tanks and other front groups that are well known for their antagonism toward regulation and devotion to "free enterprise" and "free markets." There are dozens of these organizations working on behalf of just about every significant industry in this country. Some of the ones leading the fight on behalf of corporate interests against public health and environmental regulation are familiar: the Heritage Foundation, Washington Legal Foundation, American

Enterprise Institute for Public Policy Research, Cato Institute, Competitive Enterprise Institute, Hudson Institute, Progress and Freedom Foundation, and Citizens for a Sound Economy, to name a few. Each year these think tanks, along with a host of smaller, lesser-known ones, collect millions of dollars from regulated companies to promote campaigns that weaken public health and environmental protections.

These broad public-policy groups rarely pretend to do science themselves; they generally focus on major regulatory issues. Therefore, the polluting corporations and their trade associations have also set up a different stratum of think tanks and front groups they can rely on to churn out predictable, authoritative-looking reports that cull the friendly science commissioned by the companies themselves. These reports are aimed at legislators, the press, and the public. They always question the science regarding specific hazards (generally those created by their funders). For example, the Council on Water Quality pretends to ensure that the "best available science drives government actions on setting standards for perchlorate in water."[71] As previously mentioned, this rocket fuel additive is now contaminating groundwater supplies around the nation. Lockheed Martin and other polluters that are facing the huge cost of cleaning up contaminated aquifers provide the council's funding.[72] The group is run by staff at APCO Worldwide, the public relations giant that has done similar work for Big Tobacco, so consider the source when judging the claim that "[s]cientific research shows low levels of perchlorate are harmless."[71] In fact, an analysis by the National Academy of Sciences found that perchlorate causes thyroid damage, especially in infants, at fairly low exposure levels.[18]

The Center for Media and Democracy keeps tabs on these front groups on the web[73] and in a series of invaluable books written by Sheldon Rampton and John Stauber.[74-75] One of the groups they are following is the Center for Consumer Freedom, which uses funding from the food and restaurant industries to attack studies that link fat consumption to obesity.[76] The same group started FishScam to promote the idea that mercury in fish does not pose a danger to pregnant women.[77]

Another of these cleverly named organizations is the Foundation for Clean Air Progress. This group issues regular reports showing how pristine our environment is, questioning why anyone would want to strengthen the laws responsible for such excellent air. The organization is run by Burson-Marsteller, the PR firm, using funds provided by the petroleum, trucking, and other polluting industries.[78]

The Annapolis Center for Science-Based Policy was started by a vice president of the National Association of Manufacturers for, among other purposes, fighting the EPA's Clean Air standards.[79] It is heavily funded by ExxonMobil ($688,575 between 1998 and 2005)[80,81] and large coal-burning utilities like the Southern Co. ($325,00 in 2003–2004).[82,83] A "key finding" of one Annapolis Center report states that "No one knows whether controlling [airborne particles] will actually yield net benefits to public health. Further regulation of PM is thus premature."[84] This has become the mantra of the big coal-burning power companies as they oppose further regulation of these particulates.[85,86] It is an indefensible assertion. While we cannot ethically set up a study in which we expose some people to high levels of these particulates (called PM, or particulate matter), the equivalent natural experiment happens all of the time. One of the most famous was studied by Arden Pope, a researcher at Brigham Young University who was conducting a long-term study of air pollution in Provo, Utah, in the 1980s. As his luck would have it, his research period covered a full year in which the big steel mill in Provo, which accounted for 80 percent of the region's airborne PM, was idled by a labor strike. In that year, the mortality rate and hospitalizations dramatically *decreased.* Once the strike was settled and the PM pollution from the steel mill resumed, mortality and hospitalization rates went back up.[87] The cause-effect relationship could not have been clearer.

So many studies have linked exposure to airborne PM levels and increased risk of death, hospitalization, and emergency room and clinic visits that the editor of the journal *Epidemiology,* Dr. Jonathan Samet, a distinguished scientist and chairman of the Department of Epidemiology at the Johns Hopkins Bloomberg School of Public Health, told scientists to stop submitting new studies on this topic. So many had already been published that new ones would add little of value to the scientific literature; the pages of Dr. Samet's journal could better be devoted to other topics.[88] We do not know everything about PM, but we know enough to be very confident that reducing the concentrations will prevent tens of thousands of deaths each year.[89–91]

* * *

Let's face it, the work product of the product defense industry is impressive. Carefully manicured reports and reanalyses, captured journals full of "peer-reviewed" articles, and captured think tanks hiring out their ad hoc advocacy sow uncertainty across a range of issues. Perhaps the sleaziest behavior of all, though, is their practice of denigrating scientists and studies whose findings do not serve the corporate cause. Today the most prominent and effective public face and front for this component of the attack on science is the "junk science" movement, whose sole purpose is to ridicule research that threatens powerful interests, irrespective of the quality of that research. Peter Huber, based at the Manhattan Institute, is often credited with coining the term, as I mentioned in the introduction. I would like to repeat Huber's rough-and-ready description of junk science in his book *Galileo's Revenge: Junk Science in the Courtroom:* "Junk science is the mirror image of real science, with much of the same form but none of the substance.... It is a hodgepodge of biased data, spurious inference, and logical legerdemain.... It is a catalog of every conceivable kind of error: data dredging, wishful thinking, truculent dogmatism, and, now and again, outright fraud."[92]

Orwellian indeed, as I stated in the introduction, but unquestionably the corporations and the product defense industry they fund have done a superb job in marketing the "sound science" slogan and thereby undermining the use of scientific evidence in public policy. The junkscience.com website lists a roster of "junk scientists," including six elected members of the Institute of Medicine and four recipients of the highest honor bestowed by the American College of Epidemiology, so it appears that scientists who are asked to identify *their* most outstanding colleagues do not share the opinions of the promoters of the "junk science" label.[93]

The opposite of junk science is, of course, "sound science." Rarely is the one invoked as bad without an immediate reference to the other as the ideal. The first entity to carry the official "sound science" flag was The Advancement of Sound Science Coalition (TASSC), which was "dedicated to ensuring the use of sound science in public policy decisions."[94,95] This front organization was set up by APCO Associates, one of Philip Morris's PR firms.[96] (Elisa Ong and Stanton Glantz described the founding role of tobacco in the sound science movement in the November 2001 issue of the *American Journal of Public Health*.[97]) Steven Milloy, the first executive director of TASSC, had formerly worked for Multinational Business Services, a firm run by Jim Tozzi, perhaps the premier antiregulatory tactician. Ultimately TASSC served its purpose and is now defunct, and Milloy has moved on to his own website, www.junkscience.com.

A representative "sound science" credo is this one from a TASSC press release, which quotes Dr. Margaret Maxey, director of the Clint W. Murchison Chair of Free Enterprise and professor of bioethics at the University of Texas: "More and more [science is] being used to justify preconceived agendas. Too often, public policy decisions that are based on inadequate science impose enormous economic costs and other hardships on consumers, businesses and government."[95] The usual figure provided for the annual cost of "regulations" has been in excess of $40 billion.[98] One of industry groups' favorite examples of costly policy is the Clean Air Act. Another TASSC authority, Floy Lilley, also of the University of Texas, had this to say in denouncing that regulation: "The Clean Air Act is a perfect example of laboratory science being superficially applied to reality. If it were reflective of reality, based on current government studies, medical examiners would find evidence of effects in lungs that are irreversible and life-threatening. This simply has not happened. And now we must wonder if the cost of the Clean Air Act is justified by alleged health benefits."[95]

In the fact-based world, the Clean Air Act has been one of the most successful modern public health regulations by preventing tens of thousands of illnesses and premature deaths and millions of asthma attacks.[99] Even the cost-benefit doyens of the second Bush administration, perhaps the most fervent opponents of regulation ever to occupy the White House, have estimated that its benefits outweigh its costs by somewhere between $50 billion and $400 billion.[98] But is anyone really surprised that it is subjected to ridiculous attacks? As comedian Lily Tomlin said, "No matter how cynical you become, it's never enough to keep up."[100]

6

Tricks of the Trade

HOW MERCENARY SCIENTISTS

MISLEAD YOU

Scientists who are involved in developing public health and environmental protections recognize that we do not need (and we almost never obtain) proof beyond a reasonable doubt. Our regulatory systems call for using the best evidence available at the present time. Waiting for absolute certainty is a recipe for failure: People will die, and the environment will be damaged if we wait for absolute proof.

Industry and its consultants are well aware that their use of uncertainty to challenge science exploits the very nature of science, in which knowledge is accumulated over a long period of time and the understanding of that knowledge also evolves. Scientists do not have the truth; we seek the truth. We deal not in absolute certainties but in the "weight of the evidence." We combine and evaluate information from many sources, and we apply both quantitative and qualitative methods in order to overcome real uncertainty and gaps in scientific knowledge.

Out of all scientific uncertainties, few are more complex than understanding the causes of human disease. Scientists cannot feed toxic chemicals to humans to see what dose causes cancer. Instead, we must harness the "natural experiments," where exposures have already happened in the field. In the laboratory we can use only animals. Both epidemiologic and laboratory studies therefore have many uncertainties. Scientists must thus extrapolate from the evidence to make causal inferences and recommend protective measures. In any given scientific debate involving human health, inevitably studies crop up whose findings are inconsistent, if not contradictory. For many topics of public health interest, we know enough to protect the public, but only with the acknowledgment that we may be overregulating on a given issue. This is simply the nature of the beast. In public health science, absolute certainty is rarely an option because the questions our regulatory system asks can be answered only imperfectly in most cases. For example, we know that asbestos causes lung cancer even at relatively low levels of exposure, but we cannot state with absolute certainty the precise risk of cancer associated with every given exposure. That actual question is both unanswerable and, in general, not of great interest to most scientists (who would rather spend their time on new questions) or to the funding agencies that support research.

Our regulatory programs will not be effective if absolute proof is required before we act; the best available evidence must be sufficient. Yet we see a growing trend that disingenuously demands *proof* over precaution in the realm of public health. Although industry certainly deserves the harshest denunciation, environmental activists can also be guilty of using the existence of scientific uncertainty to advance policy aims through an overzealous application of "the precautionary principle." If the weighing of potential risks and benefits is transformed into a demand for assurance that a policy or action will result in *no* harm, scientific advances or public health interventions with the potential to genuinely improve the human condition can be disparaged and delayed. Food irradiation is a case in point. This technology may genuinely improve the human condition in many developing countries where food-borne bacteria and parasites take an enormous human toll, but it has been disparaged and delayed.

By its nature, epidemiology is a sitting duck for uncertainty campaigns. Large epidemiological studies are complicated structures that require complex statistical analysis. These studies are not a matter of setting up the equations, filling in the variables, and then solving for the answer. Instead, we set up our equations *as well as we can,* fill in the variables *as well as we can,* and then solve the equations *as well as we can.* Judgment is called for all along the way, so disciplined integrity is mandatory. The nature of epidemiology and the ground rules epidemiologists use ensure that it is far more difficult to find a false positive result than a false negative one. It is relatively easy to design a study or reanalyze someone else's data in a way that ensures that the new study will find no association between the exposure and the disease in question. The joke about "lies, damned lies, and statistics" definitely pertains. The battle for the integrity of science is rooted in issues of methodology.

Except for a few very rare instances in which a disease is unique to an exposure, such as mesothelioma caused by asbestos, epidemiologists cannot state that a specific chemical exposure has definitely caused the cancer of a specific patient. The lung cancer from asbestos is indistinguishable from the lung cancer from smoking. The best that epidemiology can provide is a probability statement. In fact, this is the essence of the field: establishing probabilities that reliably pertain to a given population.

Much of what we know about the toxic effect of the more common environmental exposures, especially airborne exposures, comes from studies of workers. Workers often make up the discrete, identifiable population with the greatest exposure to any given chemical, including those that make their way into the environment at large. Studying health effects among such workers is difficult, but it is often preferable to trying to isolate those effects in the general population. Want to study the long-term effects of exposure to formaldehyde? Embalmers, mortuary workers, pathologists, and anatomists will have exposure to this chemical, so study them. (Studies of these workers find a higher than expected risk of leukemia, probably as a result of formaldehyde exposure.[1]) What about benzene? Most environmental health scientists, along with the national and international health agencies, believe this chemical increases the risk of leukemia for anyone exposed in the general population but by such a small amount that we would be unable to detect it in an epidemiologic study. However, some workers in the rubber and shoe industries have been exposed to higher levels of benzene. Study them, find higher than expected rates of leukemia (as numerous studies have), and then extrapolate to other populations with lower exposures, including the general population.

These studies of distinct worker populations, pioneered by Dr. Robert A. M. Case's investigations into bladder cancer among British dye workers, are called "historical prospective" or retrospective cohort studies. In these studies we identify the members of a population (called a cohort) sometime in the past (usually several decades earlier), follow them forward in time, and examine the illnesses they developed or died from. Cohort studies are not difficult to do; they are however difficult to do well. In fact, in many situations a good study simply is not doable. This is not to say, though, that it should not be conducted, but the results have to be carefully interpreted in this light. The main problem with most cohort studies? We rarely have accurate knowledge of the study subjects' exposure histories, so we must make what are often reasonable but crude estimations.

We are not working with laboratory animals in cages. Instead, we are trying to harness and analyze the results of what epidemiologists call "natural experiments"—not that there is anything natural about the hazardous exposures we are investigating, but they have occurred in the real world rather than in a laboratory. For one tragic example of such an unnatural "natural experiment," we know a great deal about the long-term effects of radiation exposure to humans from studies of the survivors of the events in which large numbers of people were exposed to high levels of radiation:

Hiroshima and Nagasaki. While these bombings were not planned as epidemiological experiments, scientists later capitalized on them.[2]

Most well-designed workplace studies require populations that are followed for at least twenty years, preferably thirty or more, because the cancers that most chemicals cause usually require such long periods of time to show up. Benzene is an exception; occupational leukemias start to appear among workers in as few as two years after exposure. For most chemicals, though, cohort mortality studies that examine workers whose exposures began less than twenty years earlier will not show an effect, so it is reasonable to suspect a nefarious reason for conducting such a study: obtaining negative results with which to intentionally misinform those not trained in the subtleties of epidemiology.

Thirty-year mortality studies do not actually require thirty years to conduct. Epidemiologists use extant historical records to reconstruct those years. Using all sorts of tracking systems (including Social Security data and the National Death Index, which is a list of all those who die in the United States each year, along with their cause of death), we make every effort to determine who is alive and who is dead at the end of the period under study, when they died, and the cause of death. We also obtain the best possible "exposure history" for each employee in the study. Using whatever records are available, we work with industrial hygienists to construct job-exposure matrices, which assign estimated exposure levels for the chemical in question to different job titles and different locations within the workplace. The work history of each participant is plugged into this matrix to derive a rough estimate of individual historical exposure. We compare disease rates among study participants with different exposure histories with those that would be expected of members of the general public.

Death is an extreme outcome—a crude metric for an epidemiologist to use but often the only one for which data are available. When we are studying diseases that are not likely to cause death, mortality data are even less helpful. Bladder cancer is one example. Currently, more than half of all individuals who develop bladder cancer will not die of the disease, at least within the first five years after diagnosis. If we study only mortality figures, we will miss most of the bladder cancer cases. Certain states maintain cancer registries (sometimes called tumor registries), and many of the infectious diseases are reported to state health departments, but otherwise no comprehensive database exists for illnesses in the United States. A study in a state with a cancer registry can examine the incidence of a particular cancer; otherwise, that study will be restricted to mortality and therefore less able to detect patterns of excess risk of nonfatal diseases.

Clearly, the larger the study, the better, all other elements being equal. Also ideal is the comparison of workers who have high exposures to a given chemical with workers *in the same or a similar facility* with lower or no exposure. Alas, the ideal is mostly unavailable in epidemiology since it requires large numbers of participants and rich historical exposure data. More often, epidemiologists compare the mortality experience of a worker cohort with a standard population, be it local, regional, or national. Such studies generally entail calculating the number of deaths in the worker population under study that would be expected if their mortality experience were exactly the same as that of the comparison population (adjusted for age, race, and gender). The ratio of actual deaths with expected deaths is the standardized mortality ratio, or SMR. If there are twice as many actual as expected deaths, the SMR equals 2, suggesting (but not *proving*) that these workers have twice the risk of dying from that cause.

Just as large studies are manifestly superior, small ones are inherently suspect. These studies are underpowered because they do not have the statistical power to detect a real increase in disease risk in populations. In a study of several thousand workers, a threefold risk excess is likely to be statistically significant, whereas the same excess in a study of just two hundred workers probably will not be. Competent epidemiologists use the number of people and the age distribution to determine the power of a study in advance. Too often, mortality studies commissioned by industry look at a relatively small group of workers for a relatively short period of time and fail to find any negative impact. The industry then declares that this "evidence" proves that the chemical in question does not cause disease. Conversely, in order to address criticisms of low power, industry scientists sometime add large numbers of unexposed workers to a study population, but their inclusion is largely uninformative and may help mask real effects. We will see examples in the benzene discussion to follow.

An old saying about scientific papers states that "What the discussion giveth, the methods taketh away." This is particularly true for negative studies. Generally speaking, a poorly conducted study is more likely to result in a false negative (that is, it fails to find a risk increase that is actually present) than in a false positive (mistakenly identifying an excess risk when none in fact exists). For the results from a negative study to be taken seriously, the study must be large and sensitive and gather accurate exposure data.[3,4]

Even when a study is large enough, covers a sufficient period of time (thirty years, for instance), and has access to a cornucopia of exposure data, other factors can still bedevil epidemiologists. The first is a systematic error or bias that undermines the results. An important one of this type is *selection bias,* which occurs when the worker cohort under study is not representative of the general population from which it comes and with which it will be compared. The most common selection bias is what we call the "healthy worker effect," which simply reflects the fact that the worker population was "selected" (that is, employed) because it was healthier to begin with.

In order to get and then hold a job in a factory, an employee has to be pretty healthy to start with. People who are very sick or have a disability, as well as those who are imprisoned or institutionalized, never get into the workforce. It follows that almost every study that compares the death rate of workers to that of a geographically appropriate comparison population finds that the workers have the *lower* overall risk. This is true even for workers who are exposed to asbestos, benzene, chromium, and virtually all of the other well-known, potent carcinogens I discuss in this book. Despite the cancers and deaths such occupational exposure causes, the worker cohort will *still* have a lower overall mortality rate than the unhealthier general population. (Beware, therefore, the disingenuous public affairs spokesperson or product defense consultant who claims that the overall mortality among workers in some inherently dangerous operation is lower than "expected.")

Another systematic problem that can undermine a study is *information bias,* which can take many forms, although the most common is the misclassification of exposure estimates. In fact, some degree of exposure misclassification is pretty much inevitable when dealing with information that is decades old. As it happens, both of the two most likely "mistakes"— workers with high exposure incorrectly assigned to the low or no-exposure group and workers with low exposure assigned to the high-exposure group—result in a *lower* degree of risk than in fact exists. This type of misclassification, as long as it occurs randomly, along with any sort of random error, serves to lower the risk estimate.

Yet another systematic error related to exposure misclassification is the more simple effect of *dilution.* This results when we do not have good exposure information and groups of workers with different exposures therefore get lumped together. When a small group of heavily exposed workers is diluted in a large group of other, less heavily exposed workers, a large excess for the heavily exposed workers can seem smaller than it actually is or even disappear entirely. One example is the bladder cancer cases at the Goodyear plant in Niagara Falls, which I discuss in chapter eight. Overall, the workers at that plant had a threefold excess risk, but the long-term employees in the department with the heaviest exposure to one chemical had a risk that was twenty-seven times that of the comparison population.[5]

Yet another epidemiological hazard is *confounding*—that is, the existence of a factor that is related to both the disease and the factor under investigation. Indeed, confounding is a problem for all epidemiologists and the mother lode for those whose main goal is to sow uncertainty. It is a favorite technique of industry to blame confirmed health risks on an unaccounted-for confounder—smoking. While obvious confounders, like gender or age (older and male workers may have had heavier exposures than younger or female workers, for example), will be accounted for in the design and analysis of the study, smoking is nearly impossible to account for precisely. Epidemiologists can try to obtain smoking histories on the entire population in a study or, if that is not possible, on a sample of the population. If neither of those options is open, it is sometimes possible to estimate the confounding effect tobacco might have on the results. However, in order to be a confounder, the most highly occupationally exposed workers in a population would have to be the heaviest smokers—an unlikely scenario. In some cases we have learned that cigarettes are not confounders at all; most famously, asbestos workers who also smoke have lung cancer rates far higher than either nonsmoking asbestos workers or smokers with no asbestos exposure at all. We could say that asbestos and tobacco *compound* rather than confound their risk of cancer.

If two chemicals are present in the same plant, the estimated effects of one may be confounded by that of the other. Since most workers at factories are exposed to many chemicals (often simultaneously), it is difficult to parse the respective effects. That is an instance in which the scientists make judgments by using information they import from other sorts of studies, particularly animal studies.

On top of all of these judgment calls, we have the actual results of the study that must be wisely and carefully interpreted. Again, it is not a matter of solving the equation for the "right" answer. If we have good reason to believe that in a given group of workers we should expect (based on the rates in the comparison population) ten deaths from lung cancer and our study of a given population reveals fifteen deaths, statistical tests help us decide whether the findings more likely reflect a true causal relationship or just a chance finding. Are we really seeing "too many cases," or just a fluky variation? With some signature diseases, the occurrence of just a few cases in one place is enough to establish a problem.

A well-known example is the cluster of four cases of angiosarcoma of the liver that were reported in 1974 at the B. F. Goodrich plant in Louisville, Kentucky, as I have previously related. Since only about twenty-five angiosarcomas were reported every year in the United States,[6] complex statistical analyses were not necessary here: The cause of these cancers was exposure to vinyl chloride. However, identifying instances of "too many cases" is not nearly so easy with the more common diseases or causes of death. In most situations, the identification of a genuinely increased risk depends on the size of the increase and that of the population under study. For example, if we know that exposure to a given chemical triples the risk of leukemia, three leukemia cases in a cohort of 100 workers in which only one case would be expected would not likely be statistically significant. We could not rule out chance distribution as the cause of the two excess cases. On the other hand, if the population is 1,000 workers, not 100, and we find thirty cases instead of the expected ten, it is very unlikely that the excess would be attributable to chance. In this case, we would say that the difference between the observed and the expected was "statistically significant," and we would consider an alternative hypothesis: The chemical under study is the cause of the leukemia.

As a complement to epidemiology, we have animal studies. For more than a century now, scientists have been exposing animals—especially mammals—to toxic products to predict what will happen when humans are exposed to the same substances. The logic behind these toxicology studies is simple: All mammals have similar tissues, organs, and biochemical systems. For the most part, bad news for a lab rat is bad news for all other mammals, including us. Animals studies can help explain the results of the "natural experiments" that epidemiologists study. They can also predict whether substances that we cannot study epidemiologically might cause cancer in humans.

What are the effects of different exposure levels? What are the effects of different exposure times—for example, living near a factory twenty-four hours a day compared with working in that factory for eight hours a day? What happens when exposure ceases altogether? Is there "recovery"? How about the interaction of multiple exposures or the effects on the very young, the very old, the fetus? What about new chemicals that have not been around for thirty years? Animal studies can help provide these answers because we cannot ethically subject humans, even informed volunteers, to doses of known carcinogens and powerful toxins.

The ability of a carcinogen to produce cancer at low levels of exposure was confirmed in the fabulously expensive mega-mouse and mega-rat experiments. In these studies, thousands of lab animals were randomly divided into groups that received doses of a known, potent carcinogen. The strength of the dose ranged from very low to powerful indeed. In both of the "mega" studies, the result was inescapable: There is no threshold, no minimum dose, required to induce cancer. The studies also found something that is very important in epidemiology: a dose-response relationship, which shows that the risk of disease increases as the exposure increases.[7-10]

As I have already mentioned, cancer may require many years and even decades to develop in humans—much longer than the natural lifespan of most of the small mammals used in toxicology studies. Therefore, it is necessary to study the animal throughout its entire life in order to allow the maximum time for the disease to develop. This is a problem because a study would have to follow many thousands of lab animals for their entire lives in order to detect the health effect with any confidence. That is too many.

Instead, we use a smaller number of lab animals and give them *large* doses, knowing that a substance that does not cause cancer does not cause cancer, period, not even at the highest doses. Still, this methodology is the subject of predictable criticism. It is common for the defenders of a substance that has been found to be carcinogenic in animal studies to offer as an excuse the fact that the exposure was far more than a human would ever confront.

* * *

In the end, public health and environmental protections are based not on the results of individual epidemiological or animal studies but rather on an interpretation or synthesis of the findings of multiple studies and multiple types of studies. Using their best judgment in interpreting these studies and other data, experts look for the weight of the evidence. They carefully examine and attempt to synthesize the entire picture, then make a pronouncement about causation or risk based primarily on the studies to which they have accorded more weight, perhaps because they are of better quality or are more numerous or simply more convincing. "Weight of the evidence is a subjective approach"—in other words, it is art rather than science; more accurately yet, it is art *based on* science. As a result, it is particularly susceptible to bias, whether conscious or unconscious.

Other approaches to data synthesis involve combining the results of several studies to provide numerical risk estimates. Scientists and regulators are drawn to these methods since they provide the illusion of precision, but the reality is that the results of these studies are also shaped by the assumptions and beliefs of the investigator, who decides what data to include in the new package and what to leave out. These models are therefore easily manipulated, consciously and unconsciously, to produce the desired results.

For example, a meta-analysis is a study in which the results of several similar studies are combined to provide a result that, in theory at least, should have more statistical power because it includes far more study subjects than any of its component studies. Meta-analyses can be useful when based on well-designed smaller studies, none of which would be large enough to detect a small effect by itself. However, meta-analyses are susceptible to the "garbage in/garbage out" principle: Build a meta-analysis with flawed studies, and you get a flawed result. In fact, this is a time-honored recipe for countering the results of a well-conducted study: Just mix this good study with several weak or badly designed ones, and you will get a "no findings" conclusion. The added value of this charade is that the investigator and sponsor can claim that the new meta-analysis includes the *entire literature* and therefore trumps the result of that one pesky study.

Another quantitative approach to data synthesis is model building. One particular mathematical model is the "risk assessment," which is based on a combination of data and assumptions, and it is has become the coin of the regulatory realm. Neither the EPA nor OSHA would think of issuing public health regulations without first conducting risk assessments. (These agencies must also consider the assessments conducted by the regulated industries and their consultants.) Some risk measurements are relatively straightforward exercises that use information on the known health effects associated with higher exposure levels to predict the effects at lower exposure levels. These estimations draw a curve with known data points (disease risk at higher exposure) and extrapolate to the parts of the curve that have fewer or no data points (lower exposure). The agencies construct risk assessments of this type to predict how many illnesses or deaths might be prevented, should toxic substances be reduced.

In the absence of powerful epidemiologic studies, risk assessments that attempt to measure the effects of chemical exposures are by necessity more complex, more opaque, and, as a result, more controversial. For example, an investigating team might apply untested theories about translating the risk of cancer of one organ in a rat at a certain exposure level to that of cancer of a different organ at a different exposure level in humans. The outcome would be based on the data and assumptions chosen for inclusion.

The devil here is definitely in the details. This was dramatically proved in a 1991 exercise on risk assessment conducted by the Commission of European Communities. Eleven European governments (Belgium, Denmark, Finland, France, Germany, Great Britain, Greece, Italy, Luxembourg, the Netherlands, and Spain) joined with several large corporations (including Rohm and Haas, Battelle, and Fiat) and appointed eleven teams of scientists and engineers to estimate the accident risk at a hypothetical small ammonia storage plant. The teams worked independently, developing and applying their own assumptions, which turned out to be strikingly different from one team to another. Unsurprisingly, therefore, the risk estimates for an accident were also strikingly different, ranging from 1 in 400 to 1 in 10 million.[11]

It is easy to see how mercenary risk assessments can be concocted. Change a few parameters that are buried deep in a mathematical model, and a hazardous chemical can be miraculously transformed into one that is not very dangerous at all. William Ruckelshaus, appointed by President Nixon to serve as the first EPA administrator, diagnosed the problem: "Risk assessment data can be like a captured spy: if you torture it long enough, it will tell you anything you want to know."[12]

* * *

We have seen how Big Tobacco and other industries played the uncertainty game in the preregulatory era. In the next few chapters I follow those sagas as they have played out in the regulatory era. First, however, I need to present one case study to demonstrate how industry can take advantage of the tricks of the trade introduced earlier in this chapter—the inherent uncertainty in epidemiological studies—in order to forestall regulatory action. Let's see in some detail how the scientific research that industry conducts or funds is manipulated to *mask* rather than *find* exposure-disease relationships—that is, to protect corporations, not their workers.

The chemical is benzene (distinct from benzidine, which can cause bladder cancer, as previously discussed). Benzene is still a very important chemical even though it has in many uses been replaced as a solvent by less toxic substances. Historically, though, it was used heavily throughout industry and is one of the contaminants at the majority of the nation's toxic waste sites, as listed by the EPA's Superfund toxic waste clean-up program.[13] Benzene is also a constituent of gasoline; many gas stations now have vapor recovery systems to control the release of benzene. It is also a product of combustion—that is, engine exhaust. So benzene is literally everywhere, and it is also a human carcinogen. Exposure to higher levels can cause life-threatening aplastic anemia, and what is worse is that even low levels cause leukemia, which is cancer of the blood-forming tissues (the bone marrow, most notably). The medical literature of the 1930s and 1940s repeatedly described the link between benzene and leukemia.[14–23] In 1948 the American Petroleum Institute's "API Toxicological Review of Benzene" discussed "reasonably well documented instances of the development of leukemia as a result of chronic benzene exposure." The report concluded that "it is generally considered that the only absolutely safe concentration for benzene is zero."[24]

When OSHA and NIOSH were getting started in the early 1970s, almost everyone in the field knew about the causative link between benzene and leukemia. For example, in 1973 Dr. Robert Eckardt, director of the Medical Research Division for Esso Research and Engineering, a precursor of Exxon, wrote the following: "[The] accumulation in the literature of cases of leukemia following benzene exposure leads to the inevitable conclusion that benzene is a leukemogenic agent."[25] For the first time, however, NIOSH was able to employ the emerging state-of-the-art tools of epidemiology in industrial settings. An important component of its mission was to support OSHA's standard-setting activities, and in that capacity its scientists had their pick of America's industrial facilities for harnessing the most informative possible natural experiments—factories with one predominant chemical exposure, minimal if any confounding factors, a stable workforce, and good records.

For the study of benzene, two Goodyear Tire and Rubber plants in Ohio fit the bill. The main product of these plants was synthetic rubber (rubber hydrochloride), with the Goodyear trade name Pliofilm. Other than natural rubber and soda ash, benzene was the dominant chemical in the production process, and exposure levels were readily quantifiable. Goodyear officials knew of some leukemia cases among the workers at these plants and cooperated fully with the NIOSH investigators, who were led by epidemiologists Peter Infante and Robert Rinsky.[26]

For the first time, this landmark NIOSH study of twelve hundred workers *quantified* the leukemia risk. To that point, studies had found "too many cases, something's wrong," but they had not been able to estimate the dose-response relationship that would correlate leukemia risk with exposure levels. Now the NIOSH scientists found a doubling of risk among workers exposed for up to four years, a fourteenfold excess risk among those exposed from five to nine years, and a thirty-threefold increase in those exposed for at least ten years. The authors concluded their analysis with a plea: "As a result of past failure to control benzene as a carcinogen, millions of people, without knowledge of the hemopoietic dangers, are continually being exposed to benzene at work.... We hope that our findings, which demonstrate overwhelmingly an increased risk of leukemia in workers exposed to benzene, will stimulate efforts to control occupational and consumer exposure to benzene, an agent known for almost a century to be a powerful bone-marrow poison."[26]

Published in 1977, the NIOSH study was a major factor in OSHA's decision to lower—or *try* to lower—the eight-hour average exposure standard for benzene workers from 10 parts per million (ppm) to 1 ppm (OSHA announced the new number in 1977).[27] Immediately challenged by the industry, the standard was set aside by the Supreme Court, which ruled that OSHA had not shown that its standard would achieve substantial reduction in risk.[28] This ruling established the new standard for all OSHA regulations, and it has impaired the agency's regulatory efforts to this day.

Responding to the Court's new demands, NIOSH scientists who had been working on the benzene matter went back to work. By placing every one of the twelve hundred Goodyear employees in the study on a floor plan and by establishing or estimating exposure levels for each job and location, they developed a job-exposure matrix. They refined their use of historical measures, devised rules for estimating the values of missing data points, and used weighted curves to project both backward and forward—all state-of-the-art techniques. In the end, the results of the revised NIOSH study confirmed those of the original research.[29] Dividing the worker population into four groups by exposure levels, the researchers found increased risk of leukemia ranging from 1 ppm to as high as sixtyfold for the highest exposure levels. This was a very clean and convincing dose-response curve for exposures above 1 ppm. In 1987 OSHA therefore reissued the new exposure standard of 1 ppm.[30]

Beginning in 1987, the National Cancer Institute repeated this study in China, where it used even newer epidemiological methods and better exposure data. This study reconfirmed the fact that benzene can cause leukemia even at lower exposure levels. No matter. Even before the first NIOSH study was officially released, the oil industry had spent tens of millions of dollars to cast doubt on it and the revised, updated versions with a series of analyses and reanalyses. Quite simply, the industry contended that the NIOSH study was flawed. To this day, the oil industry is still spending major money to attack the NIOSH epidemiology. All in all, this entire incident constitutes a textbook example of some of the tricks of the trade, as well as the uses and misuses of epidemiology in the regulatory arena and in litigation.

In addition, NIOSH had selected the Goodyear rubber hydrochloride plants precisely because the environment contained no plausible confounding agents. Nevertheless, one oil industry consultant immediately reanalyzed the data and suggested that since the leukemia rates at the two rubber hydrochloride plants were different, "factors other than similar exposure to a single agent are necessary to explain" the excess leukemias.[31] This we call the "divide and conquer" strategy because it looks at smaller units in order to find differences among them, then uses these differences to cast general doubt on the overall results.

An impressive number of oil companies (including Shell Oil,[32,33,34] Chevron,[35] and ExxonMobil[36-38]) have produced epidemiological studies on other, less heavily exposed worker populations—their own. These studies were essentially guaranteed not to be as informative as the NIOSH study of the Goodyear workers. Why "guaranteed"? Because they were diluted: The benzene exposures of the oil workers were much lower than those of the workers in the Goodyear rubber plants. This approach is not inherently wrong. We know that higher exposures lead to higher risk, but what about lower exposures? Let's find out more about that part of the dose-response curve. But to be useful, these studies have to have *accurate* exposure data.

Much of the work in oil refineries is performed outdoors or in distant, air-conditioned control rooms, where exposures will (almost by definition) be much lower than in enclosed factories and where it will be hard to develop accurate exposure histories and to pin down which, if any, workers are subjected to higher exposures. Therefore, the epidemiologists end up assuming that all or most of the workers received the same, low-level exposure. So, if some workers had a slightly elevated risk associated with slightly higher exposure, this would never be discovered. As I have shown, such studies commonly show little (if any) risk effect, especially when dealing with a disease such as leukemia, which is not a very common cause of death to begin with. Moreover, the overall risk of leukemia in such a study is unlikely to be significantly elevated because of the healthy worker effect.

The oil studies were both diluted and underpowered. They did not have large enough study populations to find statistically significant differences for any but the most prevalent health effects. In theory, one approach for overcoming the low power in such studies is to combine them by using the techniques of meta-analysis. These have certain advantages, but they are highly susceptible to the garbage in/garbage out problem. Specifically, in this case, putting together numerous diluted cohorts yielded only a much larger but still very diluted cohort—lots of people, but few with significant exposure. The guaranteed result: no excess leukemia. This is exactly what was reported in a meta-analysis funded by the oil industry that involved more than two hundred thousand refinery workers.[39] Yet no one took this to mean that benzene does not cause leukemia among oil workers; some of the smaller, individual studies had confirmed this fact.

If polluters are unable to deny a basic disease-exposure relationship and if their claims of uncontrolled confounders, biases, and other errors do not hold up under scrutiny, one last-ditch recourse is to claim that the disease effect is real only at the *highest* levels, while *lower* levels yield no increased risk. Although generally fallacious, this is an easy argument to make because finding a statistically significant excess risk of disease at low levels of exposure can be an impossible challenge. Unless a study is quite large, with good follow-up and exposure data, it generally has little direct information about effects at the lowest exposure levels. Regulatory science understands the problem, carries out its studies to look at the risk incurred at several higher levels of exposure, and then draws the dose-response curve. The confirmed shape of the curve at higher levels of exposure dictates the *estimated* curve for the very lowest exposures.

The oil companies commissioned a slew of analyses that claimed to detect a threshold, or safe level, for benzene exposure.[40–44] At the end of the day, however, these weak, uninformative studies, which had been set up to counter the powerful NIOSH rubber hydrochloride study, remained weak and uninformative. Why spend the money? The industry needed some "evidence" to wave in the face of OSHA and exclaim, "See! We don't find leukemia in our studies, so something must be wrong with the NIOSH study!" It's a game, and everyone knows it, but OSHA must, by law, analyze the proffered studies, file answers, analyze the answers to the answers, and so on ad infinitum. The studies served their purpose for the oil industry—they bought some time, if nothing else—but no one in the regulatory sciences was impressed. Such studies would never be enough. The industry knew this, too, and it knew it would have to go after the big dog itself, the NIOSH study.

How do you go about undermining such comprehensive work? Actually, it is easy. You selectively remove or censor cases, thereby turning a positive result—excess risk—into a negative result—no excess risk.

Simply put, the risk estimate is a fraction in which the numerator is the number of disease cases and the denominator is the study population. If you can somehow lower the numerator without lowering the denominator, an increase in apparent risk goes down. For example, ten deaths in a worker population of one hundred is a 10 percent risk, but if three of those ten deaths get excluded for whatever reason—if the numerator of the fraction is now 7, not 10—the risk is 7 percent, not 10 percent. That might not seem like a significant difference, but what about the change in *excess* risk, which is the key for regulators? Let's say the expected risk of the disease in the general population is 5 percent. When the numerator in our equation is 10, the disease risk of 10 percent is twice the expected risk of 5 percent—or 100 percent higher. When the numerator is 7, the 7 percent risk is only 40 percent higher than the expected 5 percent risk. The smaller excess risk suggests that the exposure is less hazardous. It also increases the likelihood that the results will not be statistically significant.

For regulatory purposes, lowering the numerator by a fairly small number can therefore make all the difference. With this elementary principle in mind, scientists who were working for Shell Oil and British Petroleum reanalyzed the NIOSH study and looked for disease cases that could be eliminated from the numerator.[45] One case, for example, occurred less than two years after an employee's earliest exposure to benzene. It seemed reasonable to suggest that this case was not benzene related, but subtracting that case from the numerator is still not legitimate methodology. Since you cannot distinguish between the cases that would have occurred without exposure and those that are exposure related, you have to count *all* of the cases. This particular industry critique, published in *Regulatory Toxicology and Pharmacology,* was quickly forgotten and replaced by others that were more impressive, if equally unfounded.

That first reanalysis of the NIOSH study was made before OSHA's 1 ppm standard went into effect. Several years after the standard was finally implemented, the American Petroleum Institute brought in ChemRisk's Dennis Paustenbach to reanalyze the landmark work yet again.[46] I have already introduced Dr. Paustenbach as one of the leaders in the product defense field. His scientific credentials are solid, he knows what he is doing—and his work with the NIOSH benzene study is an extreme example of how to maul a good epidemiological study and thereby defuse the results. Because there were few original measurements of benzene exposure levels in the 1940s and 1950s, the NIOSH team had made a series of estimates based on the known measurements and their own understanding of the work process. Dr. Paustenbach and his colleagues changed the exposure estimates, replacing the original ones with worst-case scenarios and eventually assuming the occurrence of levels so high that, according to the NIOSH scientists, "one would assume that such extreme exposures would produce an epidemic of serious benzene poisonings," which had never occurred.[47]

Unlikely as they were, the new exposure estimates successfully shifted the dose-response curve. When a scientist from the American Petroleum Institute constructed a new risk assessment based on Dr. Paustenbach's exposure estimates, she could assert that "occupational exposure only to very high concentrations" could cause leukemia.[41] However, the ChemRisk reanalysis nonetheless ended up with a curve that demonstrated excess leukemia risk among the workers in the lowest category of exposure. This was presumably a disappointment to the oil industry. It then hired Dr. Paustenbach (who had moved to Exponent, Inc.) to undertake yet another reanalysis. This time, the Exponent team reduced its exposure estimates for the highest categories (so they were not quite so unlikely) but not for the lower ones. The resulting new curve made it easier to claim that only very high exposures cause leukemia.[48]

Still, mercenary reanalyses and critiques would never be enough to roll back the OSHA standard—the science is strong—so why bother? First, the oil industry needs to be ready should OSHA decide to lower the standard to 0.5 ppm or even 0.1 ppm. For the moment this is a highly unlikely prospect, however; the more immediate industry concern is the EPA. Production and use of gasoline inevitably leads to the release of benzene—and if benzene were shown to cause disease at ultralow exposure levels, the EPA could force the oil companies to spend huge sums of money to reduce emissions. Then there is a third reason: litigation. I discuss this issue in more depth later, but suffice it to say here that studies of no value whatsoever in the regulatory arena can be quite valuable for corporate defendants in the courtroom. A jury might be impressed by a one-hundred-page "peer-reviewed" article that claims that all of the government science must be wrong, must be "junk science," whereas the industry's own "sound science" proves that benzene did not cause this individual's leukemia.

For the purposes of litigation protection, ChemRisk continues to churn out assessments of benzene exposure in different industries. After a Swedish study had found an increased risk of leukemia among members of the deck crews of tankers transporting chemicals and oil[49] and ExxonMobil had been sued by a seaman exposed to benzene,[50] ChemRisk then produced impressive-looking (and peer-reviewed, of course) estimates that the exposures generally did not exceed the old OSHA standard.[51] By itself, the for-hire provenance gives away the game with such studies, but other clues also suggest that these are not your normal scientific papers. One is their excessive length. In most journals, pages are a precious commodity, and editors generally strong-arm authors to shorten their submissions. Dr. Paustenbach's first reanalysis, however, ran 54 pages,[46] and his second a mind-numbing 104 pages.[48] Such triple digits do not impress scientists—most would not even consider actually reading a 104-page recalculation of exposure data from a decades-old study—but the target audience is not scientists but jurors and judges, who may be favorably impressed by the excessive length.

The first Paustenbach reconstruction of the NIOSH study generated some debate, but the second has been largely ignored in the scientific literature. Why? The debate over the correct dose-response curve for Goodyear's workers in Ohio has practically been mooted by the new research from China, where a team of researchers from the U.S. National Cancer Institute and the Chinese Academy of Preventive Medicine (NCI-CAPM) has been conducting a carefully controlled study in Shanghai since 1987. China offers the natural experiment that epidemiologists dream of: a growing industrial sector with a wide range of exposure levels for benzene; easy access to the factories; extensive exposure monitoring; and few workers lost to follow-up. The early results from this study document a doubling of the leukemia risk at exposure levels averaging only 10 ppm.[52] The NIOSH studies had reached similar conclusions by extrapolating from documented effects at higher levels, but they had too few cases among the workers exposed at the lower levels.

Then, in 2004, additional results from China were terrible news for industry because they documented blood disease—altered white blood cell and platelet counts—in workers exposed to benzene levels *below* 1 ppm.[53] The far more accurate exposure measurements possible in China allowed this much more precise assessment at exposure levels far lower than in the Ohio study. The headline in the December 2004 issue of *Science* magazine summed up the situation nicely: "A Little Is Still Too Much."[54] These results from China were perhaps not a surprise to many epidemiologists familiar with the relevant benzene literature, but they could turn out to be a body blow to the oil industry, which has spent millions over several decades attacking studies that find effects below 10 ppm. The results should put an end to the claims of the American Petroleum Institute, such as this one by API's director of Health and Environmental Sciences, Robert Drew: "We recognize that benzene can cause leukemia at high levels of exposure, say 25, 50, or 100 parts per million in the workplace. But we disagree that there is a risk of cancer at the lower levels present in the environment."[55]

The stunning Chinese result also provides further evidence that the existing OSHA standard of 1 ppm is not sufficiently protective and raises the question of whether there is any safe level of exposure to benzene at all. (Recall that the API had suggested exactly this point in its report of 1948— half a century earlier.[24]) Needless to say, oil industry product defense consultants have published papers criticizing the China study.[56,57] The criticisms were not very convincing, so the industry has taken the bolder step of producing *its own* series of studies in China. Several papers on benzene exposure and health effects have already been published by API-supported researchers working in China.[58–60] Thanks to documents unearthed in a Texas lawsuit, we now understand that the underlying rationale of the API's China initiative is to "respond to allegations" in the NCI-CAPM study. Each oil company's share of the $22 million cost of this work is to be commensurate with its share of the oil market.[61,62] A memo to the manager of toxicology and product safety for Marathon Oil points out the dangers posed for the industry. Should the toxic effects of low-level benzene exposure reported by the original China study become widely accepted by regulators, calls would soon follow for the reformulation of gasoline, for control of emissions from refineries and marketing facilities, and for the clean-up of contamination. A nightmare for the industry. And then there's litigation.

At $22 million, the study will be a bargain because the sponsors apparently know the outcome before the work has even begun. This comes as no surprise, but with this API benzene study we actually have a smoking gun that proves the point: that memo to the Marathon manager. Here is the excerpt: [63]

Project Value—How Will Research Results Enhance Industry's Ability to Achieve Objectives on Issue of Global Impact and Concern:

The planned research is expected to:

- Provide strong scientific support for the lack of a risk of leukemia or other hematological disease at current ambient benzene concentrations to the general population.
- Establish that adherence to current occupational exposure limits (in the range of 1–5 ppm) do [*sic*] not create a significant risk to workers exposed to benzene.
- Refute the allegation that Non-Hodgkins lymphoma can be induced by benzene exposure.

How could the sponsors know what the research is expected to find? Naïve question. This study will have fewer benzene-exposed workers than the original China study, so the effects at low exposure levels will be harder to see than those at higher levels. A smaller study is unlikely to find a statistically significant excess at levels below 1 ppm or even 5 ppm. Thus the scientists and their sponsors will wave their results and say, "Look, we did our own study in China and didn't find the same effect." Remember, they do not need to prove that no detrimental health effect occurs at low levels of benzene exposure. They only need to manufacture some uncertainty by raising questions about the accuracy and validity of the studies that do find an effect. Given such equal but opposite results, no definitive conclusion can be reached, no further regulation is warranted, and no verdict against the company can be entered. The oil companies win.

7

Defending Secondhand Smoke

In 1981 Horace Kornegay, a former North Carolina congressman, then president and executive director of the Tobacco Institute, was worried. It had become clear, primarily from polling data, that all of the enormous sums of money the industry had been spending in its public relations campaign were not working. Almost everyone—including smokers—believed that smoking is harmful. The social acceptability of the habit was declining, and the credibility of the industry as a source of "information or persuasion" was practically nil. Kornegay's proposed solution: fight fire with fire. "*Science* remains the fundamental problem confronting the industry. Bad press, unwarranted regulation and poor opinion are its symptoms. *Symptoms* cannot be effectively treated without attacking their underlying cause.... Industry communications must contain less of 'But *that* study is wrong' and more of 'Look what *this* study shows'" (emphasis in the original).[1]

Decades earlier—way before the first glimmer of effective regulation—John Hill of Hill and Knowlton had also urged Big Tobacco to fight the science of the antitobacco establishment with its own, better science.[2,3] In the regulatory era, the industry now had even more motivation to get proactive. Attacks on the methodology of the establishment science were not enough; the uncertainty campaign had its limitations. Maybe a little of the old mud had stuck, but now even that was drying out and chipping off. With the other option, the problem with moving onto the offensive with new science in the '80s was exactly the same as it had been in the '50s, '60s, and '70s: The industry could not produce that new and better science because the consensus science was correct.

Oh, the headaches for the industry, on top of which was a new one with multiple labels: "passive smoking," "involuntary smoking," "environmental tobacco smoke" or "ETS," "secondhand smoke." Call it what you will (I generally avoid ETS, the term coined and promoted by the tobacco industry[4]), this pollutant was becoming a veritable migraine for the industry because it necessarily caught the attention of both EPA and OSHA. The industry had seen the threat coming in the early 1970s. A confidential 1978 industry report by the Roper polling organization warned that a campaign by antismoking forces targeting secondhand smoke would be "the most dangerous development to the viability of the tobacco industry that has yet occurred."[5] In 1981 the first important epidemiologic study was published showing that nonsmoking women whose spouses smoke have a higher rate of lung cancer than those married to nonsmokers.[6] When that work garnered immediate public attention, the industry declared a red alert.

On the primary issue of smoking per se, it could still try to hide behind the "personal choice" defense, but this would not work with secondhand smoke. Such exposure was involuntary and unpleasant, as everyone understood, and if it also proved to be *unhealthy,* this could be the opening for which the most vehement of the antismoking zealots had been yearning for decades. Some even talked about prohibition. The industry would have to pull out all the stops. By 1984 thirty-seven states and the District of Columbia had already restricted smoking in some public facilities such as auditoriums and government buildings. These laws were having an impact: Internal tobacco industry documents attributed as much as 21 percent of the geographic variation in cigarette consumption to public smoking restrictions. General health concerns on the part of smokers might have been one factor, but the industry believed concern about secondhand smoke was the main culprit. These restrictions were likely to become even more numerous and more onerous in the future. Moreover, the movement to restrict smoking in workplaces was gathering steam.[7,8]

In Europe, where smoking is more prevalent, smokers are somewhat more tolerated by nonsmokers, and workplace restrictions are loosely enforced, the industry set up the "Whitecoat Project" as a way to get some friendlier science in front of the public and "restore smoker confidence."[9] Who could plausibly front for this contrived campaign? Documents from a Philip Morris presentation in London demonstrate the lengths to which the industry had to go in order to find scientists in Europe who had no "problems of attribution," that is, association with tobacco on their resumes.[10] (Some years earlier, when Philip Morris bought a laboratory in Germany, it had set up a complex scheme to hide its role, as the British medical journal

Lancet later reported. A Swedish professor served as the go-between with Philip Morris staffers in the United States, and the scientists at the tobacco-owned German laboratory "appear[ed] to have published only a small amount of its research and what was published appears to differ considerably from what was not."[11])

For the "Whitecoat Project," Dr. Myron Weinberg, founder of the product defense firm the Weinberg Group, was brought on board. Prospective scientists were asked whether they were interested in problems of "indoor air quality." Tobacco and smoking would not be mentioned. The scientists' CVs would then be used to weed out those among the positive respondents who were obviously antismoking or otherwise had "unsuitable backgrounds." Lawyers were involved in this vetting. Those who passed that preliminary smell test were then given ten hours of reading material, including articles that exonerated secondhand smoke, and asked for an independent opinion. If it was a favorable one, a Philip Morris scientist would finally emerge from the shadows and contact this individual.[10]

One of the documents concludes: "Philip Morris [would] then expect the group of scientists to operate within the confines of decisions taken by PM scientists to determine the general direction of research, which apparently would then be 'filtered' by lawyers to eliminate areas of sensitivity. Their idea is that the groups of scientists should be able to produce research or stimulate controversy...."[10]

In the United States, a Tobacco Institute document from that same time period cites fourteen academic scientists working on secondhand smoke, along with twenty-three consultants. Unfortunately for tobacco, though, the "[c]redibility of the professional consultants is limited in many instances by their willingness to work for tobacco. Academics are not immune from this problem but are less susceptible to it. . . . The nature of science prevents them from saying little more than the studies are flawed and the evidence is inconclusive."[12,13]

For every PhD there is probably an equal and opposite PhD somewhere. That's an old joke in academia, but it is not the case when Big Tobacco is involved. The industry's white coats were not nearly so white and bright and freshly starched as those sitting on the EPA's Scientific Advisory Board, for one example. The moment scientists became publicly identified with Big Tobacco, they were sullied by the stain. On the other hand, the industry felt it had a better chance fighting the scientific evidence against secondhand smoke; scientists who opposed the industry on the basic smoking question might be more willing to join them on this one. The industry argued that its studies were the target of "publication bias," banned from frontline journals with an antismoking stance. The evidence, though, does not support this charge.[14]

* * *

By the mid-1980s civil suits brought against the tobacco industry by smokers were popping up all over the country. Litigation against the asbestos companies was also in full swing by then, and these companies dragged the cigarette manufacturers into the litigation as third parties by claiming that tobacco contributed to the lung cancer of those asbestos workers who also smoked. By July 1985 there were 44 suits by smokers against just one cigarette manufacturer, R. J. Reynolds, the nation's second largest, and asbestos manufacturers had filed more than three hundred third-party claims against RJR.[15] However, RJR scientists recognized that epidemiologic studies of workers exposed to asbestos and other environmental toxins could be used to shift the blame back in that direction, and the company went to court and successfully demanded the raw data underlying the famous asbestos studies of Dr. Irving Selikoff at the Mount Sinai School of Medicine.[16] Using this information, RJR could build a model that would manipulate the data to provide whatever outcome was needed to win each particular case, no matter what the facts actually revealed. One description of RJR's "Integrated Exposure and Hazard Assessment Initiative" was explicit: Its objective was to do the following:

> Shift a portionately [*sic*] higher amount of risk (maybe all) to the asbestos defendants, particularly if plaintiff's asbestos is high; or alternatively, if smoking dose is low. . . . An example would be a case where the plaintiff's lung cancer is more likely to have arisen in another tissue and metastasized to the lung. In this case, every effort should be made to eliminate, or drive as low as possible, asbestos exposure since current evidence suggests that asbestos tumors arise principally in the lung, be they classic or mesothelioma. By contrast, if plaintiff's cancer is clearly primary to the lung, it is imperative that every effort be made to maximize occupational exposure not only to asbestos but also to other agents in the workplace.[17]

For help in constructing this model, RJR turned to Failure Analysis Associates, the California firm that would later change its name to Exponent, Inc.[18] This asbestos model was only the beginning. If lung cancer could be blamed on asbestos, why not also on radon? According to an RJR memo, the company hired Dr. Michael Ginevan, previously a biostatistician for the Nuclear Regulatory Commission, to "develop a rationale for attribution of a greater proportion of lung cancer to radiation than heretofore claimed."[19] Or why not blame the lung cancers on emissions from a power plant or chemical factory or oil refinery? How about a toxic waste dump? Tobacco tried them all.[20]

* * *

In 1987 OSHA received two petitions calling for an emergency temporary standard to prohibit smoking in indoor workplaces, one from Public Citizen and the American Public Health Association, the other from a group cleverly named for the sake of its acronym, Action on Smoking and Health (ASH). However, OSHA denied the petitions, with backing from some within the agency who believed that, even though indoor air quality standards were warranted, it was politically impossible to put them in place—and the ill-fated effort to do so would be an incredible drain on the agency's limited resources. Two years later ASH filed a lawsuit to compel OSHA to issue an emergency standard. The court sided with the agency.[21] In September 1991, still feeling some heat from antisecondhand smoke congressional members and interest groups, OSHA issued an official request for information on all problems of indoor air quality (tobacco smoke, carbon monoxide, organic chemicals, bioaerosols).[22] In March 1992, when the AFL-CIO petitioned OSHA to issue an overall indoor air quality standard, OSHA said it would consider the matter—a good way to deal with the issue in an election year. Two years later OSHA officially proposed a rule that would have required employers to either prohibit smoking altogether or construct separate, enclosed rooms that had exhaust systems to send tobacco smoke directly to the outside.[23] Clearly, most employers would choose the former, less expensive course, making life that much more difficult for tobacco addicts.

Big Tobacco saw this action as potentially do or die; it was absolutely *imperative* to discredit the link between workplace secondhand smoke and disease. [24] A July 1994 document described Philip Morris's plan to "convert the promulgation process from bureaucratic fiat to political dogfight. . . . Over the next month, if we have anything to do with it, this opposition is going to intensify and we're going to give the poobahs at OSHA a taste of what democracy is really like."[25] Over at RJR, Dr. H. Daniel Roth was on the case. Dr. Roth may be the premier, all-purpose, pro-industry reanalyzer. In 1988 he met with RJR and offered his help in attacking the NIOSH study of heart disease mortality among bridge and tunnel workers.[26] (Almost by definition, these workers are exposed to elevated levels of carbon monoxide, a significant ingredient in gasoline and diesel exhaust, and the NIOSH study showed considerable excess risk for heart disease in this population, lending support to the case against secondhand smoke, which is also rich in carbon monoxide.[27]) Dr. Roth suggested a host of ways the study could be questioned: difficulties in measurement techniques; confounding factors; the inaccuracy of death certificates in assessing heart disease; and many more.[26]

Now, in 1994, Dr. Roth pulled out all the tricks of the trade in his attack on OSHA's science in support of the rule on indoor air quality. In comments he submitted to the agency on behalf of RJR he proclaimed the following:

> OSHA neglected to include some published studies in its analyses.
>
> OSHA misrepresented the findings in other studies to suggest an ETS effect in cases where no such effect is indicated.
>
> OSHA failed to recognize that many of the studies it cited are of poor quality.
>
> OSHA failed to recognize that many of the studies it relied upon failed to adjust for confounding factors, an omission which in all likelihood led the Administration to overestimate the effects of ETS.
>
> OSHA failed to correct for the tendency of individuals to mischaracterize the smoking habits of their household members and coworkers.
>
> OSHA presented no scientifically defensible calculations to support its findings.
>
> OSHA failed to test whether the data from different studies are homogenous and could be aggregated to analysis.
>
> OSHA failed to group the data so that the overall ETS risk (if one exists) could be calculated.[28,29]

Let's catch our breath here and think about this. To the untrained eye, this indictment turns OSHA scientists and policy makers into a bunch of incompetent and/or duplicitous zealots with a presumed grudge against cigarette exhaust and a willingness to cut any scientific corner in order to regulate it and put the tobacco industry out of business. In fact, however, the OSHA analysis of 1994 was not perfect, but it was very good, and with time have come more studies—many more studies—that confirm the essential correctness of the presentation. Secondhand smoke kills.[30,31]

An ancillary benefit of any uncertainty campaign is that it is guaranteed to buy some time. This point was well made in a conference call involving Philip Morris executives, their lawyers, and Myron Weinberg (who had now started another consulting firm called WashTech). The scheme was straightforward: Overwhelm OSHA. The notes from this conference call report that "WashTech has experts in 'deductive meta analysis' that reveals confounders and identifies the real risk involved if any." Understanding the regulatory process and OSHA's obligation to respond to all comments, the conspirators planned a "line by line analysis raising scientific questions that OSHA would have to respond to.... [This] attack could take [OSHA] 2 to 3 years to respond to."[32]

The uncertainty campaign worked.[24] The tobacco industry's well-funded strategy "to put the bureaucratic machinery on overload" stymied OSHA's efforts.[25] The cigarette makers generated more than one hundred thousand letters to the agency, far more than it had received on any other issue. Philip Morris alone dispatched more than 120 witnesses to testify at OSHA's hearings. In the end, OSHA capitulated and never finalized its indoor air quality standard.

* * *

The EPA was (and still is) also a target for Big Tobacco because that agency, in 1992, categorized secondhand smoke as a Group A carcinogen—a chemical that causes cancer in humans.[33] The EPA has little authority to regulate tobacco, but any negative statement with the EPA acronym attached would be a powerful asset for localities that wanted to restrict smoking in public spaces, as well as for plaintiffs' attorneys. One industry document argued that the industry could not win a "credibility fight" with the EPA, so don't even try.[34] Another stated, "The credibility of EPA is defeatable, but not on the basis of ETS alone. It must be part of a larger mosaic that concentrates all of EPA's enemies against it at one time."[35] Acting on this advice, the industry tried to enlist as many other regulated industries as possible to front for the cause in the name of "sound science." We have already seen that this cynically named movement was the creation of Big Tobacco, initially under the aegis of The Advancement of Sound Science Coalition (TASSC), introduced in chapter five. Through the good offices of TASSC, Big Tobacco reached out to executives at Procter and Gamble, General Motors, 3M, Dow Chemical, and other corporations to serve, in the words of Sheldon Rampton and John Stauber, as "protective camouflage, concealing the tobacco money."[36]

Another industry outfit was the Center for Indoor Air Research (CIAR), which claimed that it could *prove* that the case against secondhand smoke was flawed. The idea for CIAR came from Dr. Anthony Colucci, who, before becoming R. J. Reynolds's director of Scientific Litigation Support, had collaborated with Dr. Roth in attacking EPA research into the relationship of exposure to air pollution and asthma.[37] The CIAR boasted that its talking heads had become "masters at pointing out deficiencies in study methodology. We were typically, in other words, like the guest from hell." However, the center also recognized that the guest from hell needed to present an affirmative defense, and the front group claimed to have it—three studies, the largest ever undertaken, all concluding that exposure to secondhand smoke was much too low to cause health problems and much lower than OSHA had claimed when it proposed to essentially ban workplace smoking. These studies "were and are the best available when judged in terms of scientific merit," CIAR argued. "It's hard to believe that there can be much dispute about that."[38]

It is hard to believe that someone at CIAR wrote that sentence without falling out of the chair laughing. These three studies were all based on data provided by the industry.[39] The actual game plan for CIAR's "science" was revealed in a letter in which one of the lawyers tells an executive that "CIAR does not attempt in any way to influence the substance of its grantees' published reports." However, because CIAR's value depends on the industry's "identifying research projects likely to be of value...CIAR is a credible and effective vehicle for conducting the research that is needed to buttress the industry's position."[40]

Here's how I read that contorted rhetoric: "CIAR doesn't influence studies because CIAR selects only those studies that won't need the influence."

The manipulation and selective publication of data by Big Tobacco's scientists resulted in a distortion of the literature now widely known as the "funding effect," a term used to describe the close correlation between the results desired by a study's sponsors and the results reported. We have seen evidence of the funding effect throughout these pages. It is most apparent in review articles and meta-analyses, in which an author selects a group of papers (theoretically all of the highest-quality papers on a given subject) and synthesizes an overall message or pattern. Who is surprised to learn that the funding effect is particularly strong in studies that look at the health effects of secondhand smoke and are sponsored by Big Tobacco? The CIAR had a special program to support, publish, and promote studies that found secondhand smoke harmless.[41] When researchers at the University of California examined 106 review articles, they found more than a third concluded that secondhand smoke was *not* harmful. Three-quarters of these dissenting reviews had authors who were affiliated with the tobacco industry.[42]

However, skewed literature reviews would never be enough to win the day, certainly not when the issue is cigarette smoke. The results of some studies are simply too powerful to explain away with sleight of hand; they must be attacked head on. This is where data reanalysis comes in. In all valid studies, the methods must be selected before any data are analyzed; post hoc reanalyses are clearly susceptible to mercenary manipulation since after-the-fact researchers can change the parameters of the study to yield the preferred new outcome. We have seen how this played out in the benzene saga, during which the landmark NIOSH study was subjected to three reanalyses sponsored by the oil industry. On the question of secondhand smoke, the most threatening studies for the industry were those that showed increased risk of lung cancer among nonsmokers. The early studies investigated the risk among nonsmoking spouses of smokers, specifically. The study by Takeshi Hirayama, chief epidemiologist of the National Cancer Center Research Institute in Tokyo, was the most prominent of these.[6] If it could be discredited, some of this regulatory mess might disappear, so the industry went after Dr. Hirayama's work.

One approach involved generating and slipping into the peer-review literature a competing Japanese spousal study, this one concluding that studies like Dr. Hirayama's have "little scientific basis."[43] This study was conceived and supported by the cigarette makers, but by working through Covington and Burling, a prominent Washington, D.C., law firm, they were able to conceal their intimate involvement in every aspect of the job.[44] The second approach was to attack Dr. Hirayama's study even more directly by claiming its calculations were flawed. Through the good offices of CIAR, the tobacco industry obtained Dr. Hirayama's raw data and hired another consulting firm, ENVIRON, Inc., to reanalyze the numbers.[45,46] The project was directed by Dr. Michael Ginevan, the same fellow who had worked on radon. However, RJR evidently had concerns about ENVIRON's work product, and the job was moved to Failure Analysis (before it was renamed Exponent).[47]

Initially there was a problem here with RJR, for whom Failure Analysis was working on the asbestos question, as just discussed, as well as examining another data set, this one from the large American Cancer Society study, measuring lung cancer risk among nonsmoking wives of smokers.[48] Therefore, RJR enjoyed "close control" over Failure Analysis's work product,[49] while CIAR was an industry-wide initiative, but this turf war was apparently resolved. The arrival of this new work on secondhand smoke posed potential conflict-of-interest problems at the consulting firm as well, but its scientists badly wanted to work out a suitable arrangement: "They have made every effort not to deal with other clients that represent a conflict of interest, but in turn, expected to be supported by the [tobacco] industry. *In short, they want a role in ETS*" (emphasis added).[50]

In the end, Hirayama's work has been proven correct, supported by the results of numerous other studies.[51,52] Of course, when it was first published, the results needed independent confirmation. Any single epidemiological study could be flawed, which is why we attempt to look at the same issue using different populations and dissimilar methods. In 1985, with the support of the National Cancer Institute, a group of researchers under the leadership of Dr. Elizabeth Fontham of Louisiana State University began a multicenter study designed to minimize problems that had been present in the earlier studies. One result of this research was explosive—the non-smoking wives of male smokers had an increased risk of lung cancer of 30 percent—but the second was apocalyptic for the industry: Tobacco smoke in workplaces and other locations outside the home increased lung cancer risk by 40–60 percent.[53–55]

The cigarette manufacturers now felt they had no choice. They had to discredit the Fontham study. But Elizabeth Fontham did not care to watch the industry hirelings twist her results and make her findings disappear; she refused the entreaties of the tobacco companies to give up her data. She would not cooperate, and they could not make her.[56] For the reanalysis sans raw data, the industry hired Dr. William Butler, a veteran Failure Analysis staffer who went on to start his own firm, Environmental Risk Analysis. At hearings held by OSHA and the National Toxicology Program, Dr. Butler testified that Dr. Fontham's study was inaccurate, but his reanalysis was necessarily limited to the data presented in her publications.[57,58] As it happened, Dr. Fontham's unwillingness to give up her raw data led directly to Congress's passage of the Data Access Act, also known as the Shelby Amendment, which requires all federally supported researchers to give up their raw data. Who on Capitol Hill realized that Big Tobacco was behind the Data Access Act? I return to this story in chapter fourteen.

* * *

Another key Big Tobacco initiative in Europe (and then in the United States and worldwide) was the promulgation of general epidemiological principles (GEP), which would work hand in hand with "sound science" to advance the cause of neither epidemiology nor science. Just as "sound science" is any science that serves industry and "junk science" any science that does not, so any prosmoking epidemiological study has necessarily followed GEP, while any study that does not help the cause has necessarily violated those principles.

The Chemical Manufacturers Association published the first GEP standards in 1991,[59] and Philip Morris immediately recognized the possibilities and took the lead in this field. A number of GEP seminars were held around the world, some put together by the Weinberg Group; one in England in 1995 drafted the London Principles, as their promoters labeled them.[60] (This seminar was planned by Federal Focus, a Washington, D.C., policy group whose chairman, Jim Tozzi of Multinational Business Services, had been under contract to Philip Morris for the previous two years. Tozzi, another major player in the product defense industry, had been the number-two person at the Office of Information and Regulatory Affairs (OIRA) at the White House's Office of Management and Budget during the Reagan era. Among his other credits, Tozzi played a role in delaying the warnings on aspirin with which I opened this book.[61]) Philip Morris's "Legislative Guidelines on GEP" had a single objective: "Impede adverse legislation." Since anything the tobacco industry claims has zero credibility, it would always minimize its visibility while attacking the idea that *any* but the worst environmental toxins cause disease. To this end, Philip Morris wanted to bring on board the chemical, mobile phone, computer, metal, food, packaging, pharmaceutical, and forestry/paper industries.[62]

Skillfully written by product defense experts, rigid application of these "general epidemiological practices" would make it virtually impossible to prove a causal relationship except when it came to the most powerful toxins. Exposures like secondhand smoke that increase the risk of disease by *only* 30 percent would be off the hook—yet that 30 percent is a public health nightmare.

In the 1998 decision in *Flue-Cured Tobacco Cooperative Stabilization Corp. et al. v. U.S. EPA,*[63] a federal judge in North Carolina bought the tobacco industry's claims that the agency "cherry picked" its data and threw out the risk assessment that had produced the Class A designation.[64] That took care of the EPA, despite the fact that in October 1998 the *Journal of the National Cancer Institute* published a review of several dozen secondhand smoke studies and concluded in an editorial that secondhand smoke is indeed a "low-level lung carcinogen."[65] Subsequent studies have confirmed this finding over and over again and found, perhaps not surprisingly, other effects of secondhand smoke as well. A 2005 study published in *Circulation,* the journal of the American Heart Association, reviewed twenty-nine studies of the impact of secondhand smoke on the cardiovascular system and found that passive smokers suffer a 30 percent increase in the risk of coronary heart disease.[66]

One of the authors of that study in *Circulation* was Stanton Glantz, professor of medicine at the University of California–San Francisco. On May 24, 1994, Dr. Glantz received in the mail a box of documents— thousands of pages from the files of the Brown and Williamson Tobacco Corporation (B&W), the manufacturer of Kool and Viceroy, among other brands. The return address said only "Mr. Butts."[67] As word of this incredible treasure trove spread, B&W alleged that some of the "confidential" and "privileged" papers in the collection had been stolen from one of its law firms by a disgruntled former paralegal who had had major heart surgery and wanted compensation. The documents must be returned, the company's lawyers said. However, Glantz was not the only recipient of purloined B&W material. Others had been obtained by the news media and were put to instant use, and still others became the subject of an investigation by a committee of the House of Representatives.[68] There was no shortage of these documents in circulation. The following year, two courts—one in Florida, one in California—declared that all of the documents were in the public domain because, stated the California court, "The genie is out of the bottle. These documents are out."[67,69]

After decades of "sleazy" behavior by Big Tobacco (to recall the adjective employed by Dr. C. Everett Koop, former U.S. Surgeon General[70]), this new evidence was the final straw for, among others, the Board of Directors of the American Medical Association. The AMA's esteemed journal devoted most of its July 19, 1995, issue to them[71–76] and added an editorial, signed by every member of the board, that demanded that the tobacco industry be reined in, once and for all.[77] *The Cigarette Papers,* edited and interpreted by Dr. Glantz and his team in San Francisco, was published the following year.[67] Thus, even though the science against smoking is very powerful, the behavior of the tobacco industry has been just as compelling a motivator for the antismoking forces. The B&W documents strengthened public support for the Clinton administration's attempts to expand the Food and Drug Administration's authority to include the regulation of nicotine as an addictive drug and cigarettes as delivery devices of that drug.[78] In 2000, however, the Supreme Court ruled that Congress had not given the FDA such jurisdiction.[79]

Where does everything stand today? The Federal Trade Commission has mandated advertising restrictions, the Federal Aviation Agency has outlawed smoking on commercial airliners, and federal contracts now require a smoke-free workplace, a strong incentive for many employers to ban workplace smoking. Cigarettes are taxed at the federal and state level—a type of regulation (and the main one, in the case of smoking, according to some observers). Otherwise, OSHA has backed off, the EPA has backed off, and Congress has yet to give the FDA jurisdiction over cigarettes. The most important changes in the regulation of tobacco have occurred in the states and localities, many of which have indeed passed restrictions on indoor smoking that leave people standing in the rain outside office buildings smoking their cigarettes. After decreasing for eight years, the percentage of American adults who smoke appears to have leveled at about 21 percent;[80] cigarettes are still responsible for more than four hundred thousand deaths each year and cost approximately $157 billion in annual health-related economic losses.[81] In some parts of the country, like California, the prevalence of smoking continues to decrease, which suggests that well-funded antismoking programs can further reduce smoking rates and save more lives.

On the other hand, one could live in Japan, where almost half of all men smoke (only about 10 percent of women). The Japanese government owns two-thirds of the leading cigarette makers and did not acknowledge that cigarettes are harmful to health until 1997. Predictably and inevitably, lung cancer has now replaced stomach cancer as the leading cause of cancer mortality.[82,83]

8

Still *Waiting for the Body Count*

When we left the history of workplace bladder cancer caused by chemicals used in dyes production, the big chemical companies had finally given up defending BNA, the bladder carcinogen. The BNA production lines were closed. In 1973 the newly instituted OSHA, prompted by a petition from the Oil, Chemical, and Atomic Workers Union and Ralph Nader's Health Research Group[1] moved to regulate benzidine and thirteen other carcinogens (including BNA, in case anyone tried to bring it back from the dead).[2] In response to this effort, the manufacturers finally conceded that benzidine was a human carcinogen but *still* opposed the rule. They now asserted that, while workers *had* been exposed to dangerous levels of benzidine, current workplace conditions were much improved and posed no further risk. In their testimony to OSHA, the industry executives claimed that "all of the reported instances of bladder tumors in benzidine workers of which we are aware involve employees who were exposed to benzidine before the improved production and use procedures were adopted."[3]

The meager protestations were soon moot.[4] The last two benzidine manufacturers ceased production in 1973; with the enactment of the new OSHA standard, benzidine-based dye manufacture, in which worker exposure to benzidine is virtually unavoidable, was also curtailed.[5] Eight of the nine U.S. producers discontinued operations between 1974 and 1979.[6] Today there are none. Unlike vinyl chloride, benzidine was too dangerous and had too low a profit margin to produce or even to use safely here. Once regulation began, the factories closed.

* * *

Alas, our story is not over. In February 1988 the union that represented the workers at a Goodyear Tire and Rubber plant in Niagara Falls, New York, requested that NIOSH investigate an apparent outbreak of bladder cancer among its members. Since 1957 Goodyear had been using another aromatic amine, a chemical close in structure to BNA and benzidine called ortho-toluidine (OT). Goodyear used OT in the production of an antioxidant that was added to rubber products. Union officers and their medical consultants had identified eight cases of bladder cancer among workers exposed to OT, and they feared more would be discovered with a more comprehensive search.

They were correct. The NIOSH epidemiologists found an additional 5 workers, for a total of 13 out of 1,749 employees—a 500 percent excess risk over unexposed workers. More tellingly, 6 of these workers were among only 73 who had been employed for at least ten years in the suspected OT department. The expected number of bladder cancer cases (the number that should have occurred had there been nothing unusual going on there) among those 73 employees was less than one. The NIOSH epidemiologists calculated this excess risk at more than 2,000 percent.[7]

Goodyear did not manufacture OT. It bought the chemical from, among other manufacturers, DuPont and Allied Chemical, which produced OT at the same factories where each made benzidine, BNA, and the other aromatic amines for the dye industry and where scores of workers had developed bladder cancer. Long before the Goodyear outbreak, OT had been incriminated in bladder cancer outbreaks, but it was difficult to isolate the OT risk because most of the workers in those cases had also been exposed to other powerful carcinogens.

The first indications of OT carcinogenicity in the U.S. literature had been published *fifty years* before the Goodyear episode by Wilhelm Hueper, previously introduced as DuPont's toxicologist and a giant in the field. In the 1940s researchers demonstrated that OT was capable of inducing cancer in lab animals,[8-10] and in 1951 the U.S. Public Health Service added OT to its list of chemicals found to be carcinogenic.[11] A letter from DuPont's director of medical research dated September 15, 1958, noted this fact.[12] John Zapp, who had been director of DuPont's Haskell Laboratory from 1952 to 1976, acknowledged in a deposition years later that by 1955 he was aware of the early animal studies implicating OT as a carcinogen.[13]

In short, DuPont already knew. So did Allied Chemical. In 1954 the Association of British Chemical Manufacturers, in response to an inquiry from an Allied physician, sent information from a published paper that noted that "ortho-toluidine might be expected to be a carcinogen."[14] Remarkably, the occupational health manager for Allied's operation in Buffalo,

New York, drafted a report on the carcinogenicity of OT for inclusion in the pertinent Chemical Safety Data Sheet produced by the Manufacturing Chemists Association (MCA).[15] The year was 1958. Alas, the information was rejected by the MCA's General Safety Committee, whose chairman was a representative of DuPont,[16] and dropped from the final version.[17]

The first reports of bladder cancers among workers exposed *only* to OT were published in the early 1950s—five cases at one factory where magenta (fuschine) was produced from OT.[18] No other suspect aromatic amine carcinogens were present.[19] During the next three decades, reports in the international literature implicated OT in other outbreaks of bladder cancer.[20–23] Back in the United States, two workers at the Buffalo plant who had been exposed only to OT were diagnosed with bladder cancer by 1962, but Allied Chemical did not report them in the scientific literature.[24] In 1975 DuPont's medical director noted that a worker with a history of OT exposure had developed bladder cancer but attributed the disease to BNA.[25]

Prompted by an accumulating stack of evidence in animal studies,[26,27] the National Cancer Institute (NCI) conducted its own testing, which showed definitively that this aromatic amine was an animal carcinogen.[28] That was in 1979. In 1982 the International Agency for Research on Cancer concluded that "there is sufficient evidence for the carcinogenicity of *o*-toluidine hydrochloride in experimental animals...[Thus] *o*-toluidine should be regarded, for practical purposes, as if it presented a carcinogenic risk to humans."[29] By this point, the proof was becoming redundant.

For all its scientific renown, DuPont never performed tests to determine whether OT actually caused cancer. Haskell Laboratory scientists considered OT to be an "experimental carcinogen" and recommended that "industrial manufacturing procedures and equipment should be designed to preclude employee exposure."[30] In 1977 a DuPont manager wrote to the company's customers that "tumors were observed in some rats and mice" in a "preliminary study" but reassuringly prefaced this disclosure with the assertion that "While o-Toluidine has been manufactured and processed at our Chambers Works for some fifty years, we have seen no evidence that it ever caused cancer in any of our employees."[31] A similar letter was sent to the director of NIOSH.[32] However, no epidemiological evidence supported this statement because DuPont had never conducted a full-scale epidemiological investigation, perhaps because it knew what such research would reveal: a bladder cancer epidemic among the workers at its own plant. As with benzidine, it appears this corporate giant did not want to know what it already knew.

Instead, when the results of the NIOSH study at Goodyear's Niagara Falls plant were published, the manufacturers of OT hired scientists to manufacture uncertainty about that outbreak.[33–36] A letter to the *Journal of the National Cancer Institute* from a toxicologist employed by an OT manufacturer (since acquired by DuPont) suggested that the *drinking water* in Niagara Falls could have been the cause of the excess.[37] This individual apparently did not quite grasp the obvious: All of the workers in the plant drank the same water, but only those exposed to OT developed bladder cancer.

Allied Chemical finally stopped manufacturing OT in the 1970s,[38] but DuPont continued production. Early studies should have, *at minimum,* raised serious concerns. The additional bladder cancers appearing every year among men working at the Chambers Works should have ended all debate. They did not. Those cases were always ascribed to exposure to BNA or benzidine, two substances no longer used at the plant.

Exposure continued at other plants around the country as well. Between 1981 and 1983, NIOSH estimates, almost thirty thousand U.S. workers were exposed to OT.[39]

In 1990, a year after the NIOSH report on the Goodyear outbreak, DuPont added a remarkably equivocal statement to its OT safety sheet, dated October 4, 1990: "May cause cancer based on tests with laboratory animals. . . . Results of epidemiology studies do not show a clear association between exposure to *o*-toluidine and bladder cancer. An increased incidence of bladder cancer has been shown in industries where mixed exposures to dyestuffs and their intermediates are identified."[40]

It was also in 1990 that DuPont identified the first case of bladder cancer at the Chambers Works in which OT was a prime suspect. The cancer occurred in a thirty-four-year-old who had worked in OT production and who was hired at the plant after DuPont itself reported that the use of benzidine had been discontinued.[41]

At some point DuPont simply stopped reporting additional bladder cancer cases in the scientific literature—a corporate policy that held for several decades. And there *were* additional cases. By the early 1990s DuPont had identified about 450 cases of work-related bladder cancer among the employees of the Chambers Works.[42]

* * *

Benzidine, BNA, and OT are not the only culprits among the aromatic amines. For all practical purposes, the same story pertains to dichlorobenzidene (DCB), which is structurally very similar to benzidine. Take the Upjohn Company, which manufactured DCB at its North Haven, Connecticut, plant after switching from benzidine in the mid-1960s. When OSHA proposed an exposure standard for the chemical based on animal tests, Upjohn opposed the move, pointing to the lack of human evidence. All of the cases of bladder cancer at the Upjohn plant were among workers exposed to both benzidine and DCB and therefore were "probably attributable to benzidine."[43] The company failed to acknowledge the obvious: No workers had been exposed only to DCB long enough for it alone to have caused a recognizable increase in the incidence of bladder cancer. By 1985, however, cases started appearing in workers who were first employed at the plant *after* benzidine was phased out. A study published in 1996 found an eightfold excess risk of bladder cancer among employees who began work after the production of benzidine had been terminated.[44]

Likewise, I could have gone into the details with 4,4'-methlyenebis (2-chloroaniline), dubbed MOCA or MBOCA. The opposition to OSHA's regulating this substance was fierce: Opponents asserted that OSHA's decision to rely on data from animal studies was "illogical."[45] The Polyurethane Manufacturers Association asserted that "no epidemiological or clinical evidence exists to even hint at carcinogenicity in humans even though studies have been undertaken covering in excess of eighteen years of human exposure to [MOCA] at the DuPont Company."[46]

Although the MOCA standard that OSHA proposed was never finalized, U.S. producers of MOCA ceased operations by 1979. Later on, NIOSH researchers conducted a screening program at one of the facilities and found that 3 employees, among 385 screened, had developed tumors of the bladder. Two of the men were nonsmokers under the age of thirty; one of them had been exposed to MOCA for eight years and the other for eleven before the cancers were diagnosed.[47,48] MOCA causes cancer. Could the manufacturers really not have known this?

It seems to me that the companies knew almost everything all along. The German dye industry discovered that aromatic amines caused human bladder cancer in *1895*.[49] With the publication and dissemination of the 1921 report by the International Labour Organization, the uncontrolled exposure of dye workers to these carcinogens should have been eliminated.[50] *Eliminated.* Instead, the corporations' modus operandi was the same as it always is. Attack the science. Ignore the science. Demand of the science something neither it nor any institution possesses: absolute certainty. Erring on the side of protecting people's health when the potential harm is great (death from cancer would seem to qualify) is a fundamental public health principle. It should not be too much to ask of our great industrial corporations, but apparently they disagree.

In defending their right to expose workers to any and all of these carcinogenic aromatic amines, manufacturers argued that the scientific evidence used by public health authorities like OSHA was wrong or irrelevant. They asserted the nonexistence of adequate proof that these chemicals would cause cancer at the current levels. In each case subsequent research proved them wrong. While the body count continued to mount, the dissemination of scientific information about bladder cancer outbreaks to chemical manufacturers had little impact on the decision-making process of corporate managers. Instead, each manufacturer went through its own discovery process, ignored well-publicized warnings, and allowed uncontrolled exposure to occur until the human cost became so obvious that it was no longer acceptable, at least in terms of public relations.

The saga of OT illuminates the limits of the ability of the regulatory enterprise. Despite the earlier accumulation of scientific evidence (animal studies, case reports of individual workers with bladder cancer, structural similarities to known human carcinogens), OT was identified as a human carcinogen only by counting the bodies in the morgue. By then it was too late; the presence of a national workplace safety and health regulatory apparatus in the 1970s and 1980s did little to prevent the bladder cancer outbreak at Goodyear.

Although many of the carcinogenic aromatic amines are virtually banned in the industrialized countries, the developing world, where workplace and environmental regulations are weak or nonexistent, is awash in these chemicals. Any developing nation that manufactures dyes or rubber products using aromatic amines now faces outbreaks of bladder cancer, the virtually unavoidable toll associated with these chemicals. Reduction of exposure levels will limit the numbers, but only the elimination of exposure to these deadly chemicals will completely protect the workers. The most alarming proof of the point is provided by China, where benzidine production did not begin until 1956 (although it had been imported since the 1930s).[51,52] Until its production was ended in 1977, more than one hundred thousand tons were produced in the cities of Tianjin and Jilin for use in sixteen dye production facilities, half in Shanghai and half in Tianjin.[52] A study of workers employed in Shanghai factories reported that bladder cancer risk among those exposed to benzidine was an astounding seventy-five hundred times that of unexposed workers.[51]

Beginning in the late 1970s, by which point U.S. production had been stopped and China had had enough, India, Mexico, Egypt, Poland, and a few other countries ratcheted up their benzidine dye production and were shipping the colors to the United States.[53]

This tragedy of the aromatic amines should never have happened here and should not be happening now in these other countries. But it did, and it is.

9

Chrome-Plated Mischief

In the old days, veteran employees at chromium-processing plants introduced new workers to the peculiarities of the job by inserting a dime in one nostril and withdrawing it from the other. A parlor trick? They could only wish it was. Chromium dust—hexavalent chromium oxide, to be precise, also known as chromium 6—had eaten away the nasal septum. This toxic oxide is rare in nature but a common by-product of the production processes that incorporate the raw ore into metal alloys for stainless steel and chrome plating. The ore itself has not been mined in this country for many decades, but various industries import hundreds of thousands of tons.[1] In 2006 OSHA estimated that more than half a million workers in this country alone were exposed to chromium 6.[2]

The downside of working with this metal was self-evident early in the twentieth century, but such manifestations of danger as an extra hole in the nose were about as far as the knowledge of the day had taken researchers. By midcentury, industry's voluntary exposure limit was 52 micrograms in each square meter of air in the workers' breathing zone (written as 52 $\mu g/m^3$), based on a 1943 recommendation by the American National Standards Institute. This recommendation was based on reports from the 1920s, when the risk of cancer was not yet recognized. When OSHA was starting out in the early 1970s, the cancer risk was understood, and no one, not even the industry, pretended that the old standard was fully protective of the workers—or even close. The new agency adopted the old voluntary limit but recognized that a change was mandatory. In 1975 the National Institute for Occupational

Safety and Health (NIOSH), the research agency set up to work side by side with OSHA, urged a limit of 1 $\mu g/m^3$—a figure surely much closer to the correct mark. The agency based this recommendation on dozens of epidemiological studies, which were remarkable at the time for their focus on this single carcinogen.[3] As a petitioner stated in a later court filing, "Hexavalent chromium is unusual in that the primary evidence of its carcinogenicity comes not from animal studies, but from 50 years of epidemiological studies. . . . In short, the principal evidence is actual human body counts."[4] The landmark study was that by Thomas Mancuso and Wilhelm Hueper, which found elevated risk of lung cancer mortality among the workers at a chromate plant in Painesville, Ohio, who had been hired between 1931 and 1937. These two giants of occupational health published their study in 1951;[5] Mancuso then continued to follow the group for almost five additional decades and documented excess lung cancer in updates published in 1975[6] and again in 1997.[7]

Confronted in the midseventies with the excellent Mancuso-Hueper study and many others, NIOSH really had no choice but to recommend the drastically reduced exposure standard for chromium 6.[3] In a statement for the record, Dr. Morton Corn, OSHA's chief at the time and a former professor of chemical engineering and occupational health at the University of Pittsburgh, said, "I think first of all the agency has an obligation, one which I feel very strongly, to state in a standard the scientific facts—what is the safe level based on the best available evidence. That obligation cannot be ignored and . . . should be in the forefront of anything OSHA does."[8] In the May 1976 *Federal Register*, Dr. Corn then posted notice that OSHA was preparing to bring the chromium standard in line with the best scientific evidence: "OSHA has concluded that a comprehensive occupational health standard is *urgently needed* to protect employees from the harmful effects of exposure to chromium 6. Consequently, OSHA hereby announces its intention to commence a rulemaking proceeding. . . . In order to complete the rulemaking proceeding in the *shortest possible time*, OSHA is encouraging public participation at an early stage of the proceeding"[9] (emphasis added).

Despite these good intentions, OSHA did not manage to introduce a rule in 1976, and the efforts later fell prey to a larger backlash against regulation. In 1977 Dr. Eula Bingham, professor of toxicology at the University of Cincinnati, took over as head of the agency. Dr. Bingham came to the job armed with an ambitious regulatory agenda, including a proposal for a generic carcinogen standard: Any chemical found to cause cancer in either one human study or two animal studies would be regulated as a human carcinogen until science proved the initial designation wrong. Bingham folded the new chromium standard into this generic carcinogen standard, which perhaps made sense at the time. However, this bold and badly needed generic standard was stalled by the Supreme Court's "benzene decision," which required OSHA to perform a specific risk assessment for every new chemical standard,[10] and then derailed by the election of Ronald Reagan in 1980. Derailed along with it was a new standard for chromium 6.

In the end, it was thirty years after Dr. Corn's statement of urgency before OSHA finally issued a standard for occupational exposure to chromium. This action in February 2006 was forced on the agency by a livid federal judge.[11] For decades the old worthless standard inherited from the 1920s had remained in effect—although its beneficial effect was minimal when the issue was cancer. Over the past decade, particularly, the saga of bureaucratic inertia and corporate malfeasance that protected the worthless standard degenerated into low farce. As a direct result, industry employees died from lung cancer caused by exposure to chromium 6. How many? Hundreds? Thousands? The exact number is unknown—and irrelevant to the point: Congress mandated OSHA to set standards so that *no employee* suffers material impairment of health.[12]

In 1993, with Bill Clinton in the White House, the watchdog group Public Citizen teamed with the Oil, Chemical, and Atomic Workers International Union (now part of the United Steelworkers of America) to petition OSHA to issue an emergency temporary standard for chromium 6 of 0.5 $\mu g/m^3$.[1] The petition politely noted that OSHA had acted to protect workers from other chemicals whose cancer risk was similar. Now it should protect chromium workers. In response, OSHA agreed that chromium 6 is a carcinogen and admitted that exposures that met the existing limit could nevertheless cause cancer and other illnesses. However, it denied the petitioners' request for emergency action, citing "the extremely stringent judicial and statutory criteria" that must be met before issuing an emergency order.[13]

Now the farcical aspect of this story begins to take shape, even with Bill Clinton in the White House and a new team in charge of the Labor Department and OSHA—all in all, a group with more of a regulatory instinct than the Reagan and Bush administrators had manifested over the previous twelve years, I believe it is fair to say. After turning down the request for emergency action, OSHA said it expected to post a Notice of Proposed Rulemaking by March 1995...then May 1995...then December 1995... then April 1996...then July 1996.[13–18]

In 1995 in Washington, D.C., OSHA commissioned a risk assessment that would help determine how stringent the new workplace standard for airborne chromium 6 should be. The conclusion: A forty-five-year career working with chromium at the exposure standard in force at the time would result in somewhere between 88 and 342 *excess* cancers per 1,000 workers— an extraordinarily high number.[19] (While few if any workers will actually work for forty-five years in such exposure conditions, regulations should be set with built-in safety factors. The aim of a protective standard is to find the exposure level at which few or no workers will get sick and then to add a safety factor on top of that level in order to take uncertainty into account.)

Breathing chromium 6 increases everyone's risk of lung cancer, not just workers'. In the late 1980s the EPA commissioned epidemiologists at Johns Hopkins University to conduct a new epidemiologic study that would measure the risks associated with lower levels of exposure. The most obvious group to study the effects of lower exposure levels were the workers at a chromate plant in Baltimore that had been constructed by Allied Chemical *after* publication of the first studies that showed that chromium 6 could cause lung cancer. The company attempted to keep exposures in Baltimore lower than those in the Painesville plant studied by Dr. Mancuso. It also set up systems to constantly monitor exposure levels, which provided invaluable data (more than seventy thousand airborne measurements) for future studies. Epidemiologists at Johns Hopkins University (located a short distance from the factory) had done a mortality study in the 1970s but they did not use the existing exposure measurements in the analysis and they did not attempt to take each worker's smoking history into account.[20] In addition, since the factory opened in 1952, relatively few deaths had occurred among the twenty-three hundred workers in the study population. By 1988 the EPA decided a more in-depth, longer-term study would be useful and contracted with Hopkins epidemiologists to undertake the research that would use precise exposure measures and also address the main confounding issue, smoking.[21]

The Chrome Coalition, the trade association representing chrome producers and consumers—companies whose workers had high exposure levels—was starting to panic, knowing OSHA might eventually be forced to issue a new, more protective standard. In November 1995 the association's members were told that the EPA-Hopkins study was finding "a clear dose response relationship with increased risks even at exposure levels below the current OSHA limit."[22] The coalition needed help countering the regulatory agencies' efforts. In February 1996 the trade group's leaders met to plan the counteroffensive with Dennis Paustenbach and his staff from ChemRisk, who had already been working with some of the largest chromium-producing companies to reduce the cost of cleaning up chromium contamination in New Jersey (see chapter 5). Also in attendance was William Butler, the epidemiologist who had spearheaded the tobacco industry's attacks on Dr. Elizabeth Fontham's secondhand smoke study.

The minutes of the meeting document the predictable strategy, which was taken right from Big Tobacco's playbook: Reanalyze old studies, and commission new ones that would yield better results. Quickly get some studies into peer-reviewed journals, and make points to influence OSHA's deliberations. Get the data from the not-yet-published EPA study to "do a proper analysis" (estimated cost: "$500,000+"). Another project: "Develop an anti-Mancuso manuscript," and publish it in a peer-review journal ($40,000).[23,24]

In hiring ChemRisk, then later Exponent, Inc. (when many of the former firm's employees switched employers), the Chrome Coalition employed one of the tobacco industry's standard tactics: It hired the consultants through the coalition's attorneys, so that materials produced by the consultants could be shielded under the attorneys' work product and attorney-client privileges.[25-27] Since 1996 at least eighteen epidemiological studies, risk assessments, or reviews of the health effects of chromium 6 have been published by scientists working for these two consulting groups, and all of them have minimized the risk of disease associated with chromium 6 exposure.[28-45]

* * *

The chromium producers and their consultants settled on the threshold theory as the best way to avoid stronger standards—the idea that a level existed below which chromium 6 did not cause cancer. The problem was that all of the epidemiological studies found an elevated cancer risk for workers with higher exposures, and none had had enough workers in the low-exposure group to merit confidence in the suggestion. The industry decided to commission a study of workers at several of the newest facilities, where exposure levels were much lower. Chosen to conduct the study was Applied Epidemiology, a consulting firm that was a ChemRisk subcontractor on chromium projects.[46,47]

The original March 1997 protocol was designed to combine the data from *six* plants—the two in the United States (Castle Hayne, North Carolina, and Corpus Christi, Texas), two in Germany, and two in England. (These last two were eventually dropped for logistical reasons.) The Castle Hayne group had previously been studied, but it was a small population with a short follow-up and therefore uninformative.[48] This problem would be addressed by the proposed Applied Epidemiology study; creating a large study population with workers from multiple plants was crucial, explained the firm's protocol, "to improve statistical power and the inferential value of the results."[46]

* * *

In March 1997, two years after OSHA's first promised deadline for proposing a new rule, Public Citizen and the union asked the agency for a commitment to a timetable.[49] The following month the agency set a target date of September 1998.[50] *Another year and a half?* Public Citizen went to court and asked for a judicial review of this latest unconscionable delay.

OSHA's timeline continued to stretch out:

1998: The court declined to compel action, having found that competing policy priorities were a reasonable cause for delay.[51] Then OSHA indicated that it would issue a proposed rule by September 1999.[52]

1999: When the September deadline had come and gone, OSHA announced a new one in November: June 2001, eighteen months down the road. It cited other rule-making activity as partial explanation.[53]

2000: The long-awaited EPA-Hopkins study on the workers in Baltimore was finally published, and it reaffirmed the utter inadequacy of the old exposure level: Workers who had been exposed well below the old standard were at increased risk of lung cancer.[21] No surprise there, and Public Citizen urged OSHA to finally take action in light of the new study. The only reply was yet another target date for a preliminary rule: September 2001.[54]

2001: September came and went, and in December 2001 the Bush administration removed chromium 6 from OSHA's calendar entirely.[55] Officially it nominated the metal for "long-term action" with the date for a proposed rule "to be determined," but that was just a charade. The agency was trying to kill the process. Among the new priorities that would take precedence over a new chromium standard were revision of the rule on highway signs and adoption of clearer language in the existing rule on emergency exits. In a way, this novel approach to the chromium question by the new administration had the merit of relative honesty. Over the previous decade or so OSHA had missed at least ten deadlines. The agency now said it was through with such games and cited several reasons for its new stance, including the terrorist attacks and the fact that "the day the [Bush] Administration took office, it instructed the agencies that any new regulatory actions must be reviewed and approved by a department or agency head appointed after January 20, 2001." In addition, OSHA stated that it "believes that the information now available is inconclusive on important issues, such as whether the epidemiological studies . . . apply to all [chromium 6] compounds and the utility of the data to establish a dose-response relationship."[11] In a word: uncertainty. After more than fifty years, numerous epidemiologic studies, and who knows how many lung cancer deaths, the agency pointed to problems with the latest study as an excuse for further deferral.

2002: In February, Public Citizen and the union returned to court yet again to petition the court to order OSHA to proceed with rulemaking. (My friend, colleague, and former student Dr. Peter Lurie was now the chromium 6 point man for Public Citizen.) The advocates' petition pointed out that none of these new priorities cited by OSHA had anything to do with protecting workers against significant health risks. "[A]t some point," the petition argued, a court must tell an agency "that enough is enough."[4]

Clearly worried about the effect of the EPA-Hopkins study, the Chrome Coalition commissioned Exponent, Inc., now home to most of the Chem-Risk scientists experienced in chromium 6, to critique the paper. Exponent faced a challenge, however; the industry had not yet obtained the raw data from the EPA-Hopkins study. The Exponent team, led by Dr. Paustenbach, did not allow that to stop them, however. The scientists developed a simulated data set, derived from the totals in each of the tables given in the study, then ran new analyses that allowed Exponent to advance a classic "uncertainty" argument. The argument, which attacks virtually every aspect of the EPA-Hopkins study, is so over the top that I want to quote it at some length:

> These exposure estimates are not reliable for many reasons. . . . The value of these data for quantitative cancer risk assessment seems to be overstated. . . . The findings of this study should be judged cautiously because of the many uncertainties in the information presented. . . . Risk estimates for lung cancer at the lower levels of cumulative [chromium 6] exposure may be inaccurate for several reasons and should not be relied upon for health risk assessment. A review of the raw data is currently on-going. . . . There are several significant concerns with the data, and the analyses that were used to evaluate them, which directly affect any risk estimate derived from these data and severely limit their utility. . . . Findings at the lower dose levels are highly questionable and extrapolation of the risks due to short-term exposures to long-term cumulative exposures is not scientifically defensible. . . . While these data do present an opportunity for improved quantitative cancer risk assessment, further data analysis and more complete data presentation are required to ensure confidence in the findings.[56]

Finally beginning to stir in August, OSHA issued a "Request for Information Regarding Occupational Exposure to Hexavalent Chromium," in which it asked the public to comment on the studies done to date, as well as the agency's risk assessment.[57] The chromium industry again turned to Exponent, which prepared two submissions, including a new reanalysis of the EPA-Hopkins study, this time using the real data, which had been obtained from the EPA. In this reanalysis Exponent changed several aspects of the study: Instead of four exposure groups, it made six (each smaller, thus making statistical significance more difficult to achieve), and it selected a different comparison population. As if by magic, the reanalysis made it appear that only the most heavily exposed workers were now at increased risk for lung cancer. The original EPA-Hopkins conclusion—that exposure levels below the current standard were not safe—must be wrong![58] (In 2004, while working on behalf of a different trade association, Exponent *praised* the EPA-Hopkins study.[59] Whatever serves the interests of a given client—that's the rule for the product defense firms.)

In December 2002 the court at long last agreed with Public Citizen and the union about OSHA's delaying tactics. Enough really was enough. The delay had "exceeded the bounds of reasonableness." The court told the industry that it could mount its uncertainty campaign during the formal regulatory procedure, but it could not use that campaign to forestall the procedure altogether. Judge Edward Becker, chief judge of the U.S. Court of Appeals for the Third Circuit, wrote the following: "Nor do we find persuasive OSHA's broad assertion that the Hopkins study 'does not answer all of the technically complex questions . . . that OSHA would need to resolve in developing a [chromium 6] rule.' . . . This is obviously true, but without more it is irrelevant, for the Occupational Safety and Health Act does not require scientific certainty in the rulemaking process. Indeed, read fairly, the Act virtually forbids delay in pursuit of certainty—it requires regulation 'on the basis of the best available evidence,' . . . and courts have warned that 'OSHA cannot let workers suffer while it awaits the Godot of scientific certainty.'"[11]

In October 2004, as required by the court ruling, OSHA officially announced its intention to regulate chromium 6 as a human carcinogen with a proposed new workplace exposure limit of 1.0 $\mu g/m^3$, a decrease of 98 percent from the existing standard (52 $\mu g/m^3$) and one that would, at long last, protect chromium workers. In its justification and risk-assessment analysis, the agency cited the classic research by Thomas Mancuso on lung cancer among the workers in Painesville, Ohio, the first installment of which had been published *fifty-three years earlier*.[5] The announcement was accompanied by a general request for additional scientific evidence and a specific appeal for epidemiological data about the workers at the plant in Castle Hayne, North Carolina, where exposure levels were typically low— below 10 $\mu g/m^3$—and therefore presumably more representative of the exposure levels found in workplaces today. Although OSHA knew about the earlier mortality study of this population,[48] it did not know of the four-plant study (including Castle Hayne) commissioned by the chromium industry. The agency now requested all "updated analyses."[60]

As it happened, a mortality study of the Castle Hayne workers and another group in Corpus Christi, Texas,[61] was accepted for publication by the *Journal of Occupational and Environmental Medicine (JOEM)* in October 2004,[62] the same month OSHA proposed its rule and asked for all new information. (I introduced *JOEM* in an earlier chapter as one of the peer-reviewed journals that has published some shoddy papers by product defense specialists.) The authors' affiliation for the new study was listed as ENVIRON International Corporation, the consulting firm that had purchased Applied Epidemiology, Inc., the group that had actually conducted the study. The sponsor of the research was listed as the Chromium Chemicals Health and Environmental Committee of the Industrial Health Foundation (formerly the Industrial Hygiene Foundation), the industry trade group that had been sued for its alleged involvement in the asbestos cover-up (see chapter two) and had gone into bankruptcy as a result.

I later did some digging and discovered that this study was part of the four-plant study commissioned by the industry in 1997. It was completed and submitted to the industry sponsors in September 2002 but was never given to the government agencies that could use it to protect workers. In June 2002, when officials of the Chrome Coalition met with NIOSH to discuss the agency's chromium recommendations, the chrome officials said not a word about the study, which by then was almost completed. When they received the study three months later, they did not submit it to OSHA (or to the EPA, even though the Toxics Substance Control Act requires manufacturers to submit newly gathered information about toxic effects). Nor did they present it to OSHA two years later—October 2004—when the agency put forward its specific request for any updated analyses of the Castle Hayne workers. Nor did they submit in February 2005, when OSHA held eleven days of public hearings on the proposed new chromium 6 standard, during which industry representatives repeatedly suggested that OSHA should really be relying on data from groups with lower levels of exposure. (The National Association of Manufacturers, for example, attacked OSHA for not using newer data and claimed that "OSHA is relying on 30- to 50-year-old exposure profiles and outdated cancer estimates that are not reflective of today's modern workplace conditions."[63]) Instead, it was published in *JOEM* in April 2005, where it appeared just weeks before the close of OSHA's official "comment period."

Of course, the study appeared to be favorable to the industry's contention that a threshold existed below which chromium exposure did not increase the risk of lung cancer. The authors found no elevated risk of lung cancer in the two worker populations in Castle Hayne and Corpus Christi and offered the preliminary conclusion that "the absence of an elevated lung cancer risk may be a favorable reflection of the [lower-exposure] environment."[61] So what was going on here? If the results of this study were so supportive of the industry's position and important enough for publication, why had neither the sponsors nor the authors overnighted the results to

OSHA way back in 2002? Why did they not speak up during the hearing *three years later?*

The answer has two parts. The first stems from the simple fact that the published work was deeply flawed. Not a single employee at the Castle Hayne plant had been followed for more than 18 years (the average was 10 years), and 40 percent of the workers at the Corpus Christi plant had been followed for fewer than 10 years. As noted in the earlier discussion, good epidemiology assumes that no effects from exposure to a carcinogen (except for leukemia) will become apparent until at least 20 years after exposure began. If chromate exposure *doubled* the risk of lung cancer starting 20 years after the first exposure, this industry study would not have picked up this salient fact. It also has little statistical power, with just 27 deaths overall and only three from lung cancer.[64] (By way of contrast, the EPA-Hopkins study of the workers in Baltimore included 855 deaths overall, 122 from lung cancer, with a follow-up period ranging from 18 to 42 years.[21])

To a scientist or regulator, such underpowered work says essentially nothing and provides no information as to whether lower levels of chromium exposure cause lung cancer. In short, this is just another of the many studies that have been trumped up for self-serving purposes that are proliferating in certain journals associated with occupational and environmental health. The belated publication ensured that the study was *not* included in OSHA's initial literature review, where it would have been dismissed for its abysmal design. Moreover, this tardy submission allowed the chrome industry and its allies to portray the worthless work as an important, late-breaking study that OSHA had not addressed. Further delay in the rule-making work would therefore be required!

Three trade associations made reference to this inadequate study in their last-minute official comments to OSHA.[65-67] The Specialty Steel Industry of North America stated that it had "very recently" learned of the study, and "while we have not had any opportunity to examine this study ... [it] contains potentially incredibly significant data which would allow the development of a dose response relationship based on actual, experienced exposures, as opposed to the modeled exposures upon which OSHA currently relies to set the PEL. Indisputably, this would be much more relevant and appropriate data upon which to establish a risk-based regulatory limit." (The study had been concluded two and a half years earlier, but this group, a member of the Chrome Coalition, claimed that it did not know about it until "very recently.") Furthermore, the group stated, OSHA's failure to consider these results would be "arbitrary and capricious."[66] In the regulatory field, such language is a coded warning that failure to address these "new" findings would be grounds for a legal challenge.

The study was flawed but could still serve to muddy the waters. I believe that is one reason it was published. The second reason takes a turn toward the lower depths, which I entered by happenstance late one night in June 2005, when I Googled the Chrome Coalition and the Industrial Health Foundation (IHF), the trade group listed in *JOEM* as the sponsor of the study. One of the items that caught my eye was a bankruptcy hearing. Apparently the IHF was closing up shop, and two closely connected trade associations, one of them the Chrome Coalition, asserted their rights to a collection of IHF file cabinets because, they stated, the IHF was simply a "third-party administrator" of the two trade associations."[68] Now I knew for certain that we were dealing with a chrome industry study and that the industry wanted those file cabinets. In the end, it got them, but by cold-calling another party to the bankruptcy proceedings I was able to obtain a trove of other industry documents, including two versions of the original study protocol submitted by Applied Epidemiology[46,47] and the final report.[69] All are smoking guns.

In contrast to the published paper, the final report on the four groups of workers (the two in the United States and the two in Germany), which was completed and submitted to the trade group in September 2002, found a significantly *elevated* risk of lung cancer mortality associated with exposure to chromium 6 in the newer, relatively low-exposure facilities. In one analysis, workers in the highest exposure group had twenty times the lung cancer risk of the workers in the lowest exposure group. That was not such a surprise. The finding of greater regulatory interest was that workers in the intermediate exposure group, whose exposures were only slightly higher than the new level of 1 $\mu g/m^3$ (which OSHA had proposed in 2004), had an almost fivefold excess risk of lung cancer mortality.[69] Clearly, this result was no good for the industry. It was *terrible* for the industry (and for the workers, of course). How could they allow this result to see the light of day? Clearly they could not, and the report was therefore never submitted to OSHA and never published—never published, that is, *in its entirety.*

Instead, the ENVIRON authors simply separated the U.S. and the German results and published the U.S. results separately—despite the repeated emphasis in the protocol of the strength of the combined study population. So, instead of a bad result for the industry based on data from four plants, the hired guns at ENVIRON issued a skewed version based on data from just two plants. In a response to a letter we sent to *JOEM*, the authors stated that the German component of the study had not been published because it was rejected by the journal to which it had originally been submitted. They defended breaking up the original study on grounds that different exposure measurements were used in the different countries.[70]

(According to the original protocol, the methods were chosen "so that the data may be combined validly and analyzed as a single multi-plant [and multinational] cohort."[46] In epidemiology, changing your methods after you have seen your results is extremely bad form, especially if it changes those findings. This raises questions as to whether you are manipulating the data to get the result you want.) In June 2005 I gave copies of the study protocol and the final report of the *complete* four-plant study to Public Citizen, which entered them into the OSHA docket—the legal file of all of the materials the agency has received.

There's more. In October 2005 ENVIRON's researchers finally submitted the German component of the study to OSHA, accompanied by a letter stating that the paper had been accepted for publication in *JOEM*.[71] To our amazement (but not surprise; there's a difference), the finally published German study omitted the key analysis that had yielded the damning results in the four-plant study that the authors had dismembered. Instead of comparing the intermediate-exposure with the low-exposure group (which showed that the intermediate group had greater lung cancer risk), they combined the low- and intermediate-exposure groups to use as the new baseline or control group. They then compared the high-exposure group with this new not-so-low combined exposure group. By doing this, they were able to claim that lung cancer risk was elevated only in the highest-exposure group. Furthermore, by combining the two lower-exposed categories, the estimated increase in risk from lung cancer mortality in the highest-exposure category dropped from 2,000 percent to 700 percent, making chromium appear less potent as a carcinogen. That intermediate group—the population that would help OSHA set a safe level—disappeared. It was swallowed up in the combined group.[72]

In summary, the chromium industry repeatedly criticized OSHA for relying upon data about workers in high-exposure factories; without informing the agency, it commissioned a study of four low-exposure factories. Although the combined results would have confirmed the elevated cancer risk even for these workers, the product defense specialists split the study into two parts and changed the exposure categories and, as a result, the most important finding disappeared.

* * *

On February 28, 2006, OSHA at last issued a final rule for chromium 6—a workplace exposure limit of 5 $\mu g/m^3$, significantly weaker than the 1 $\mu g/m^3$ proposed at the start of the rule-making period. The standard went into effect beginning in November 2006 for businesses with twenty or more employees; engineering controls were not required to be implemented until May 2010. According to OSHA's own estimates, exposure at 5 $\mu g/m^3$ will result in 10–45 lung cancer deaths per one thousand workers over a lifetime of exposure; the rule also eliminates the proposed training requirements and limits some employee notification of exposure monitoring results. The aerospace industry (which hired Exponent to try to influence OSHA's final rule) was a big winner—OSHA granted it a PEL of 25 μg/m^3, based on the reasoning that it was too difficult for these companies to reduce exposure to 5 μg/m^3.[2] The outdated standard has finally been replaced—but by an insufficiently protective new one. The behind-the-scenes lobbying by the chrome industry and its allies seems to have been effective. Public Citizen has sued OSHA yet again, and the saga will probably continue for many more years.

10

Popcorn Lung

OSHA GIVES UP

The fact that OSHA issued a chromium 6 standard only after a federal judge ordered the agency to do so is hardly news. When it comes to issuing rules that reduce on-the-job hazards and thereby prevent workplace illness, the agency has pretty much stopped working. The most conclusive proof I can offer for this assertion is the popcorn-lung issue, which first came to wide attention in the public health world in May 2000. At that time, Dr. Allan Parmet, an occupational medicine specialist in Kansas City, Missouri, contacted the Missouri Department of Health to report eight cases of *bronchiolitis obliterans* among the workers at the Gilster–Mary Lee microwave popcorn–processing plant in Jasper, Missouri.[1]

This devastating lung disease is characterized, as its name suggests, by an "obliteration" of the pulmonary airways; a lung transplant is often the only hope for these patients. The disease is also rare, so multiple cases in a single workforce is a loud alarm calling attention to some powerfully toxic agent. We call these "sentinel" cases. In Missouri, the state health department's immediate preliminary investigation confirmed ten cases of the disease at this one plant, three of whom were awaiting lung transplants at that time. Another twenty, perhaps thirty, workers showed less severe but still notable respiratory symptoms.[2] This was nothing less than an epidemic; many of the workers were both young and nonsmokers. Something bad was clearly going on.

The Missouri officials considered conducting their own epidemiologic investigation of the disease cluster, but obtaining medical releases and physicians' reports would take some time, and time was of the essence here. They therefore notified both OSHA and NIOSH and implored OSHA to inspect the facility immediately in view of the fact that "[a]s a regulatory agency . . . [OSHA] can more promptly address this situation, and if there is an obvious hazard to workers, address it quickly."[2]

A few days later, an OSHA inspector visited the popcorn plant. According to the inspector's notes, the company had become "concerned that there might be some environmental problem at their facility so they had their [workers' compensation] insurance carrier come into their plant and conduct environmental sampling for total nuisance dust."[3] The company's records indicated that the insurance carrier had taken those air samples in 1996, *four years earlier.*[4] The inspector now collected no additional dust samples and offered his "professional opinion that it would be ludicrous to re-sample the area again." He did collect samples of oil mist in the air the workers were breathing, but the OSHA lab in Salt Lake City discarded them because the agency's sampling method applies only to petroleum-based oils, not vegetable oil. In August 2000, three months after Dr. Parmet's report of eight cases of a rare, often deadly lung disease in the factory, OSHA decided there was no problem. The inspector, according to his own notes, "determined the company to be in compliance and closed out the case file since there were no other OSHA sampling protocols at his disposal to test further at the plant."[3]

That same month, NIOSH scientists—whom the Missouri health officials also contacted—inspected the popcorn factory and found the volatile organic compound diacetyl, which is predominant in popcorn's butter flavoring—present in concentrations up to one thousand times higher than in the office and outdoor areas at the same plant. (This compound occurs naturally in many benign foods, including milk, coffee, and vegetables, but for commercial purposes it is made in an industrial process at a chemical factory.) Working independently of OSHA, NIOSH also conducted health assessments of nearly 90 percent of the Gilster–Mary Lee employees and discovered rates of chronic cough and shortness of breath that were 2.6 times the national average, adjusting for both smoking and age. Twice as many workers as expected reported being told by their physicians that they had asthma or chronic bronchitis; lung function testing revealed that three times as many workers as expected had obstruction to airflow.[5,6] In December, NIOSH issued interim recommendations suggesting that all workers wear respirators pending the implementation of engineering controls to eliminate exposure to the artificial butter flavoring.[1]

The following year, NIOSH tested artificial butter flavoring and released the unambiguous results in 2002. Exposed to airborne concentrations for a single, six-hour period, the lab rats manifested, in the words of the study's lead investigator, "the most dramatic cases of cell death I've ever seen."[7] This is rather solid proof that inhaling diacetyl is tantamount to inhaling acid, and the diacetyl levels to which the rats had been exposed—285–371 parts per million—were "not extraordinary when compared with levels measured in the workplace."[8] (One of the real tragedies in this story is the fact that BASF, the German chemical manufacturer, had conducted a quite similar animal study years before—in 1993—with comparable results. A single four-hour period of exposure to diacetyl resulted in an "abundance of symptoms indicative of respiratory tract injury."[9] The results of that study were never published in the scientific literature and never reported to any government or health agency, including NIOSH and OSHA.)

As it was conducting the animal studies in 2001, NIOSH continued to monitor the health of the microwave popcorn employees in Missouri and worked with the company in planning and implementing control measures. In September, its staff returned to the factory to inform workers about the latest research and distribute materials that included this ominous warning: "There is a work-related cause of lung disease in this plant. We at [NIOSH] believe the problem is continuing even after the company made changes that we recommended."[10] Following this very unusual warning, an attorney representing several of the ill workers filed a complaint with OSHA because NIOSH can evaluate workplace hazards and it can even (with a court order) obtain forced entry, but its inspections have no teeth. *Only* OSHA can issue regulations that require employers to meet safety requirements, and *only* OSHA can enforce these conditions. The attorney's complaint alleged that NIOSH had not done enough to improve ventilation in the plant, as evidenced by the fact that "one employee lost half of his lung capacity working in the plant *after* the remedial measures that NIOSH suggested were taken" (emphasis in original).[11]

This complaint prompted OSHA to send a different inspector to visit the plant.[12] The man stayed for forty minutes. He did not conduct an inspection.[13] In a letter to the attorney who had filed the complaints, OSHA denied any need for further investigation at the plant: "[T]he hazard which you brought to our attention has been corrected and . . . Glister [*sic*] Mary Lee is complying with the recommendations of NIOSH. . . . The hazard does not fall within OSHA's jurisdiction because there is no Permissible Exposure Limits [*sic*] for the food blend chemicals of concern that are used at the factory."[14]

Remember, this is the agency that was created to ensure that workplaces in the United States are, in the words of Congress, "free from recognized hazards that are causing or are likely to cause death or serious physical harm."[15] In the congressional hearings that led up to passage of the OSHA legislation, workers, union leaders, and scientists described numerous outbreaks of work-related disease about which nothing was done until a sufficiently large number of workers had died.[16] Tony Mazzocchi, then legislative director of the Oil, Chemical, and Atomic Workers Union (and the extraordinarily dedicated individual who recruited me and dozens of other scientists and physicians into the occupational health field) called this "the body in the morgue approach."[17]

Congress wrote the law to give the agency a great deal of leeway in identifying hazards and setting protective exposure limits to enable the agency to act *before* workers became sick or injured and certainly before their bodies were shipped to the morgue. It instructed OSHA to develop standards based on the best scientific evidence available. To initiate the regulatory process established by Congress, OSHA is required to make a determination that a regulation would reduce or eliminate a "significant risk" for workers exposed to the hazard. In its landmark benzene ruling of 1980, the U.S. Supreme Court stated that the risk Congress envisioned must be "quantified sufficiently to enable the Secretary [of Labor] to characterize it as significant in an understandable way." However, the justices emphasized that it was not the Court's intention to place OSHA in a "mathematical straightjacket." Consequently, it permitted the agency significant flexibility in quantifying health risks.[18]

Faced with that new, apparently narrower but still somewhat ambiguous mandate, OSHA has invested a great deal of time and resources over the last twenty-five years preparing detailed, quantitative risk assessments for its health standards. Estimating the risk of disease associated with exposure to various substances is difficult and often involves extrapolating from high to low doses and from animals to humans. I have discussed these technical difficulties, but at least the agency occasionally grappled with them in years past. In many other cases, including the one involving diacetyl described earlier in this chapter, OSHA has simply taken a pass—in complete and utter contravention of its mission.

One of the agency's extremely important enforcement tools is—or should be—the "general duty clause," which outlines the obligation of employers to provide safe working conditions. Until a few years ago, OSHA inspectors who encountered obvious hazards for which no applicable OSHA standard existed would cite this clause as the legal basis for their enforcement actions. Nowadays this is rarely done. The clause has not been invoked in the case of diacetyl even though this notorious airborne hazard, which has caused dozens of workers at numerous facilities to contract a serious lung disease, appears to be a logical candidate for such action. Instead, OSHA officials have clung to the position that hazards for which no existing OSHA standard applies do "not fall within OSHA's jurisdiction."[14]

We have not set a standard; therefore, the issue is not within our jurisdiction.
How's that for a catch-22 excuse for inaction? It is time to set a standard for diacetyl, like the ones issued for asbestos, benzene, vinyl chloride, and other substances this book discusses. Moreover, no lengthy, complex epidemiological studies are required. A real hazard is indisputably causing a disease with rapid onset and a clear range of disabling respiratory effects. Two approaches to the regulation would be plausible. When the story broke in 2000 (with many questions still unanswered), OSHA could have established inhalation exposure levels for *all* butter flavoring vapors at microwave popcorn plants until more was known about the cause or causes of the bronchiolitis obliterans outbreak. Such a regulation would have protected workers from exposure to all potentially hazardous chemicals. In 1976 OSHA had embraced this approach for protecting coke oven workers when it required reductions in exposure to *all* airborne chemicals (known as coal tar pitch volatiles) in the working environment rather than attempting to identify the precise cancer-causing agent among the myriad substances in the coke oven emissions.[19]

One problem with this blanket approach is that it would not protect workers employed in the flavorings factories and snack food plants that also use the *specific* chemical or chemicals that cause the disease. However, OSHA could therefore have moved to regulate exposure to the single most likely cause of the illnesses while researchers conducted additional research. Through the early years of the decade, more and more evidence pointed to an excellent candidate: diacetyl.[20] Yet OSHA did nothing. Today OSHA has even more powerful evidence that diacetyl is a prime causal agent in the development of bronchiolitis obliterans among workers at all sorts of facilities that use the artificial butter flavoring, not just the microwave popcorn plants.[21] It has animal studies, epidemiological studies, and devastated lungs—the equivalent of bodies in the morgue.

In December 2003, NIOSH issued a warning to four thousand companies because it was apparent by that time—to anyone who wanted to see—that workers in a wide variety of plants that used artificial butter flavoring in their products (including candy, pastries, and frozen foods) had incurred lung damage as a direct result of their exposure to diacetyl.[22] One treating physician told me of diagnosing bronchiolitis obliterans in a worker who mixed the flavors for dog food. In Missouri, Dr. Parmet reported damaged lungs in two workers at a plant that made large commercial popcorn machines for movie theaters. These two workers tested the device that squirted the cooking oil into the big pot—butter-flavored oil, made with diacetyl. None of the other workers in this plant had unusual lung damage.[23]

The weight of the evidence leans *heavily* toward the culpability of diacetyl. No one can honestly deny this. In fact, there is *no* evidence leaning the other way; nothing suggests that diacetyl *cannot* be the cause of bronchiolitis obliterans. Thus, a prudent public health approach would support severely restricting airborne exposure to diacetyl unless and until it is shown to be safe. "Prudent"? That approach is not in the cards today. Uncertainty is all the rage, and this policy gives OSHA all the cover it needs to do nothing. If OSHA should actually move to regulate diacetyl, the product defense consultants will likely swing into high gear and deny the validity or the applicability of the NIOSH studies. They will presumably argue that unknown confounders are the cause of bronchiolitis obliterans. In their view, there will never be sufficient proof of any direct cause and effect between diacetyl and the disease.

Uncertainty is the basis of the strategy in the court cases in which the popcorn workers with destroyed lungs have sued flavor manufacturers. In one of these cases, a consultant toxicologist for International Flavors and Fragrances testified that any purported evidence is insufficient.[24] The NIOSH scientists must be mistaken. By and large, judges and juries have given more credence to the NIOSH science by approving settlements and awarding plaintiffs a total of more than $100 million. Given the inability and/or unwillingness of the regulatory apparatus to address workplace hazards, litigation may be the only means of compelling employers to protect their workers. When I told the popcorn-lung story at a "Science for Judges" conference, one jurist suggested that the judicial system has become the last resort for these public health issues. Where else can employers and manufacturers be penalized for permitting exposures that result in workplace disease? Perhaps these large awards will motivate them to ensure that workers are provided with adequate protection. Still, the judicial system is no substitute for a robust OSHA.

Instead of such an OSHA, however, we now have one that ignores NIOSH's research. Despite everything, OSHA maintains that "a cause-effect relationship between diacetyl and bronchiolitis obliterans has not been established. Food-processing workers with this lung disease were also exposed to other volatile agents."[25] (Meanwhile, California's own OSHA has fined at least one offending flavor company $45,000.[26])

Unwilling to sit by as more and more workers become sick, a group of public health activists have tried to push OSHA into taking some action. In July 2006, the United Food and Commercial Workers and the International Brotherhood of Teamsters petitioned OSHA to finally issue an emergency temporary standard for diacetyl.[27] Dozens of the nation's leading occupational health physicians and scientists signed a letter to the Labor Department presenting the scientific evidence supporting the petition.[20] The unions also asked OSHA to start formal rulemaking on all flavoring chemicals. After all, the Flavor and Extract Manufacturers Association, the manufacturers' trade association, regrettably known as FEMA, estimates that more than 1,000 flavoring ingredients pose potential respiratory hazards to workers, but OSHA has issued workplace exposure limits for less than five percent of these—46 at last count.[28]

We shall see what happens. I am not wildly optimistic. So far, instead of effective action, OSHA has been content to enter into an "alliance" (OSHA's term) with the popcorn manufacturers, whose organization is called the "Popcorn Board," in order to "help foster a culture of prevention."[29] That was back in September 2002. Under the presidency of George W. Bush, such alliances have replaced any effort to strengthen weak standards and improve inspections. Bluntly put, OSHA has moved from a regulatory to a collaborative/consultative model. By design, these agreements "do not include an enforcement component."[30] Instead, OSHA says, let's cooperate and voluntarily develop and share information regarding worker health and safety. That's fine, but it is no substitute for enforcement. It is only a slight exaggeration to say that these alliances are little more than a way for the agency to look busy. By March 2007, 467 alliances had been formed.[31] My personal favorite is the agreement with the International Society of Canine Cosmetologists to "provide pet care professionals with training and knowledge that will help them stay safe and healthy on the job."[32]

According to the alliance agreement with the Popcorn Board, the trade association would provide OSHA with a mailing list of member companies engaged in microwave popcorn packaging so that OSHA could send these firms "recent information on the potential adverse health effects of employees' exposure to artificial butter flavoring compounds." There was no mechanism for participation by exposed workers, their representatives, or the public health community. Another provision allowed the industry to "review and provide comment and input on a draft OSHA 'Hazard Information Bulletin' to be developed for internal distribution to OSHA's compliance officers in the field."[29] This alliance was put together in 2002 and then concluded in March 2003. As of July 2007 the hazard bulletin that would supposedly help OSHA inspectors understand the butter flavor hazard and conduct effective inspections had not been issued.[33]

It appears that it will literally take an act of Congress to force OSHA to issue a diacetyl standard. In April 2007, committees of the House of Representatives and the Senate held hearings on OSHA's failure to protect workers from diacetyl and other serious hazards. Eric Peoples, one of the Gilster–Mary Lee popcorn workers now on the waiting list for a lung transplant, was a witness at the House hearing.[34] I testified at the Senate hearing.[35] Congressional hearings force agencies to at least make it appear they are trying to do their jobs. In his testimony at the House hearing, Edwin Foulke, the head of OSHA, announced a "National Emphasis Program"—OSHA would finally start inspecting popcorn factories.[36] The problem with OSHA's new initiative was that most popcorn factories had already started addressing the problem, and that new cases of bronchiolitis obliterans were now turning up in flavor factories around the country. A few months earlier, I had given OSHA a soon-to-be-published study that found several cases of bronchiolitis obliterans among the workers in a Dutch diacetyl factory—not a plant that makes or uses flavorings but one that produces pure diacetyl.[37] Furthermore, diacetyl is used in making Twinkies[38] and many other snack foods. OSHA would make no effort to find out what exposures were occurring in these factories.

Members of Congress, it seems, have had enough. In June 2007, the House Committee on Education and Labor passed a bill giving OSHA 90 days from final passage of the bill to issue an interim standard for diacetyl in popcorn and food flavoring facilities, and two years to develop a standard for any workplace where workers are exposed to diacetyl.[39] Although OSHA opposed the legislation,[40] the bill was supported not just by labor unions and public health advocates, but also by FEMA, the flavor manufacturers' trade association.[41] FEMA leadership had seen the human carnage and had set up a comprehensive but voluntary program to help flavor manufacturers reduce diacetyl exposure. But a voluntary program would never be sufficient; FEMA needed OSHA to step in to ensure that responsible employers would not be undercut by the fly-by-night operators who were unwilling to invest in safe work practices.

Incredibly, when the bill was introduced, House Republicans rose in opposition, raising the predictable uncertainty arguments. ("There is no clear scientific evidence that diacetyl alone causes 'popcorn lung' disease . . . I cannot—and will not—sacrifice sound science for the sake of political expedience."[42]) Once their statements were recorded, they backed down and allowed the bill to be voted out of committee on a voice vote, probably so they could avoid being on record as opposing the legislation.[43]

Every episode in this book so far has included an appearance by the product defense industry, manufacturing uncertainty to slow regulation and victim compensation. "Flavor Workers' Lung Disease," as it is now called, is no exception. The experts at ChemRisk, employed by defendants in diacetyl lawsuits, presented their analysis in a poster at the 2007 Society of Toxicology Meeting. I have never seen a ChemRisk analysis which does not highlight the flaws and limitations of studies suggesting a relationship between any chemical and a disease. This leads to the inevitable finding of uncertainty: "While it is possible that elevated exposures to artificial butter may have been related to the incidence of respiratory disorders in some popcorn workers, the data collected to date do not appear to be sufficiently robust to draw any firm general conclusions." Predictably, they call for

NIOSH to release the raw data from its studies so the mercenary reanalyses can begin.[44]

Diacetyl exposure is not only a concern in factories, of course. What about the vapors consumers inhale while opening the steaming bag of microwaved popcorn? After all, NIOSH has recommended that when quality control workers at the popcorn factories open bags of microwaved popcorn, they wait for the bags to cool and open them under a fan that pulls the air away from them.[45] There are few studies that shed light on this topic; the Environmental Protection Agency announced in the middle of 2003 that a study of emissions from microwaved bags of popcorn was under way and that results were expected by the end of that year. The study has been completed, but the EPA turned down my request under the Freedom of Information Act (FOIA) to release the study's results. However, through the FOIA request, I was able to obtain letters to the agency from ConAgra, which produces the Orville Redenbacher popcorn brand, discussing ConAgra's research into consumer exposure to artificial butter flavor.[46,47] That didn't surprise me, since dozens of current and former employees at the Orville Redenbacher plant in Marion, Ohio, are reported to have developed diacetyl-related lung disease.[48] But ConAgra isn't releasing their research results either.

As a case study in the failure of the regulatory system, diacetyl implicates multiple agencies. It is the FDA that is charged with ensuring "the safety of the nation's domestically produced and imported foods."[49] Back in 1980 the FDA convened a panel of scientists who reviewed the literature, found no danger in eating diacetyl in the small quantities used to flavor food, and included diacetyl on its list of "generally recognized as safe," or GRAS, food additives.[50,51] But what about *inhaling* diacetyl? How could it be "generally recognized as safe" in the face of compelling evidence that breathing diacetyl vapors causes lung disease and with *no* evidence of a safe exposure level? When I inquired at the FDA, I was told that since the NIOSH studies showed only workers getting sick, the FDA had no reason to do anything, including investigating whether breathing the stuff at home was dangerous. Catch-22. No evidence, so there is no reason to look for evidence. In September 2006 I petitioned the FDA to remove diacetyl from the GRAS list.[52] My objective was not to pull diacetyl from the market but to goad the agency into doing its job and determining whether it was safe to breathe the low levels of diacetyl released when we microwave popcorn at home.

Eight months later, Representative Rosa L. DeLauro went even further, calling on the FDA to remove diacetyl from the market until adequate testing is done.[53] While the FDA could ignore me, they could not ignore Ms. DeLauro, who chairs the House appropriations subcommittee that funds the FDA. But their response was typical of an agency that has its head in the sand: "At this time, the agency does not have evidence that would cause it to take immediate action with respect to diacetyl."[54] In other words, even though diacetyl is killing workers, we have never attempted to determine if home exposures are dangerous. Therefore there is no reason to do anything about home exposures.

In September 2007 I broke the story of the first reported case of "popcorn lung" found in a consumer of microwave popcorn. Earlier that summer, Dr. Cecile Rose—the chief occupational and environmental medicine physician at National Jewish Medical and Research Center, the most prestigious lung disease hospital in the country—wrote to the FDA, CDC, EPA, and OSHA, informing the agencies of a patient she had recently identified who had what was likely a case of bronchiolitis obliterans.[55]

Wayne Watson, a Colorado furniture salesman, was having a great deal of difficulty breathing and was referred to Dr. Rose. She did a thorough examination and history but could not identify any possible cause of his illness. Fortunately, Dr. Rose was a consultant to FEMA and was one of perhaps a dozen or two physicians in the entire country who have seen patients with popcorn lung. His symptoms did seem like those seen among the diacetyl-exposed popcorn and flavor industry workers. At the end of the work-up, Dr. Rose said to him, "This is a very weird question, but bear with me. Are you around a lot of popcorn?" Mr. Watson's jaw dropped, and he replied, "How could you possibly know that about me? I am Mr. Popcorn. I love popcorn."[56]

It soon became clear he had "popcorn lung." A CT scan and lung biopsy showed that Mr. Watson's lungs looked just like those of the popcorn workers. National Jewish researchers then measured the diacetyl levels in his home when he microwaved popcorn, and found them comparable to the levels in some factories where workers had gotten sick. He stopped making popcorn and his lung function stabilized.

Alarmed by her finding, Dr. Rose wrote to the FDA, CDC, EPA, and OSHA, informing them of the case.[57] None of the agencies did anything to investigate her report. The FDA's only response was to ask Dr. Rose to formally submit her letter to the public docket containing my petition to remove diacetyl from the GRAS list.[55]

Once the letter was in the public domain, I posted it on my blog, "The Pump Handle." Almost immediately, the national media blanketed the country with the story. A few days earlier, Pop Weaver, one of the major popcorn manufacturers, had announced that its popcorn would no longer be flavored with diacetyl.[58] ConAgra and the other major companies followed suit.[59] Manufacturers of other snack foods that use artificial butter flavoring have remained silent about their diacetyl use, though, so their employees may still be at risk.

* * *

Workers wait for OSHA at their peril. It is as simple as that. New workplace health standards are rare, and it makes little difference whether the White House is in Democratic or Republican hands. In the last ten years OSHA has issued workplace standards for a total of two new chemicals. Two. Indeed, since its inception it has issued comprehensive standards for only thirty toxic materials. Additionally, the agency enforces permissible exposure limits for fewer than two hundred of the approximately three thousand chemicals the EPA characterizes as high-production volume (HPV) because more than a million pounds of the substance is produced or imported each year. Of these OSHA standards, all but a handful were borrowed whole from the voluntary levels established by industry consensus groups prior to the agency's creation in 1971. Many are now hopelessly, dangerously out of date; new science has had no impact on these regulations. Because OSHA has been so beaten down by the opponents of regulation, it has virtually given up on developing new regulations or strengthening outdated ones.

On the other hand, OSHA has had plenty of extra help in its obstructionism when the Republican Party has controlled Congress. To see how this works, let's now consider not toxic chemicals in the workplace but ergonomics—work-related musculoskeletal conditions and repetitive strain injuries (RSIs). In 1990 OSHA issued voluntary ergonomic guidelines for the meatpacking industry, and then Secretary of Labor Elizabeth Dole introduced them by explaining that "These painful and crippling illnesses now make up 48 percent of all recordable industrial workplace illnesses.... We must do our utmost to protect workers from these hazards, not only in the red meat industry, but all U.S. industries."[60] In 2001, the last year in which the information was collected, a meatpacking worker was thirty times more likely to develop an RSI than the average private sector worker.[61] The problem has not disappeared. What happened?

Two years after issuing the meatpacking guidelines, OSHA published official notice of intention to issue a regulation to protect all workers from ergonomic hazards.[62] This would be an actual regulation with teeth, not a toothless guideline. Clearly, the economic implications of an ergonomics rule would be huge; many industries, not just meat packers, would be required to change their employees' work practices to prevent the crippling conditions Elizabeth Dole described. United Parcel Service, for one, must have envisioned a mandated change in its policy that requires employees to lift boxes weighing up to seventy pounds without assistance. Opposition to any ergonomics rule was instantaneous, organized, and well funded. Thus UPS, the American Trucking Association, and their allies devised a brilliantly simple strategy: no more debating the merits of an ergonomics rule;

make Congress prohibit the agency from issuing any standard at all. This was political hardball, plain and simple. Forget OSHA. Forget the injuries.

When the Republicans took control of both houses of Congress in 1994, this congressional strategy became that much easier to implement. In each of the following three years Congress prohibited OSHA from issuing an ergonomics rule. The '96 version of the prohibition that passed the newly radicalized House of Representatives actually banned the agency from even collecting statistical data on repetitive strain injuries. Having no data is the ultimate in uncertainty; without numbers, OSHA would have a hard time justifying a new standard. However, such a data blackout was overreaching even for that time and place, and the 1998 legislation backed off a little. Nevertheless, OSHA was still barred from acting on ergonomic hazards, but Congress did ask the National Academy of Sciences (NAS) to review the scientific evidence on the work-relatedness of musculoskeletal disorders.

And so it did. In August 1998 the NAS convened a two-day meeting in which sixty-five experts from around the world reviewed the evidence on ergonomic injuries and the effectiveness of workplace interventions. Their conclusions, published in October 1998, were the following:

- There is a higher incidence of reported pain, injury, loss of work, and disability among individuals who are employed in occupations where there is a high level of exposure to physical loading than for those employed in occupations with lower levels of exposure.
- There is a strong biological plausibility to the relationship between the incidence of musculoskeletal disorders and the causative exposure factors in high-exposure occupational settings.
- Research clearly demonstrates that specific interventions can reduce the reported rate of musculoskeletal disorders for workers who perform high-risk tasks. No known single intervention is universally effective. Successful interventions require attention to individual, organizational, and job characteristics, tailoring the corrective actions to those characteristics.[63]

The panel found more than enough evidence for OSHA to move forward, but the opponents had other ideas. There is no evidence that they were using the debate over the science as anything more than a delaying tactic. Indeed, Congress now appropriated a million dollars for the NAS to conduct another, more in-depth, time-killing study. However, the opponents could not get around the fact that Bill Clinton was president, and he eventually threatened to veto any more appropriations bills that prohibited OSHA from issuing a regulation. As the NAS was conducting its second study, OSHA, now allowed to move forward, developed and circulated for public comment a preliminary new rule. As a consequence, UPS and other employers faced reengineering their workplaces to eliminate the back-destroying jobs that involved the continuous lifting of heavy items. This was just the beginning, however; the regulatory process is tedious and complex in the best of times. The Small Business Regulatory Fairness Act, one of the few components of Newt Gingrich's Contract with America that became law, allowed small businesses (and their large business allies) to have an early crack at the proposal, which was scrutinized under the interagency review system, thus giving every agency its own crack. Not surprisingly, internal opposition came from the two agencies that most represent business interests: Treasury and Commerce. The strongest support came from the Department of Health and Human Services. I represented the Energy Department at the interagency meetings; we supported the proposal as a way to reduce the RSI toll we were seeing among the workers in the nuclear weapons complex.

In November 1999 OSHA issued its proposed standard.[64] The new standard was a complex document, probably too far reaching. Rather than limiting its rule to meatpacking and other industries with high rates of RSIs, OSHA elected to issue a generic standard that covered all industries. This approach could have led to a reasonable policy debate about starting instead with the highest-hazard industries or perhaps implementing a series of pilot programs, but the anti-ergonomics forces did not want such a debate. Perhaps this was because they were led by employers with major ergonomic hazards, like UPS, who would be covered by a rule that included only high-hazard industries. So they went after the science, with the objective of no rule.

The attack was led by Eugene Scalia, the son of Supreme Court Justice Antonin Scalia. Scalia fils founded and ran the National Coalition on Ergonomics, a group of trade associations opposed to an OSHA regulation. For this duty he was nicknamed the "godfather of the anti-ergonomics movement" by Molly Ivins and Lou Dubose in their book *Bushwhacked: Life in George W. Bush's America.*[65] In an analysis published by the Cato Institute, Scalia claimed that OSHA's proposed regulation was based on "junk science."[66] He coaxed readers to "appreciate the folly of ergonomic 'science' and regulation" and asserted that "leading physicians and medical organizations dispute that [repetitive motion injuries] actually occur."[67]

Is the National Academy of Sciences nothing but a bunch of deluded junk scientists? Apparently so, because the report of the second NAS panel, this time composed of nineteen nationally recognized experts, reads as if written to explicitly dismiss the unsupported ravings of Scalia and his coalition. Here are a few choice quotes:

There is no doubt that musculoskeletal disorders of the low back and upper extremities are an important and costly national health problem. . . . In 1999, nearly 1 million people took time away from work to treat and recover from work-related musculoskeletal pain or impairment of function in the low back or upper extremities. Conservative estimates of the economic burden imposed, as measured by compensation costs, lost wages, and lost productivity, are between $45 and $54 billion annually.

The panel's review of the research literature in epidemiology, biomechanics, tissue mechanobiology, and workplace intervention strategies has identified a rich and consistent pattern of evidence that supports a relationship between the workplace and the occurrence of MSDs of the low back and upper extremities.

The panel concludes that there is a clear relationship between back disorders and physical load; that is, manual material handling, load movement, frequent bending and twisting, heavy physical work, and whole-body vibration. For disorders of the upper extremities, repetition, force, and vibration are particularly important work-related factors.[68]

Little good it did. Once again, as in the midnineties, the opponents' strategy was to play the political card. On January 16, 2001, OSHA's ergonomics standard, the last health standard the agency has issued without being forced to by a federal judge, went into effect.[69] It never was enforced, and two months later Congress repealed it with the full support of the new Bush administration.[70] The new president took the anti-ergonomics effort even further and appointed Scalia solicitor of the Department of Labor, where he would serve as OSHA's chief lawyer and defender. In the six years since Congress overturned the ergonomics standard, OSHA has issued voluntary guidelines—but not enforceable regulations—for employers to use to prevent ergonomic injuries in three industries: poultry processing, retail stores, and nursing homes. In March 2003 OSHA came up with an extremely effective way to control the rate of reported RSIs: The agency revoked a planned regulation that would have required employers to report annually the number of musculoskeletal disorders occurring among their employees. In other words, just don't collect the data, and the injury numbers will go down drastically. Obviously OSHA must be doing a great job.[71,72]

11

Defending the Taxicab Standard

On the issue of manufactured uncertainty, I began the discussion with Big Tobacco because it showed the way. Half a dozen other industries picked up Big Tobacco's strategy and have developed it further in their usually successful attempts to foil regulation. I now conclude this part of my argument with the incredible story of the beryllium industry, which carries the torch high and proud.

Beryllium is a remarkable metal, lighter than aluminum yet stiffer than steel. Its alloys and compounds exhibit a host of unusual technical characteristics. This is one reason it is a useful metal in industry—but perhaps also the reason it is almost unimaginably toxic to the human lung. At some point in almost every production process involving beryllium, the metal or its compound must be transformed into a fine dust or fumes. Breathing the tiniest amounts of either can cause disease—a fact that became all too clear in the 1940s on the production lines of the fluorescent lamp industry, an early industrial use of beryllium. Almost immediately, some of the lamp workers developed a form of chemical pneumonitis caused by the body's immune reaction to the unwanted atoms of beryllium deposited in the lungs. Symptoms included labored breathing, coughing, and chest pain, and they manifested within days.[1] A shockingly high ratio of these victims—30 percent—died. Rather quickly, the lamp manufacturers decided that beryllium was just too dangerous, and they developed an alternative process.[2]

At the same time, however, scientists who were working on the Manhattan Project discovered another use for the metal, one for which there was no plausible work-around. Beryllium turns out to be a splendid "neutron moderator" for atomic bombs because it slows down the colliding uranium neutrons in order to sustain the necessary chain reaction. The metal is invaluable—indispensable, really—for increasing the power of nuclear weapons, and once production of these weapons became a national priority with the advent of the Cold War, the health hazards associated with beryllium came to the forefront again. Physicians soon realized that beryllium causes not only acute beryllium disease but also a chronic version (CBD), whose symptoms are similar but have a slower onset.

Both manifestations were diagnosed among scientists, technicians, and line workers in the new nuclear weapons industry—and even among residents who only lived *near* the facilities, especially around one particular plant in Lorain, Ohio.[3] Since the weapons complex was now the nation's primary consumer of beryllium products, the Atomic Energy Commission (AEC)—the agency responsible for the Manhattan Project—tacitly assumed responsibility for researching the health perils the valuable metal posed. In a 1947 report, entitled *Public Relations Problems in Connection with Occupational Diseases in the Beryllium Industry*, the AEC openly acknowledged problems of both "obvious moral responsibility" and public relations, the latter exacerbated by the fact that, unlike the remote research and bomb-making facilities, some of the beryllium-processing factories were located in more populous areas. The 1947 report states bluntly, "There is no doubt at all that the amount of publicity and public indignation about beryllium poisoning could reach proportions met with in the cases of silicosis or radium poisoning." It also noted that the industry was already reporting problems recruiting workers "because of local prejudice . . . engendered by actual and rumored experience with beryllium poisoning."[4]

The AEC took the extraordinary step of X-raying 10,500 citizens of Lorain, one-fifth of the city's population. When eleven CBD cases were discovered in individuals who had never set foot inside the production plant, the agency tentatively set an exposure limit for these residents of .01 micrograms per cubic meter—an infinitesimally small amount. In 1949, though, the agency set the permissible exposure limit (PEL) for its own and its vendors' workplace facilities much higher: 2 $\mu g/m^3$. This exposure level is now known as "the taxicab standard" for the simple reason that it had been reached a year earlier during a discussion in the backseat of a taxicab that took place between Merril Eisenbud, an AEC industrial hygienist, and Willard Machle, a physician consulting with the company that was building the Brookhaven Laboratory on Long Island. Dr. Eisenbud tells the story in his autobiography and frankly admits that the number was established "in the absence of an epidemiological basis for establishing a standard."[5] The two men did not pull the 2.0 figure out of the air exactly, but they had no idea whether it would be fully protective. No one knew. How stringent is 2 μg? It is the equivalent of the amount of dust the size of a pencil head floating in a six-foot-high box the length and breadth of a football field.

The new "tentative" standard was reviewed annually for seven years before permanent adoption. That is not to say, however, that the AEC had developed solid science to back up the standard. It had not. In 1971, when the newly created OSHA adopted the taxicab standard for all industries working with beryllium, the state of knowledge was *still* rudimentary. It was widely recognized that employees could not safely work with beryllium without respiratory protection, and everyone knew that abrasive work processes (such as high-speed grinding and sanding), which released beryllium into the breathing zone, were extraordinarily dangerous. But no one really knew whether the taxicab standard was fully protective.

Nevertheless, the technology and workplace systems that producers had put in place decades earlier had had an immediate and positive impact. Through 1977, 887 cases of beryllium-related illness had been submitted to a registry maintained in Massachusetts, but virtually no *new* acute cases had been reported, and new cases of the chronic disease had been curtailed.[6] The regulation was a notable—though not complete—success because this was the Cold War, after all, and weapons production was the highest priority of the military-industrial complex. The history of the beryllium industry during that anxious period is replete with instances in which the AEC and the producers gave priority to production to the detriment of the workers, who were sometimes exposed to beryllium levels exponentially greater than the taxicab standard.[7]

Even when stringently enforced, was the standard *fully* protective? Doubt was growing.[5,6] By 1972 at least twenty of the cases reported to the Massachusetts registry were workers who had started employment *after* 1949, when the new standard had nominally gone into effect.[8] In the 1966 text *Beryllium: Its Industrial Hygiene Aspects,* Herbert Stokinger of the U.S. Public Health Service wrote the following: "Numerous cases of the chronic disease have occurred from exposures to seemingly trivial concentrations of a beryllium compound that at higher levels produced no effect. . . . There is a peculiar hypersusceptibility to the chronic disease form whose mechanism is unknown. . . . Some individuals have developed [CBD] after dosages of a very few micrograms of beryllium compounds, whereas far larger doses of the same substance have failed to elicit a response in others."[9]

In other words, a straightforward dose-response relationship—the higher the dose, the greater the risk—does not seem to apply to this strange substance, beryllium. Disease was reported in individuals whose only exposure was laundering the clothes of beryllium workers or having a milk delivery route near a beryllium factory or tending graves in a cemetery near a factory or simply having relatives who worked in the factories—cases just like those of the "bad old days," except these were no longer the bad old days.[8]

In 1972 the one-year-old NIOSH issued a full review of the beryllium literature, including a list of workers who developed chronic disease after relatively short exposures; one machinist had been diagnosed ten years after an exposure of less than three months. The NIOSH document concluded that "There has been no comprehensive, long-term control study relating environmental beryllium concentrations with a cause-and-effect relationship to beryllium disease; therefore, the level to which a revised standard could be recommended is largely one of conjecture."[8]

Then, in 1974 a contingent from the Japanese beryllium industry stunned the government agencies and the U.S. industry with data that showed that exposures at levels *below* the taxicab standard resulted in chronic beryllium disease. The Japanese met with representatives of several U.S. beryllium firms, including Brush Wellman and Kawecki-Berylco, as well as with the agencies. A letter dated August 9, 1974, confirmed five CBD cases afflicting workers exposed to levels below the $2\,\mu g/m^3$ standard.[10] Similar cases occurred at U.S. plants, including four cases among workers at a single metal refinery who were consistently exposed to beryllium below $2\,\mu g/m^3$.[11]

* * *

Then there was the other problem: cancer. Suspicions that beryllium could cause not just acute and chronic beryllium disease but also cancer dated all the way back to 1946, with the surfacing of the first reports of the metal's ability to cause the disease in lab animals.[12] These AEC-sponsored studies were then discussed at a symposium at the famous Saranac Laboratory in upstate New York. At that meeting Dr. Willard Machle, of "taxicab standard" fame, remarked that "the startling uniformity with which sarcoma [a type of tumor] can be reproduced by a variety of beryllium compounds in one species of animals is a significant observation. . . . We are again in a state of unknown hazard with respect to the human population."[13]

With generous AEC funding, the state of knowledge on this question developed rapidly. By 1954 Saranac researchers were so confident of their findings and their technical expertise that they applied to the Tobacco Industry Research Committee for funding to expose rats to both beryllium and tobacco to determine whether tobacco increased or decreased the known rate of beryllium-induced tumors. In their application, the researchers acknowledged one important problem: Beryllium was so dangerous to humans that "elaborate circumspection" would have to be used to protect everyone involved.[14]

Laboratory studies with animals could take the case for the carcino-genicity of beryllium (or any other substance) only so far. The first indi-cations of beryllium-related cancer in *humans* were reported in 1969 by none other than Dr. Thomas Mancuso, whose ground-breaking work has come up time and again in this book.[15,16] As chief of Ohio's Division of Industrial Hygiene from 1945 to 1962, Mancuso had worked on the Lorain, Ohio, study that confirmed the cases of chronic beryllium disease among residents who had never been inside a beryllium factory. When he joined the faculty at the University of Pittsburgh, the AEC selected him to conduct the largest occupational mortality study ever conducted—half a million workers in the nuclear weapons complex. (It was Mancuso who demonstrated that records collected by the Social Security Administration could be effectively used to understand the patterns of death among factory workers.[17,18]) In 1969 his preliminary analysis of the workers employed by two beryllium producers found indications of increased risk for lung cancer. However, recognizing the limitations in his study design, Mancuso called for further research. He continued this work into the 1970s, as did several scientists at the newly formed NIOSH; together they eventually published several analyses that found elevated lung cancer risk among beryllium fac-tory workers.[19,20]

The 1970s were the halcyon days of occupational epidemiology. During that era NIOSH had hired a cohort of sharp young epidemiologists who initiated studies in many of the smokestack industries then plentiful in the United States. In some ways this was low-hanging fruit; the evidence was there for the taking. As part of their work, NIOSH epidemiologists documented increased risk of cancer among workers exposed to benzene, vinyl chloride, acrylonitrile, and cadmium. Although in this period NIOSH and OSHA worked together as the enabling legislation had envisioned, they no longer attempt to do so. First NIOSH collected and distilled the research, conducted more when needed, and then recommended new stan-dards to OSHA, which tried to promulgate them.

Weighing the evidence on beryllium, NIOSH did what it was supposed to do. It recommended action. In a letter dated December 10, 1975, its director informed OSHA that "beryllium poses a carcinogenic risk to man" and recommended that occupational exposures be reduced to a minimum.[21] Formally alerted, OSHA decided to take action. Its legislative mandate in fact gave it no choice. In October 1975 the agency proposed reducing the beryllium exposure limit by 50 percent—from 2.0 $\mu g/m^3$ to 1.0.[22] As the evidence continued to accumulate, in 1977 NIOSH recommended an even lower limit: 0.5 $\mu g/m^3$.[23]

The beryllium industry had a simple answer: Forget it. It denied the pos-sibility that beryllium was a carcinogen and argued that anomalous working conditions—shop floors that were not up to code, for instance—were responsible for beryllium disease. It admitted the necessity of a comprehensive upgrade across the industry, including environmental engineering controls, work practice controls, monitoring of airborne beryllium levels, personal protection, and worker education. What it adamantly *opposed* was the lower exposure level. The old taxicab standard was sufficient, and industry would defend it to the bitter end.

Regarding the suggestion that beryllium was a carcinogen, Brush Wellman, the largest of the manufacturers, said bluntly in an internal memo, "If beryllium is determined to be a carcinogen and so labelled [*sic*] and so regulated it would only be a matter of time until its usage would shrink to a point where it would no longer be a viable industry. . . . Loss of invested savings for stockholders [is a real suffering that has] to be equated against the hypothetical nature of an unproven health hazard to employees."[24]

In effect, the industry drew *two* lines in the sand. It would prevent any workplace exposure limit more stringent than the taxicab standard of 1949, and it would prevent the labeling of beryllium as a carcinogen. Quite simply, it was going to protect both its market and its profit, which it felt, correctly or otherwise, would be threatened by the new regulations. It devised a strategy of cloaking its obstructionist campaign in the guise of objective science.

In his testimony at an OSHA hearing in August 1977 Edward J. Baier, deputy director of NIOSH, stated, "Probably no compounds known to man give so consistent a carcinogenic response in so many animal species as do the compounds of beryllium. . . . Some beryllium compounds have been shown to cause lung cancer at doses lower than that for any other pulmonary carcinogen. . . . Based upon these observations, beryllium compounds are considered to be among the most potent carcinogens that have ever been tested in animals."[23] Industry would have none of it. Led by Brush Wellman, it hired two academic toxicologists to identify methodological flaws in the numerous animal studies done to date and to challenge the whole idea of extrapolating from the results of animal experiments to human experience.[25]

Neither the Mancuso nor the NIOSH study was perfect, and no one claimed they were. As is often the case in interpreting results, some disagreement about interpretation surfaced within NIOSH itself, but the senior scientists who were looking at the weight of the evidence saw a convincing beryllium-cancer relationship. Indeed, subsequent studies have *all* confirmed the initial findings of those early studies.[26–28]

Again, the industry would have none of it and demanded that NIOSH provide the raw data used in its analyses, including data from Dr. Mancuso, who was not a government employee, in order for the industry to reanalyze everything. The manufacturers commissioned Drs. H. Daniel Roth and Brian MacMahon, who at the time was the chair of the Epidemiology Department at the Harvard University School of Public Health, to review and reanalyze NIOSH's work.[29] Dr. Roth is the renowned reanalyzer whose work on OSHA's secondhand smoking studies I have previously cited. These two consultants concluded that "[the NIOSH study] should not be considered in making a determination about the carcinogenicity of beryllium"[30] and "[it] adds nothing to a scientific assessment of the question of whether this group of workers experienced an excess risk of lung cancer because of exposure to beryllium."[31]

No surprise. Wrong, but no surprise. To my knowledge, reanalyses by industry scientists virtually never confirm a cancer link for *any contested carcinogen*. Funny—or not so funny—how that works. And this knee-jerk response by industry is not because regulators are bound and determined to find such links. If they were, their agencies' lists of known carcinogens would be far longer than they are.

The industry accused OSHA of engaging in "an arbitrary and capricious misuse of regulatory authority."[32] It enlisted eight scientists to sign a letter that opposed the cancer label for beryllium and accused the government of "shocking examples of shoddy scholarship and questionable objectivity."[33] Questionable objectivity? Six of the eight signers worked as consultants to the industry, but none had disclosed the fact in the letter, which had cited only their academic affiliations.[34]

Joseph Califano, secretary of Health, Education, and Welfare and therefore responsible for NIOSH (though not for OSHA, which is under the Labor Department), appointed a panel of independent scientists to review the evidence.[35] This panel's conclusions concurred with OSHA and NIOSH. Dr. Carl Shy, a professor of epidemiology at the University of North Carolina, recommended additional studies to examine the suggested association with cancer, but he added, "It would be imprudent from a public health perspective to delay our judgment about beryllium exposure of current workers, until these studies were completed."[36]

On March 7, 1978, the *Wall Street Journal* featured a report titled "Beryllium Firm Optimistic on Fight to Keep Metal off Carcinogen List."[37] The firm—Brush Wellman—was right. The beryllium industry won that battle in the late 1970s, but not on the merits. They were mooted by the politics. In the Carter administration, Secretary of Labor Ray Marshall acceded to the demands of Secretary of Defense Harold E. Brown and Secretary of Energy James R. Schlesinger to halt the agency's rulemaking on beryllium.[38]

Years later, reporter Sam Roe revealed the whole story in his award-winning six-part history in the *Toledo Blade*. Using the argument that a label of carcinogenicity and a lower exposure standard would force producers out of business and imperil beryllium supplies for weapons production, Brush Wellman had engineered the intervention by the Department of Energy (DOE) that blocked OSHA's new standard. As the sole remaining supplier of the metal in 1979, the corporation received from DOE a one-time 35 percent price increase, a promise not to seek alternative suppliers, and a commitment to oppose a more restrictive exposure standard.[7]

* * *

End of story? Hardly. In 1975 OSHA's announcement of the proposed change precipitated a battle between regulators and manufacturers that continues to this day—a classic case study of the struggle to control science and to regulate workplace safety. Combined with the political clout of the weapons agencies, the repeated and well-funded assertions of methodological flaws and inappropriate analyses had defeated OSHA in Round One, but Brush Wellman could not rest on its laurels because the science that supported carcinogenicity and a tighter exposure standard was relentless.

In 1980 the International Agency for Research on Cancer (IARC), a unit within the World Health Organization, published a monograph that evaluated the carcinogenic risk of various metals, including beryllium.[39] IARC relied on several of the same studies NIOSH and OSHA used and concluded that "the experimental and human data indicate that beryllium should be considered suspect of being carcinogenic to humans."[39] The following year, the National Toxicology Program's Second Annual Report on Carcinogens included, for the first time, beryllium and some beryllium compounds described as "reasonably anticipated to be a human carcinogen."[40] Moreover, NIOSH planned to conduct additional epidemiologic studies. The EPA was unlikely to ignore the accumulating evidence in its regulation of air and water contaminants. In addition, California was moving to implement its own environmental regulations.

For the industry, it was ominous news on every front, and throughout the 1980s Brush Wellman kept its epidemiology consultants busy churning out reports and testimony to counter any study anywhere that implicated beryllium as a carcinogen and suggested the exposure standard needed to be lower.[41–44] How about a friendly textbook? In a 1987 memo, two Brush Wellman executives wrote the following:

> The literature on beryllium published in the last twenty years has been very damaging. The literature is constantly being cited, either to our doctors at medical meetings in rebuttal of the Brush experience, or by potential customers as the cause of their unwillingness to use our products. Federal Government regulatory agencies, such as OSHA and

EPA publish much of this material and then in the absence of good data, cite these erroneous documents to support regulatory activities.

What is needed to combat this situation is a complete, accurate and well written textbook on beryllium health and safety. It will have to be financed by Brush (or Brush and NGK?) and the bulk of the work done by Marty Powers and Otto Preuss [the authors of the memo]. To be fully accepted and credible, however, it will have to be published under the auspices of some not-for-profit organization such as a university or medical group. . . . In addition to the book, we should have a number of medical papers published in prestigious medical books.[45]

Among the proposed chapters was this one: "'A Critical Review of the Recent Literature Associating Beryllium with Increased Lung Cancer Rates.'. . . Preferably, the primary authors should be Drs. MacMahon and Roth. However, most of the work on this paper would have to be done by Brush Wellman."[45]

This book was not a pipe dream. *Beryllium: Biomedical and Environmental Aspects* was published a few years later, edited by the two former Brush Wellman staffers, Powers and Preuss, along with a respected academic physician from the University of Pennsylvania.[46] Dr. MacMahon is listed as the sole author of the chapter "Assessment of Human Carcinogenicity."

In 1989 the industry took the predictable course and contacted Hill and Knowlton. Pitching for the new business, this firm wrote the following:

Beryllium undoubtedly continues to have a public relations problem. We still see it cited in the media, as well as in our conversations with people who should know better, as a gravely toxic metal that is problematic for workers. This situation is indeed ironic since beryllium is in fact one of the true success stories of industry's responsible management of a potentially hazardous material. Unfortunately, the misperceptions about beryllium endure.

We would like to work with Brush Wellman to help change these common erroneous attitudes. We envision a public relations program designed to educate various audiences with the facts about beryllium and reinforce these facts consistently over time to dispel myths and misinformation about the metal.[47]

The proposal did not mention Hill and Knowlton's successful work for Big Tobacco specifically, but it boasted about the firm's extensive experience advising clients (including manufacturers of asbestos, dioxin, lead, vinyl chloride, and fluorocarbons) whose situations were "akin to the beryllium situation because in each case entire industries were threatened as a result of misperception, fear, uninformed reporting, and organized opposition." Matt Swetonic, the staff person proposed to direct its beryllium activities had been a key player in Hill and Knowlton's efforts on behalf of R.J. Reynolds Tobacco to convince the public that second hand smoke was harmless[48] and to "create a favorable public climate" that would help defeat laws suits filed by smokers with lung cancer.[49] Swetonic had previously performed public relations work for Johns-Manville, the asbestos producer, and had been the first full-time executive secretary of the Asbestos Information Association, an organization founded by the asbestos industry to counter the evidence of that mineral's deadly properties.[50]

In 1990, following the model of the independent-looking scientific panel developed by Hill and Knowlton for Big Tobacco, Brush Wellman and other interests set up the Beryllium Industry Scientific Advisory Committee (BISAC), whose members were scientists who had worked for the companies. A 1993 document outlined the strategy: "BISAC will provide the scientific basis for our cancer strategy by: a. Breaking the link, if possible, between animal and human experience . . . c. Examining cancer risk assessment methodology. . . . We see cancer as posing not a true medical threat, but rather a perceived threat. . . . Therefore, we have formed a cancer strategy group which will deal with the combined medical, legal, operational, and promotional aspects of beryllium as a suspect carcinogen. . . . In a worst-case scenario beryllium could ultimately be classified as a human carcinogen, which might result in limited end use opportunities in consumer markets."[51]

Meanwhile, NIOSH researchers were engaged in two new epidemiology studies that would provide evidence to either confirm or dispute the earlier studies. One, published in 1991, found an elevated risk of lung cancer mortality among chronic beryllium disease patients.[26] The next year NIOSH published a large mortality study that included workers at two plants in Pennsylvania and four in Ohio. The research found elevated risk of lung cancer for the overall population, with statistically significant excesses at the plants in Reading, Pennsylvania, and Lorain, Ohio.[27]

As a public agency, NIOSH was willing to share its preliminary analyses with the industry, and it did so with both of these studies. The Brush Wellman higher-ups immediately swung into action. In a scathing letter to Dr. Donald Millar, director of NIOSH, Brush's president and CEO, Gordon Harnett, wrote the following: "Prior to publication of the study containing its present conclusion, I request we be given adequate advance notice of the publication journal. This will allow us to contact the editor and request publication of our rebuttal in the same issue. . . . Dr. Millar, we are fast approaching a situation painfully reminiscent of that of the late 1970's [*sic*] with its acrimonious public debate over the scientific objectivity and competence of NIOSH studies.... [A]ttachment of the current conclusion to the analysis, and then its publication, with no more scientific support than is in the study, would be difficult to explain short of a malicious effort to harm the industry."[52]

To its everlasting credit, NIOSH refused to be intimidated, and the study appeared in the *Journal of the National Cancer Institute*, as prestigious as any such publication. It was accompanied by an editorial in which IARC's Rodolfo Saracci asserted that the results "go one step forward toward reinforcing the causal interpretation of the association between occupational exposure to beryllium and lung cancer."[53]

The industry demanded the raw data used in the studies and again brought in Dr. Roth, who had reanalyzed the NIOSH studies fifteen years earlier. Once again Dr. Roth and his colleagues plugged in new assumptions about smoking and comparison populations and the excess cancer risk in the beryllium workers disappeared.[54] There was no particularly good justification to use the new smoking assumptions, except that they yielded more cancers for smokers and therefore relatively fewer for inhalers of beryllium. It would have been equally valid to choose assumptions about smoking that yielded *fewer* cancers from smoking and therefore *more* cancers due to beryllium.

Any competent epidemiologist can employ particular tricks of the trade when certain results are desired. Roth et al. finished the analysis in 1991 (even before the study it was meant to challenge was published) and circulated it widely, if unofficially, often claiming that it was in the process of publication.[55–57] (In fact, it did not see the light of day for more than ten years, which suggests some difficulty in finding a journal to publish it.) Industry scientists worked feverishly to discredit the NIOSH work,[57–59] but their arguments were rejected by the panel of independent scientists who reviewed the analysis for the National Toxicology Program.[60] The task would not have been an easy one because the industry's own consulting scientists—BISAC—had concluded that "while the results are arguable, the analysis was sound."[61]

In 1993 IARC officially reclassified beryllium and beryllium compounds as Group 1 carcinogens (that is, carcinogenic to humans based on sufficient evidence in both epidemiological and animal studies).[62] Undeterred and unashamed, BISAC responded with a major effort to support a new claim, while evidently discarding Dr. Roth's assertions about the wrong comparison population and smoking adjustments. Now the elevated cancer rates at Brush Wellman's Lorain, Ohio, plant must have been the result of confounding—that is, the plant really did have too many cases of cancer, but they were caused by exposure to some factor other than beryllium, thus confounding the analysis. As a way to reverse the IARC decision, BISAC member and Harvard epidemiologist Dimitrios Trichopoulos suggested this approach. In some previous monographs, IARC had labeled a *process* rather a specific chemical as the carcinogen; if the process at Lorain was carcinogenic, then the product, beryllium, would be exonerated.[63,64] What factor could serve the industry as a plausible confounder?[65] An engineering consultant was hired to come up with something that made the Lorain plant different. His answer: sulfuric acid mist—because "Lorain was the only commercial extraction/reduction operation which used the sulfate process to open the ore . . . without health and safety precautions."[66]

Beryllium executives and their consulting scientists then spent the next several *years* discussing this new hypothesis and considering the pros and cons of advancing the case for sulfuric acid mist. The voluminous exchange of internal memos and letters is fascinating reading (for the specialist, at least). Engineers were brought in to estimate the historical level of acid mist exposure. Brush Wellman's vice president for Government Relations wrote the following to Dr. Trichopoulos: "The one bit of documentary evidence that is lacking is actual measurements on sulfuric acid mists. However, we can paint a picture of a plant that had ventilation that was barely adequate to control the acid fume to the level of tolerance of the employees, but sufficiently inadequate to cause the employees to avoid the sulfating mill, if at all possible."[67] The initial picture painted of horrific working conditions was over the top, however. According to the minutes of a BISAC meeting, Dr. Trichopoulos reported that the engineering data showed exposure levels "too high for human endurance." The engineers had over-massaged the data. "Accordingly, [Trichopoulos] made some assumptions and drafted a summary for Brush review and concurrence" before he would even submit the paper to BISAC for review.[68]

A review of the BISAC minutes and memos does not reveal a group of scientists trying to determine whether beryllium exposure actually increases cancer risk. These documents contain not even such a pretense. The only purpose was to determine whether they could use these various strategies to sow some timely uncertainty and thereby buy some time. In this they succeeded. The industry's big rebuttal to NIOSH was finally published in the *Journal of Occupational and Environmental Medicine* in March 1997.[69] Now, *JOEM* is not a prestigious journal, but getting the rebuttal into the peer-reviewed literature was a coup for the industry.

In a moment of irony, one consultant later brought in to influence the EPA's assessment of beryllium sent a memo to Brush Wellman. The note highlighted articles from the literature that showed that sulfuric acid mist does not cause lung cancer at all.[70] The evidence he cited—a review of sulfuric acid mists and respiratory track cancers—was developed by scientists consulting for the European Sulfuric Acid Association, which was eager to convince regulators that sulfuric acid mist was not a lung carcinogen.[71]

* * *

As we have seen, the Department of Energy was complicit with the beryllium industry and the Department of Defense in killing OSHA's attempt to lower the exposure level in the late 1970s. In the eighties the industry had its hands full with all the new science, but the antiregulatory fervor of the Reagan years gave it a wide margin for error. That fervor then cooled, beginning with the presidency of George H. W. Bush, who took office in 1989 and whose appointments of Gerard F. Scannell and William K. Reilly to head OSHA and EPA, respectively, worked to strengthen the commitment of those agencies to public health. The secretary of energy, Admiral James D. Watkins, positively embraced the regulatory model. Former chief of naval operations and former head of President Reagan's Commission on the HIV Epidemic (also known as the Watkins Commission), the admiral was appalled by what he found at the Department of Energy—a bureaucracy with little regard for environmental or occupational health issues. The DOE's official historians report that Watkins:

> criticized DOE's antiquated "back in the fifties" management systems that fostered lack of accountability. "Every time I asked who was responsible for something," he later recalled, "each person pointed to the one at his left." Watkins castigated DOE's operational culture with its "heavy emphasis on achieving production goals, made within an atmosphere of collegial secrecy." Environment, safety, and health problems had "backlogged to intolerable levels" and been "hidden from public view," he noted, so that "we are now paying the price for this long-term cultural misdirection."[72]

Watkins dispatched "tiger teams" to conduct wall-to-wall inspections of the nuclear weapons plants. He told the DOE staff to make sure the workers and the environment were better protected. Armed with such unaccustomed support from above, the staff proposed reducing the permitted exposure level of beryllium to 1 $\mu g/m^3$ (the level that OSHA had tried to establish for private industry in the late seventies). The beryllium industry could live with a new standard that applied *only* to the weapons facilities themselves, but it feared a domino effect. In a letter dated Jan 10, 1992, a Brush Wellman executive wrote the DOE, "We would be less than forthright if we did not express our disappointment that DOE did not see fit to accept most of our recommendations which we feel are supported by our experience of over half a century. We are grateful for the insertion of language clarifying that the standard is applicable to GOCO [government-owned, contractor-operated] contractors only and not to suppliers such as Brush Wellman...We regret that DOE apparently still intends to abandon the existing standard of over 40 years standing with no evidence, either that the existing standard is unsafe or that the new proposed standard affords any greater degree or [sic] safety."[73]

No evidence? There was already plenty of evidence. In an internal memo written only two months later, that same Brush executive asserted that, with regard to an Ohio facility, "Despite significant investment in metallic beryllium manufacturing at Elmore, not all of the processes are capable of operating within the 2-μm/m^3 standard. Increasing CBD is causing fresh doubt about the efficacy of the 2-gm standard; DOE facilities are in the process of reducing the standard to 1-gm. I don't need to repeat the long list of environmental challenges which we face."[74]

Even with support from Admiral Watkins at the top, the DOE's effort was slowed by internal opposition. Money spent protecting workers would mean less money for arms production. An internal battle raged for almost a decade as the weapons production offices blocked the health and safety offices from going forward with the proposed change. They had plenty of assistance from the beryllium industry, which promoted its own negative studies that purported to demonstrate that workers who have low exposure to beryllium do not develop CBD. At a DOE-sponsored public forum, Brush Wellman's director of Environmental Health and Safety read a prepared statement. The Department of Energy's notes paraphrased the remarks thusly: "'Brush Wellman is unaware of any scientific evidence that the standard is not protective. However, we do recognize that there have been sporadic reports of disease at less than 2 μg/m^3. Brush Wellman has studied each of these reports and found them to be scientifically unsound.'"[75]

This was the industry's primary argument, and its logic was fatally flawed. It was not difficult to go back into the work history of anyone with CBD and estimate that at some point the airborne beryllium level must have exceeded the standard. Brush did this and then reasoned that the 2 μg/m^3 must be fully protective since everyone who had CBD had at some point been exposed to levels above the standard.

Brush needed a more convincing argument, and so it hired the product-defense firm Exponent, Inc., which proceeded to do what it does best: manufacture uncertainty. Maybe *different forms* of beryllium do not pose the same health hazard. Maybe *particle size* is what is important. Maybe *skin exposure* is more significant than we thought. Whatever is going on with beryllium is very complicated, according to this line of reasoning, so we need to do more research, more research, more research. In a paper first given at a symposium in September 1999 Exponent Inc.'s Dennis Paustenbach summarized the new strategy: "At this time, it is difficult to identify a single new TLV [threshold limit value] for all forms of beryllium that will protect nearly all workers. It is likely that within three to four years, a series of TLVs might need to be considered. . . . In short, the beryllium [PEL] could easily be among the most complex yet established."[76]

Brilliant in its way. Give Exponent an A+ for manufactured uncertainty. Just do not forget the bottom-line message to exposed workers: Yes, we now admit the current exposure limit may not be safe, but since we do not know how low the limit should be, it is best to leave the old, inadequate standard in place until the scientific evidence emerges to help us determine the appropriate limit. This campaign was no doubt worth every penny of the $1.5 million the industry paid Exponent.[77]

For its part, however, the Department of Energy forged ahead. As assistant secretary, I ran the process that that considered whether DOE—on its own, without OSHA—would lower the exposure level for its workers and those of its contractors. At a hearing I chaired in February 1999 I took testimony from an industry representative who stated that "important research is under way which may provide a scientific basis for a revision to the occupational standard for beryllium"—the Exponent gambit. The gentleman pointed to studies on particle size, particle number, and particle surface area.[78]

We listened carefully, but we did not base our new standard on particle size, number, or surface area. Instead, we applied the measure that scientists have used for years: airborne beryllium exposure by weight. We felt that at some time in the future we may understand the relationship between these characteristics and CBD risk and that this understanding may influence the appropriate standard, but these factors provide no information that is useful in protecting workers *today* from this potentially fatal disease. In the end, after years of internal dispute and a thorough review of the literature, the DOE set an "action level" that triggers the use of respirators and other mechanisms to prevent exposures above $0.2\,\mu g/m^3$, a tenfold reduction from the previous standard of $2.0\,\mu g/m^3$.

Subsequently, OSHA acknowledged that DOE was doing the right thing with its radically restrictive beryllium standard and planned to follow suit. The Assistant Secretary of Labor with responsibility for OSHA wrote that "we now believe that our $2\,\mu g/m^3$ PEL does not adequately protect beryllium-exposed workers from developing chronic beryllium disease, and there are adequate exposure and health effects data to support this rulemaking." The letter continued: "Cases of chronic beryllium disease have occurred in machinists where 90% of the personal exposure samples found levels of beryllium to be below the detection limit of 0.01 μg/m^3.... Viewed from OSHA's regulatory perspective, these DOE study results document.... risk of chronic beryllium disease to machinists of 94 per 1,000 [exposed workers]."[79]

Those are red-alert numbers. Ninety-four per thousand is a lifetime risk of almost 10 percent. Once again OSHA committed itself to issuing a more protective standard, this time by the end of 2001.[80] In 2001, early in the first term of the George W. Bush administration, the agency did a quick about-face and announced that the agency needed "a substantial amount of information" before it would consider new regulation.[81] Today the federal government finds itself in the somewhat embarrassing position of explaining why the employees of DOE and its contractors are now protected by a workplace rule ten times more restrictive than the one covering workers in the private sector.

In the several years since DOE issued its new standard, NIOSH and industry scientists have completed and published the research the industry's consultants had predicted would be the basis of a type of new standard, one based on beryllium form or particle size.[82–88] These studies provide compelling evidence that the old standard was not protective: Numerous cases of CBD were found in workers who were never exposed above the old level. Unfortunately for Brush Wellman but perhaps not surprisingly, the new studies provide little if any of the evidence that Exponent and the beryllium industry had promised.

The link between beryllium and lung cancer has also been confirmed in more recent studies, specifically a case control study published in 2001 that addressed the issues raised by the reanalyzers of the major report on carcinogenicity issued almost a decade earlier.[28] NIOSH consulted with industry scientists while the study was planned and executed.[89–93] The new study used "internal" comparisons, with lung cancer cases compared to noncases at the same workplace, thus eliminating questions about a proper comparison population. It better controlled for smoking than the earlier investigations. It is an excellent study, one that was put together with input from the industry, but no matter. The industry still attacked the results because they confirm—yet again—that beryllium exposure causes lung cancer.[94]

In November 2002 OSHA actually took a step backward, implicitly accepting the industry's approach when it issued a new Request for Information (RFI) for additional data on—what else?—the relationship of beryllium disease to, among other things, particle size, particle surface area, particle number, and skin contact.[95] That is where matters still stand today—and are quite likely to stand for years to come.

In short, when the accumulation of scientific evidence became so great that it was no longer credible to deny the existence of CBD cases caused by levels below the old standard, the industry came up with new reasons to delay the issuance of a stronger standard. No matter what a study's results, the industry conjured up reasons for yet more studies. They manufactured still more uncertainty.

* * *

There you have it—the beryllium story at some length, but actually in brief. Product defense triumphed over public health not once but twice: first in killing the proposed OSHA standard in 1978 and then in stopping the agency almost twenty-five years later. The scientific uncertainty these consultants manufactured was not particularly convincing, but it was sufficient to provide scientific cover for the beryllium industry to employ its political power to successfully defend an inadequate workplace exposure standard for decades.

Now for the real irony: Brush Wellman has instituted *exemplary* worker protection programs. Exposures to beryllium in its facilities are very low already, and I believe Brush engineers could easily meet any new standard OSHA might reasonably adopt. The metal has now been designated as a "known human carcinogen" by the National Toxicology Program[96] and the International Agency for Research on Cancer,[62] but the company nevertheless continues its long, hard fight against change in the standard or any label of carcinogenicity. Why do they keep it up?

For two reasons, I believe. With the end of the Cold War, the government needs far fewer nuclear weapons and is purchasing less beryllium. The industry has been trying to find new markets (e.g., golf clubs, computer disk drives), while customers, both retail and wholesale, tend to prefer products that do not carry the carcinogen label. Small wonder. If other companies fear they cannot work safely with beryllium materials, they will look for less toxic substitutes. Thirty-one workers in Canadian recycling plants have recently been diagnosed with CBD.[97] If beryllium-containing products are barred from recycling, they become financially less attractive to make in the first place. A Brush Wellman document from the 1970s draws an analogy with the besieged asbestos industry. It states, "Asbestos is being designed out of many applications and its usage will decline rapidly in coming years. The decline in beryllium usage would be accelerated by the presence of warning labels and signs."[98] Note the utter lack of concern for whether the warning labels and signs were justified.

The second fear is litigation. A new, lower exposure standard would be used as proof that workers were made sick at levels Brush Wellman had claimed were safe. The company's 1991 Health, Safety, and Environmental Strategic Plan summarized the strategy: "Employ legal means to defeat unreasonably restrictive occupational and emission standards and to challenge rulemaking and other regulatory activities that seek to impose unreasonable or unwarranted changes. Resist an attempt to make the existing occupational exposure standard of two micrograms/cubic meter . . . more restrictive. The standard is safe, it is one of the most stringent standards, and it is fundamental to our product liability defense."[99]

In the late 1990s dozens of workers with CBD, some of them crippled by the disease, sued Brush Wellman, and the company (along with the U.S. government, often a codefendant because the exposures took place at nuclear weapons plants) spent large sums defending itself. As I explain in chapter sixteen, the federal workers' compensation program that I conceived and shepherded through Congress now provides both cash payments and medical costs for such workers, but only if they drop their lawsuits. Most have, and the initiative has saved the beryllium industry millions of dollars. In the first five years since the program began, it has provided more than $270 million in compensation to sixteen hundred workers with CBD and another thousand who had been sensitized to the metal.[100]

Nevertheless, old habits die hard. In early 2003 Ohio Representative (and now Governor) Ted Strickland introduced legislation to add lung cancer to the list of beryllium-caused diseases compensable under that federal program.[101] Attempting to derail the effort, a lobbyist for Brush Wellman circulated a newly published article from a scientific journal that asserted that "the most recent published and peer-reviewed analysis" concludes "there is no elevated cancer rate for beryllium workers."[102] That "most recent science" was not new science at all. It was the same ten-year-old reanalysis[54] of the seminal 1992 NIOSH study.[27]

In Europe, where regulators still attempt to label cancer-causing chemicals, the beryllium industry has mounted an uncertainty campaign to stop a Norwegian proposal to classify beryllium as a carcinogen; in support it provides strong statements from three scientists described in the industry's submission as "independent": Drs. Roth, MacMahon, and Trichopoulos.[103]

12

The Country Has a Drug Problem

Many of the health risks I have discussed in the previous chapters are concentrated among people who are *involuntarily* exposed to the hazards in question—and to their detriment. Scientists who are studying the effects of this exposure cannot ethically or practically set up experiments to find out, once and for all, what effect a given level of exposure to, say, molecules of beryllium has on the likelihood of lung cancer. With prescription and over-the-counter drugs, however, the benefits and risks of usage accrue to the people who choose to take them. As a result, clinical researchers in the pharmaceutical field *can* examine the effectiveness and safety of medicines in controlled laboratory experiments involving people. These clinical trials present researchers with a wonderful tool that beryllium and asbestos and diacetyl and chromium researchers can only dream about.

There is a catch, however. Under the U.S. system, the pertinent regulatory agency—the Food and Drug Administration (FDA)—grants licenses for new medications based on its review of the various laboratory tests and clinical trials reported *by the companies themselves.* The FDA can study the data and the results as reported, but it has neither the staff nor the resources to duplicate the work itself. Without the oversight agency's imprimatur, the companies cannot sell one pill; with it, they sell billions. The critics of the status quo include the editors of the major U.S. medical and biomedical journals, almost without exception. These journals are supported, by and large, by the advertising and reprint payments from the manufacturers, and yet the editors stand united in revolt against their main source of support by demanding controls on the way the companies conduct and report their research.

It is not my intention in this chapter to write a broad critique of Big Pharma, a commonly used collective name for the largest drug companies. The "disease mongering," the knockoff drugs that add nothing new to our fight against disease, the co-optation of the medical profession, and the apparently unmatched political and marketing clout that lamentably accompany the invaluable discovery of remarkable medicines are not my subject here. Professionally, this is not my main field, nor could I hope to match in one chapter the host of excellent, eye-opening books published in recent years.[1-5] As I have with the other industries, I concentrate instead on statistical issues.

Randomized clinical trials are as close to perfect experiments as we can get, yet the deceptions the manufacturers perpetrate in these studies are brazen indeed. If this manipulation of science is not the root of the problems in this industry, it is nevertheless a major one. Address it, and we would have a much better system for delivering the best drugs to the most people. Ignore it, and nothing substantive will ever change. I join in applauding the wonderful new drugs that have saved and improved so many lives over the past half-century or so—without a doubt, Big Pharma employs many of this nation's best scientists—but its claim that we enjoy these benefits *thanks to* our wonderful system of drug research and testing ignores significant flaws inherent in this system.

Having a financial stake in the outcome changes the way even the most respected scientists approach their research and interpret the results of experiments. Common sense says as much, and certainly no one is surprised to learn that the studies that Big Tobacco paid for over the decades disproportionately reported whatever result was best for the manufacturers. Many lay observers (but no longer the editors of the medical journals) are shocked to learn this is how it works even with medicines, but we have overwhelming evidence that such is the case. When a scientist (or the scientist's employer) is hired by a firm with a financial interest in the outcome, the likelihood that the result of that study will be favorable to that firm is dramatically increased. This close correlation between the results desired by a study's funders and those reported by the researchers we now call the "funding effect."[6,7]

The documentation that links pharmaceutical industry sponsorship with pro-industry conclusions began to appear in the 1990s. In 1994 a group in Boston led by Dr. Paula Rochon examined the clinical trials testing non-steroidal anti-inflammatory drugs (NSAIDs)—a class that includes aspirin, ibuprofen (Advil), and naproxen (Aleve)—used in the treatment of arthritis. The researchers discovered that, when trials of these drugs were funded by manufacturers, they almost always reported that the manufacturer's drug was better than, or at least comparable to, the comparison drug—but the claim was often not supported by the actual data.[8] Another of the first important revelations was written by a group led by Dr. Henry Thomas Stelfox of the University of Toronto. Numerous papers in the literature had been debating whether calcium channel blockers (a category of drugs used to treat hypertension) increased heart attack risk. Intrigued, the Canadian scientists examined the financial ties to the drug manufacturers of the authors whose published articles addressed the question. The results startled the scientific community: Ninety-six percent of the authors who supported the use of calcium channel antagonists had a financial relationship with manufacturers of these drugs, compared with 60 percent of authors who were neutral on the controversy and 37 percent who were critical of the drugs.[9] A wave of subsequent papers has demonstrated the same correlation between sponsorship and conclusions on the subject of oral contraceptives[10] and drugs meant to treat schizophrenia,[11] Alzheimer's disease,[12] cancer,[13] and a host of other conditions.[14–17]

Within the scientific community, there is now little debate about the funding effect, but the exact mechanism through which it plays out has been a surprise. At first, it was widely assumed that the misleading results associated with corporate sponsorship were the product of shoddy studies done by mercenary researchers who manipulated methods and data in order to reach a preordained conclusion. Such scientific malpractice does happen, but close examination of the manufacturers' studies showed that their quality was usually at least as good as, and often better than, studies that were not funded by Big Pharma.[15,18]

This discovery puzzled the editors of the medical journals, who generally have strong scientific backgrounds and pride themselves on their ability to analyze research papers. On the other hand, the drug makers have almost unlimited financial resources and more experience in conducting clinical trials than any one else. Who could be better at skillfully and surreptitiously stacking the deck with studies that *seem to be* excellent work? The recently retired editor of the *British Medical Journal (BMJ)*, Dr. Richard Smith, has stated that he required "almost a quarter of a century editing . . . to wake up to what was happening. . . . The companies seem to get the results they want not by fiddling the results, which would be far too crude and possibly detectable by peer review, but rather by asking the 'right' questions—and there are many ways to do this . . . many ways to hugely increase the chance of producing favourable results, and there are many hired guns who will think up new ways and stay one jump ahead of peer reviewers."[18]

Simply put, the manufacturers have strong motivation to promote the *certainty* that the drug is effective, while downplaying any possible risk.

When such a risk is indicated, however, the strategy flips, and the new objective is to create *uncertainty* about the *danger*. Product defense experts may be called in to save the day, as we will see. Let's now look at how this dynamic works out in the clinical trials that are the bread and butter of the pharmaceutical industry.

These trials proceed in three phases. Phase One trials involve a small number of healthy volunteers. This stage identifies dosage issues, side effects, and other safety matters. If justified by the results of this preliminary investigation, Phase Two trials gather preliminary information on the effectiveness and safety of the new product by using as many as a couple of hundred volunteers with the target condition. If still justified, Phase Three is the well-controlled, usually "randomized" clinical trial—the gold standard, in theory, involving usually hundreds of volunteers, often thousands, all of whom have the condition or risk factor in question. The "randomization" in the randomized clinical trial does *not* mean that participants are chosen at random. Far from it. They have to have the condition that the new drug targets, and they generally have to meet specific age, sex, and health status characteristics as well. The randomness comes into play as the volunteers who fit each required profile are randomly divided into at least two groups, one receiving the new drug of interest, the other receiving either an established treatment or a placebo. In some trials the study is divided into multiple arms that involve several groups, each of which receives different doses or treatment regimens. These trials are also called "double blind" because neither the participants nor the researchers know which participants are getting which treatment.

During the Phase Three clinical trial, the bad science can and all too frequently does infiltrate the process. One way this happens involves the "loaded" selection of those people included *and excluded* from participating. Most drug trials involve middle-aged adults. The companies prefer not to test their drugs on very old people or on patients with several medical conditions, perhaps because the results of trials in these populations are less likely to show efficacy and more likely to suggest the existence of safety concerns. Some of the same researchers who studied the NSAID drugs discovered that only 2 percent of the subjects in those trials were sixty-five years of age or older, even though these are the patients most likely to be given the drugs once they are approved by the FDA. The drugs are also likely to have a higher incidence of side effects in elderly people.[19] Even in the trials for Viagra, men with uncontrolled diabetes or angina or with a history of recent stroke or heart attack were *excluded,* thus guaranteeing the nonavailability of information about risk in this large population.[20] Extrapolating from the results of these studies on healthier people, doctors are forced to guess the nature of the risks and benefits of taking a drug by someone much less healthy.

The drug companies do not like head-to-head competition between their proposed new drug and an established one because the new drug *might lose* and thereby compromise opportunities for touting superiority or at least comparability—"no drug is better than this one"—in advertisements. Trials against placebos are therefore ideal, but in the case of NSAIDs, a field that has proven performers, including generic aspirin, head-to-head clinical trials are required. These are tricky matters for the researchers. In such trials, the devil is in the details. Take rofecoxib, much better known as Vioxx. Both it and Celebrex were the most popular painkillers (often targeting arthritis) in what became dubbed the "COX-2" category. (The older, basic NSAIDs such as aspirin and naproxen [Aleve] blocked the action of two enzymes that contribute to inflammation and pain, which were labeled COX-1 and COX-2. The problem with those older medications is that blocking COX-1 may also cause gastrointestinal (GI) complications, including bleeding and ulcers. For this reason, some patients simply cannot tolerate them. It would therefore be great to have a drug that blocks only the COX-2 enzyme. However, aspirin also *reduces* the risk of cardiovascular problems. Therefore, the challenge for the drug companies was to find a painkiller that proved superior with regard to GI side effects by inhibiting only the COX-2 enzyme without looking inferior to aspirin on the cardiovascular question. Such a drug could be marketed not just to patients who are sensitive to COX-1 inhibitors but also to just about everyone. The market would be enormous.)

In 1999 Merck and Company initiated a major, eight-thousand-participant clinical trial to demonstrate Vioxx's ability to reduce both pain and GI side effects. The company's scientists had to set up this study very carefully. Their first decision was to veto aspirin as the competition because Vioxx would almost certainly not be able to meet aspirin's proven cardiovascular benefit. The second decision was to exclude anyone with a high risk of heart problems. The third decision was to prohibit participants from taking aspirin on the side. And, of course, participants could not have existing gastrointestinal problems because the whole point of the trial was to demonstrate the superiority of Vioxx in controlling GI problems while keeping reports of heart problems to a minimum.

In the end, Merck chose naproxen (Aleve) as the competition for the trial. This popular product was not known to reduce heart attack risk, as aspirin was. We can imagine the shock with which the Merck executives greeted the results of the trial, which became available to them in early 2000: Participants who took their drug for an average of nine months had *four times* the risk of heart attack as those taking Aleve.[21] This was a catastrophic number for Vioxx and therefore Merck. Or was it? Couldn't Merck turn the results upside down and construe them to show not that

Vioxx increased the risk by 400 percent but that naproxen *reduced* the risk—and by an astounding 80 percent? Granted, that result would have made naproxen several times as effective as aspirin in this regard—a rather unbelievable result, especially since there was little prior evidence that naproxen conferred any such benefit.[22] Moreover, the FDA already had in hand data that suggested that Vioxx could increase the risk of heart disease.[23] Several independent scientists (that is, not on Merck's payroll) had also raised red flags.[24] The FDA had mostly ignored these alerts up to this point, but could Merck expect the agency to still go along when it reviewed Merck's application for Vioxx in mid-1999?

It could and did. Merck chose the interpretation that implausibly credited naproxen over the one that much more plausibly indicted its own drug, and it embarked on a four-year defense of this almost ridiculous hypothesis. Representative Henry Waxman (D-CA) subsequently issued a report that documented in detail how Merck developed its marketing campaign to mislead physicians into underestimating the heart attack risk associated with Vioxx.[25] The company attacked the detractors at every opportunity and threatened the careers of academic physicians who questioned Merck's position on the safety of its drug.[26] When Harvard researchers working under a Merck contract found the drug "associated with an elevated relative risk" of heart attacks compared with Celebrex or no related painkiller at all, Merck asked them to modify their conclusions. They refused, and lead researcher Daniel Solomon said, "We made a decision that we should let the science rule the day."[27]

It is now clear that the correct interpretation of the Vioxx clinical trial was that the drug is a powerful cause of heart attacks; the significant questions raised in 2000 were definitively answered when the results of a new placebo trial were announced in 2004. This trial was almost an accident of history because it is rare for a drug to be compared first with another drug in its category and then subsequently with a placebo since it is unethical to withhold a proven effective treatment from the patients who get the placebo. However, even though Vioxx could not be compared with a placebo for the purpose of pain relief, Merck wanted to find out whether it might have value in preventing colon polyps, which are precursors to colon cancer. Since no medication is known to prevent these polyps, a study that compared Vioxx with a placebo was ethically legitimate.[28]

This trial turned out to be a bad mistake for Merck, but one that ended up saving thousands of lives. Merck scientists reported that participants in the new trial who took Vioxx for more than eighteen months suffered twice as many heart attacks and strokes as those who took a placebo—seven excess heart attacks per thousand users *per year*. The correct interpretation of the original study was now beyond question: Vioxx causes heart attacks.

These dramatic results were front-page news around the world. Scientists at the FDA estimate that Vioxx caused between 88,000 and 139,000 heart attacks, probably 30–40 percent of them fatal, in the four years the drug was on the market.[29,30]

Subsequent litigation uncovered memos that document that Merck executives were concerned about the increased risk of heart attacks associated with Vioxx but downplayed these concerns in their communications with physicians and resisted the FDA's efforts to add warnings to Vioxx's label. Then the editors of the *New England Journal of Medicine (NEJM)* reported that Merck scientists had not counted all of the heart attacks among the group taking Vioxx in one of the key studies. Who was responsible for the original submission? It is well known in the medical world that drug industry writers actually pen many of the papers signed by academic scientists. When the editors of *NEJM* retrieved the diskette with the original data for the study, they found that three heart attacks had been removed from the data set on a Merck computer.[31,32]

This revelation was soon followed by a reanalysis sponsored by *NEJM* that debunked Merck's demurral that the increased risk for heart attacks pertained only to those patients who took the drug for eighteen months.[33] The fact that Vioxx increases heart attack risk relatively quickly was then confirmed by another clinical trial comparing Vioxx to a placebo, this one conducted by scientists at Oxford University in Britain.[34] These findings did not come as a surprise to many independent observers, since there was no biological reason the effect would only occur after eighteen months. In fact, an analysis that examined the computerized medical records of 125,000 Quebec residents reported that heart attack risk increased by 67 percent in the first *two weeks* of taking Vioxx.[35]

As this story unfolded in 2004, it was hard for me to imagine that the company's scientists were deliberately promoting a drug they knew was unsafe and would result in disease and death for a considerable number of people. At first I thought their original interpretation that naproxen prevented heart attacks (rather than that Vioxx caused them) was the result of the unconscious workings of the funding effect. On the other hand, as revelation followed revelation, I found it harder and harder to believe that this was merely a case of well-meaning scientists unintentionally misinterpreting the data. It was almost painful to read the scientists' public statements suggesting that naproxen had powerful cardioprotective effect. No drug has ever been shown to reduce heart attack risk by 80 percent. If the scientists honestly believed their claim, they should have lobbied the government to pour Aleve directly into the nation's water supply. Still, I had trouble believing that scientists would knowingly promote such a dangerous drug. When I presented this theory at a meeting, an editor of one of the leading U.S. medical journals criticized me for hopeless naiveté. Industry scientists know the truth and simply lie about it, he said.

Perhaps the most outrageous part of the whole Vioxx debacle is that most of the patients who were prescribed the drug (as well as those getting Celebrex and the other COX-2 inhibitors) did not need them because they were at little or no risk for stomach bleeding. Aspirin or some of the other analgesics work just as well and at far less cost than the COX-2 drugs. For many patients, Vioxx would be more likely to cause a heart attack than to prevent a gastrointestinal event. Millions of patients were being prescribed drugs they did not need; thousands had heart attacks that were 100 percent avoidable.[36]

* * *

In the last few years several distinguished scientists have published commentaries that describe and sometimes ridicule other ingenious ways drug industry researchers design clinical trials to make their drugs look better than they are.[18,37-40] Here are some of the more widely used tricks of the trade:

1. *Test your drug against a treatment that either does not work or does not work very well.*

   The manufacturer of a new antifungal medicine, fluconazole, wanted to show that the drug was more effective than another treatment, amphotericin B. Instead of using intravenous amphotericin B, the standard treatment, the manufacturer's researchers chose to compare fluconazole with an oral version of the medicine, which is poorly absorbed and not an established treatment.[41] Similarly, in several trials for drugs to control hypertension, the manufacturers compared their drugs with a beta-blocker, even though diuretics have proven to be more effective for the same condition.[42]

2. *Test your drug against too low a dose of the comparison drug because this will make your drug appear more effective.*

   In the studies of NSAID painkillers discussed earlier in the chapter, the comparison drugs were often given at lower doses than were the sponsors' medications.[8]

3. *Test your drug against too high a dose of the comparison drug because this will make your drug appear less toxic.*

   At least eight studies sponsored by three different drug companies compared their newer antipsychotic drug to unusually high doses of the older, comparison drug, thereby ensuring that the new drugs would have fewer side effects.[40]

4. *Publish the results of a single multicenter trial many times because this will suggest that multiple studies reached the same conclusions.*

The manufacturer of a drug for treating postoperative nausea and vomiting sponsored nine trials but published the reports in twenty-three papers without telling readers that many of the subjects were included in multiple papers. Combining all of the published studies resulted in a 23 percent overestimation of the drug's effect.[43]

5. *Publish only that part of a trial that favors your drug, and bury the rest of it.*

In September 2000 *JAMA* published the results of a major clinical trial for the COX-2 painkiller Celebrex and stated that the drug was associated with a reduction in reported ulcers over a six-month period.[44] This was major news for doctors and patients and lauded by an accompanying editorial, one of whose authors was Dr. M. Michael Wolfe, a gastroenterologist at the Boston University School of Medicine.[45] Pharmacia, the manufacturer of Celebrex, had duped Dr. Wolfe, though. The company had conducted its trial over twelve months (most arthritis patients take their chosen medicine for years), and this more valid period of time showed absolutely no benefit in reducing ulcers. In the *JAMA* article, however, Pharmacia reported data on only the first six months of the trial, during which a small ulcer-reducing benefit appeared (but which disappeared by the end of the year-long trial). Dr. Wolfe discovered the real story only while serving on the FDA's arthritis advisory committee the following year.[46]

6. *Fund many clinical trials but publish only those that make your product look good.*

An examination of 178 trials for treating acute stroke found that analyses in which the treatment was found to be safer were more likely to be published than those that showed it to be harmful. In addition, it found that if a study concluded the treatment in question did not work, it was less likely to be published than a study that concluded the opposite.[47]

In my experience, newcomers to the issues this book confronts are invariably astonished to learn that the drug companies can get away with these tricks, amazed that they can submit journal reviews on their clinical studies that are so incomplete as to be dishonest, and astounded that they are not necessarily breaking any law when they do so. On the other hand, the companies can be caught, at least some of the time, because the FDA (in stark contrast to most federal regulatory agencies) demands manufacturers' raw data so that the agency's scientists can do their own analyses.

As a rule, the FDA ignores the papers submitted to scientific journals because it knows they can be either incomplete or filled with more spin than substance. So while the government may be well informed about the minutiae of the clinical trial, physicians, who base treatment decisions on what they read in the medical literature, are left in the dark. It is a remarkable system. Taking full advantage of it and hoping to convince the FDA and the investment community of the efficacy of their new product, drug manufacturers go to great lengths to report positive results in clinical trials. A last resort may be "data dredging," which is also known as "Texas sharpshooting." Fire a bullet at a blank wall, draw a bull's-eye around the hole, and then claim this had been your target all along. Such corporate-sponsored "research" is found in many industries, but Big Pharma specializes in the practice: Conduct a study and shuffle the numbers until a good one comes up. With a sufficiently large database, a good researcher should be able to concoct *something* deemed statistically significant. Dredge deep enough, wide enough, long enough, and then announce your new finding as a fantastic breakthrough. By any name, this is bogus science because legitimate statistical analysis requires that you state your hypothesis in advance.

A good example comes from the quest for an AIDS vaccine. In the clinical trial for a vaccine known as AidsVax, developed by VaxGen (a biotech company in Brisbane, California), the results were negligible overall but had a statistically significant effect among the blacks in the study. The vaccine did not work for Asians, but so few Asians participated in the trial that they could be added to blacks and yield a "blacks and Asians" category that was still technically significant. In fact, "others" could be added without ruining the count, so "blacks and Asians and others" was *still* statistically significant. Ideally, Hispanics could have been added to the group, and the vaccine might then have been touted for "nonwhites," but the study showed no benefit for Hispanics, of whom there were many in the trial, so the "nonwhite" category was no good. It is possible that the test had turned up something of interest, but the only way to know for sure was to report honestly that the vaccine did not work for whites or Hispanics but did show some statistical benefit for blacks—and then consider the feasibility of more research, perhaps a new clinical trial. However, since "blacks, Asians, and others" was the best the company could do, that is what it went with.[48] When the vaccine received its next real test—a large clinical trial in Thailand—it failed miserably.[49]

Parenthetically, a second VaxGen initiative failed more recently. Not long after the AidsVax debacle, the Bush administration gave VaxGen an $877 million contract to produce 75 million doses of anthrax vaccine. In December 2006 the government cancelled the contract, citing VaxGen's failure to begin the clinical trials necessary to test the drug.[50]

* * *

The Food and Drug Administration is one of our oldest regulatory agencies, created early in the last century (even though drugs did not even require a physician's prescription until 1951). Its seniority is of no avail, however. Like all of the other regulatory agencies, it is simply outgunned, with a budget of $643 million to review new drugs in fiscal 2004 matched against the $216 *billion* in drug sales in the United States alone.[51] The agency does get the raw data from the clinical trials, but the companies apply pressure every way they can. They have designed to their advantage the Prescription Drug User Fee Act (PDUFA), which requires the drug companies to pay user fees with each application for review. This legislation seemed like a good idea when it was first passed in 1992 because it gave the FDA a larger budget, compliments of the industry, and therefore allowed it to hire more staff and speed up the review process in its Center for Drug Evaluation and Research (CDER). Concerned that life-savings drugs were stalled in the bureaucracy, AIDS activists became a major political force behind the legislation. And in this respect the plan did work. The mean review time dropped significantly. It had to: With PDUFA, each new application brings in $300,000, but the FDA staff was now given tight deadlines to complete the reviews.

Then came the unintended consequences (if they *were* unintended by the industry lobbyists who cooperated in the drafting of the legislation; only the truly naive would be surprised to learn that the drug makers' money comes with strings attached). First, the new system skewed the FDA's efforts toward approving new drugs, not postmarketing safety surveillance of previously approved drugs. Under PDUFA, the FDA can spend the user fees to send drug reviewers to conferences or to get additional training, but it cannot use that money to fund work on drug safety. Furthermore, the new law ensured that the FDA would get a certain amount of industry money, but only if it continued to spend the pre-PDUFA budget for new drug application review, adjusted for inflation. Perhaps predictably, with user fees flowing in, Congress cut the FDA's budget. Thus, in order to meet the PDUFA criterion and qualify for Big Pharma's contribution, the agency has had to shift funds out of ongoing safety surveillance and into the review process. When this consequence was finally understood, PDUFA was reauthorized in 2002 to put a small percentage (5 percent) of the user fee income into surveillance of the safety of drugs *after* they have been approved, although that spending was restricted to use on drugs that were recently approved. Comparing the situation today with that of the pre-PDUFA period, the agency reviews more drugs at a faster rate, but by prioritizing the speedy review of new drugs over safety studies, the agency's ability to ensure the safety of the drugs we take has been damaged.[52,53] A recent analysis by Harvard professor Daniel Carpenter links the accelerated approval process, including the PDUFA deadlines imposed on FDA staff, with subsequent agency regulatory actions, including requirements of stronger warnings and even removal of drugs from the market. Dr. Carpenter's analysis suggests that if the FDA had not been rushed to meet the PDUFA deadlines, the agency reviewers might have gotten it right the first time.[54]

PDUFA has also left the agency with fewer resources with which to conduct the postmarketing safety studies vital to identify the risks associated with long-term use of any medicine. As with Vioxx, postapproval revelations led to the withdrawal from the market of Baycol (a cholesterol-lowering drug that caused hundreds of cases of rhabdomyelosis, a toxic breakdown of muscle fiber); Bextra (a COX-2 drug that was associated first with potentially fatal skin reactions and subsequently with increased risk of heart attacks); and Propulsid (heartburn medicine that caused cardiac arrhythmias). In each case, the FDA had failed to act on early indications of the problems. Two important investigations were launched. Congress asked the Government Accountability Office to look at the FDA's postmarketing decision making and oversight, and the FDA itself requested the Institute of Medicine to undertake a similar investigation. Both inquiries reached similar conclusions: Major changes were needed to fix the FDA's system for examining the safety of drugs already on the market.[52,53]

The problem in this regard is straightforward. For the most part, the initial clinical trials that were conducted to gain the FDA's approval to sell a drug are too small to detect many of the adverse reactions (or side effects) caused by taking the drug. This is not shocking. The hypothetical clinical trial in which one hundred participants were given a drug could not detect an adverse reaction that occurs in one in a thousand patients and, for statistical reasons, might even miss the one in a hundred adverse reactions. Even a larger Phase Three trial might include just a few thousand subjects, but once the drug is placed on the market, tens or hundreds of thousands of individuals will take the drug. Some of these hazards will be detected only by continuing to study them *after* licensing. A 20 percent increase in heart attacks would be a public health disaster, but this phenomenon could not be detected in anything other than the largest and longest clinical trials.

Moreover, most clinical trials are quite short, lasting just weeks or a few months. The raft of new antidepressant drugs was approved after a series of trials that lasted typically *six weeks*.[1] Six weeks for powerful drugs that treat complex conditions with complex brain chemistry? Depression does not come and go like a stomach ache, nor is it cured like a stomach ache. For many chronic diseases, patients may take certain drugs for decades, but clinical trials will not detect any effects that require an exposure longer than the length of the trial.

I am not suggesting that randomized clinical trials should go on forever. That is not feasible, and once a drug is found to be effective and safe, especially if it is a first treatment for a condition, it would not be ethical to deprive patients of its benefits—both those trial participants who are taking the placebo and the market at large. On the other hand, the FDA could require the company to continue to follow the participants from the original studies—that is, actively monitor them for side effects instead of passively waiting for them to turn up and be reported. Clearly, the only study that will tell the full story is the real-world experience after the drug hits the market. But the agency rarely does what it eventually did with Vioxx, which was to analyze a really big data set—the members of the Kaiser Permanente HMO—to look for telltale relationships. All of the big managed care companies now have tremendous databases that hold extensive information about who took which drugs and who got sick and when. This is the future of postmarketing drug safety studies, and the FDA has slowly begun to mine these data sets to learn what really happens when millions of people, over many years, take a drug that may have been tested on a few hundred people for a few months.

In describing the overall problem with safety testing, two members of the investigative panel of the Institute of Medicine, Bruce Psaty and Sheila Burke, have written the following about the FDA's Center for Drug Evaluation and Research (CDER):

> [The CDER] lacks a systematic approach to identifying possible pre-marketing drug-safety problems and translating them into high-quality post-marketing studies. Without an organized system to identify potential safety signals, the studies needed to resolve them may not be performed. The post-marketing commitments that are requested by the FDA are often hastily assembled by sponsors, who may not have a symmetric interest in safety and efficacy. Even so, once a drug is approved, CDER lacks the authority to force sponsors to complete agreed-upon post-marketing commitments or to require sponsors to initiate new studies. As a result, hundreds of agreed-upon studies remain "pending" in perpetuity. Since CDER lacks the resources to conduct its own studies, when a new drug is launched, the current regulatory system creates *"an evidence-free zone."*[55] (emphasis added)

As I write this, Congress has given the FDA the authority to require manufacturers to conduct postmarketing safety studies. A few manufacturers had agreed to undertake these studies as a condition of approval, but the vast majority remained unfinished, and the FDA could do nothing about it. Once a drug was licensed, what incentive did the manufacturer have to identify *and reveal* the side effects? Only one: avoiding liability. The industry now wants to take care of this problem with a federal law that states that no company can be sued for damages if the FDA has approved the drug. Let's see now. Many studies and books have documented the lies and legerdemain the companies have used to get approval and the studies they have tried to bury, but the manufacturers argue that once they have tricked or cajoled the FDA into approval, they should have retroactive immunity from all legal liability. That's nerve.

Other than liability issues, there is no reason whatsoever for the companies to find problems with an approved drug. Business-wise, it would be insane. British Professor Edwin Gale, who first applied the descriptor "evidence-free zone" for the period during which a new drug is launched, explains that "companies need to market aggressively during this period because the countdown on the life of their product license has already begun. Even the most ethical company will be reluctant to launch studies which might discredit a marketing claim based on weak evidence."[56] Yes, the companies are required to report instances of adverse reactions to the FDA, but they cannot report what they do not know, so the less they know, the better. In the well-chosen words of Carl Pope, executive director of the Sierra Club, "strategic ignorance" is their wisest policy.[57] Pope is referring to industrial polluters—we have seen numerous examples of the strategy—but the adage pertains to the drug industry as well.

Physicians are not required to report adverse reactions, and they do so only irregularly. Rare events, such as a massive stroke in a young woman shortly after she takes an appetite suppressant might get reported (this is not a hypothetical example; more on this shortly), but physicians would be hard pressed to identify the heart attack in an older man as an adverse reaction to Vioxx, even if the small print on the label says something about cardiovascular events. Heart attacks are simply too common, and even though Vioxx may have caused one hundred thousand or more, physicians were never told enough to associate them with the drug their patients were clamoring for.

Even when there *is* evidence of postapproval problems, the suspect drug will not necessarily be expeditiously withdrawn. Warner-Lambert's diabetes drug Rezulin was pulled off the shelves in this country two and a half years after it was taken down in Britain. (In Europe, the follow-up on safety is on the whole much more aggressive than here.) David Willman of the *Los Angeles Times* won a Pulitzer Prize in 2001 for his investigation of the tragedy in which hundreds of patients died from Rezulin-related liver failure. It turns out that the drug was approved by the FDA in the first place only after its lead investigator, who opposed approval because the drug was associated with inflammation of the liver, was removed from the application process.[58]

Now let's return to the young women who suffered strokes shortly after taking an appetite suppressant, occurrences so unlikely that they *were* reported to the FDA by physicians. Some readers probably know that the drug is phenylpropanolamine (PPA) because this infamous episode was widely reported in the news media. Since the early seventies PPA had been used as a decongestant and an appetite suppressant in over-the-counter medications (by 1999 *six billion* doses annually[59]), and reports of hemorrhagic strokes in young women who were taking PPA had been circulating for many years. In 1991 the FDA finally raised its own questions. In 1993 the reports reached a critical mass, and the agency proposed removing the drug from category I ("safe and effective") until additional data were gathered. The industry said no way. It knew that pseudoephedrine (marketed as Contac and Sudafed, among other names) is comparable to PPA in its action, but pseudoephedrine costs a bit more and has a bitter taste that has to be masked, especially for children's products. The industry wanted to keep PPA on the market. Eventually, both agency and industry reached a compromise. The manufacturers would select an investigator and fund an epidemiologic study whose design would be approved by the manufacturers and the FDA. The industry chose Dr. Ralph Horwitz, a professor of medicine and epidemiology at Yale University School of Medicine.

Almost ten years later, the study confirmed the causal relationship between PPA and hemorrhagic stroke: Women who used PPA as an appetite suppressant had sixteen times the risk of hemorrhagic stroke as other women.[60,61] The benefits of this chemical—minimal, with Sudafed a ready-to-go alternative in hand—did not come close to outweighing this risk. Did the manufacturers do the decent thing and withdraw PPA, which by then had annual sales of more than $500 million? No. Instead, they turned to the Weinberg Group, specialists in product defense, veterans of the tobacco wars with a proven willingness to defend virtually any product under siege. According to emails uncovered during litigation, the industry's scientists originally hoped to reanalyze Yale's raw data but did not have adequate time. Instead they chose to "look for bias and areas of concern related to the proper understanding of the results."[62] In other words, it was the usual uncertainty campaign. Meanwhile, industry attorneys put the Horwitz team through grueling legal depositions. David Kessler, ex-head of the FDA and now dean of the San Francisco School of Medicine of the University of California, said, "With the amount of hassle and harassment that [the Yale scientists] had to endure, I'm sure the next time they're asked to undertake something like this, they'll wonder if it's worth the cost."[63]

Despite the industry's (and the Weinberg Group's) best efforts, they lost this war. Armed with powerful epidemiologic evidence, the FDA finally forced the manufacturers to stop marketing PPA. Internal industry documents show that the company hoped to ward off action at least through the 2000–2001 cold season. Their strategy for preserving their market share was partially successful: By the time the FDA told them to remove PPA-containing products from distribution in November 2000, they had a PPA-free alternative ready to ship.[63]

The debate over the PPA science was lengthy; thirty years had passed since the first reports of hemorrhagic strokes. The FDA estimates that, before it was withdrawn, PPA may have caused between 200 and 500 strokes per year among 18- to 49-year-old women: 6,000 to 15,000 strokes in all.[59] Is the Weinberg Group embarrassed that it may have slowed the FDA's attempt to take PPA off the market? Far from it. Until I wrote about this episode in *Scientific American,* the firm *advertised* its contribution to the ten-year delay in the FDA's cancellation of yet another drug.[64]

* * *

The manufacturers do conduct postapproval trials, but not for the purpose of confirming long-term safety. The idea behind these trials is to establish the drug as a treatment for conditions other than those initially approved by the FDA. (It was Merck's subsequent trial to determine whether Vioxx prevented colon polyps that inadvertently brought the drug's heart attack propensity to everyone's attention.) One important reason for these efforts is the promotion of off-label use, although the manufacturers have to be careful because they are forbidden from explicitly encouraging off-label use. In any event, these postapproval clinical trials are published *only* if they legitimately demonstrate—or can be massaged post-hoc style to "demonstrate"—*exactly* what the companies want them to.

Now, what if a postapproval clinical trial uncovers results with negative import? No law says they must be honestly and accurately reported to the medical profession. In the industry, such trials are known as "phantom papers" because they effectively disappear.[65] Perhaps the most notorious example of such selective release of postapproval Phase Four studies is the case of the drugs used to treat depression, called SSRIs (selective serotonin reuptake inhibitors). Study data showed that SSRIs increased the risk of suicidal behavior among teenagers who were taking these drugs. The results were provided to the FDA but labeled "commercial confidential" by the manufacturers, which made it a criminal offense for FDA scientists to disclose them. Meanwhile, industry-funded academic scientists withheld the studies from publication. Only under pressure from New York attorney general (now governor) Elliot Spitzer's consumer fraud suit did Glaxo-SmithKline release the results. The company contended that it had complied fully with the law—and perhaps it had. That's the shame of this system. The FDA's belated analyses of 372 published and unpublished adult SSRI trials confirmed the increased risk for "suicidality" in young adults between 18 and 24 years of age.[66,67] The agency then required the addition of a "black box" to the label, which warned of the increased risk.[68]

In a separate civil suit, parents whose children committed suicide while taking one of these drugs, called Zoloft, sued its manufacturer, Pfizer. The parents brought Welsh researcher Dr. David Healy to testify. Dr. Healy had researched SSRIs and warned his colleagues that their use in children could be dangerous. The defendant challenged his testimony. The judge ruled in February 2002 that Dr. Healy's opinion that SSRIs increased suicidal behavior was a "distinctly minority view" and could not be presented to the jury.[69] What irony. His was indeed a distinctly minority view, but only because the company had hidden the data from the majority of researchers and physicians! (In the lingo of the day, Dr. Healy was *"Dauberted"* in that trial, but he was permitted to testify in two others.[70,71] The very important *Daubert* issue is the subject of the following chapter.)

It is difficult to know how many studies commissioned by the manufacturers are deep-sixed or selectively published, but an ingenious group of European researchers took on the challenge of finding out. They utilized the records of the two institutional review boards in Denmark, through which all clinical trials conducted in that nation must be registered and approved before data collection starts. Their study found that more than half of all outcomes originally promised in the protocols were reported incompletely or not at all. Further, one-third of the trials reported positive outcomes that were never mentioned in the original protocol.[72] This suggests that the investigators found the good news after the fact and then tried to pawn it off as part of the original and controlling protocol for the trial. That is, the investigators dredged their data.

The medical community was up in arms over the highly publicized scandal about the SSRI deceit. Congress regularly considers legislation that requires mandatory public registration of all clinical trials. The American Medical Association has endorsed this idea.[73] Big Pharma predictably has argued that registration could reveal information the manufacturers consider proprietary and give competitors an idea where research is leading. Compelled to do something, however, the industry has established a voluntary database. Not good enough, say its critics. The editors of the leading medical journals have announced that they will no longer publish the results of studies that have not been properly registered,[74] and several have subsequently complained that the manufacturers have submitted little new information to the registry.[75-77]

Should we be surprised by any of this? Not really. How could this system in which the companies that are paying for the research and have so much riding on the outcome *not* result in all manner of suspicious outcomes and therefore taint the honest results with mistrust? Or, as I wrote in my introduction about the industry's campaign to prevent the labeling of aspirin consumption by children as a dangerously high risk factor for Reye's syndrome, if a medication that carries a likely risk of disease and death in children is considered fair game for a corporate cover-up, *what isn't?*

In September 2001 the scandals reached the tipping point when the editors of a dozen of the most influential medical journals, including both *JAMA* and *NEJM,* published a joint statement admitting that the "precious objectivity" of the research published in their journals was under direct threat by the commercialization of clinical research.[78–80] The editors were sick of clinical trials bought, paid for, designed, conducted, and analyzed by Big Pharma, and then used as marketing tools. Such work made a "mockery" of science, they wrote.[81] In April 2004 Dr. Drummond Rennie, deputy editor of *JAMA,* said, "This is all about bypassing science. Medicine is becoming a sort of Cloud Cuckoo Land, where doctors don't know what papers they can trust in the journals, and the public doesn't know what to believe."[82]

The bottom line is that the sum total of all of the clinical trials in any given category generally do not tell doctors and patients *which drugs are the best.* From the perspectives of both the public health and economics, this should be the whole point of the system, but as it stands now, no one—certainly not the prescribing doctors, perhaps not even the researchers or the FDA—may know if there are even significant differences in efficacy and safety of different drugs prescribed for the same condition.

Nonetheless, sometimes we do know. Surprisingly often, head-to-head competition finds that new, expensive drugs are no better than the older, cheaper ones they are supposed to replace (because they are going off patent).[83,84] In such unfortunate cases, the challenge for the manufacturers' scientists is to provide the data in such a way that the sales force can convince physicians to move patients from the older drugs anyway. In the invaluable newsletter "Worst Pills Best Pills," Dr. Peter Lurie of Public Citizen tells the fascinating story of Prilosec and Nexium, two blockbuster heartburn drugs made by the British manufacturer AstraZeneca. Prilosec is a combination of two isomers of a single generic drug called omeprazole: "What is an isomer? It is, chemically speaking, a molecule containing identical atoms to another molecule, but differently arranged: a mirror image, to be precise. Consider two isomers of a certain molecule to be like a pair of gloves—same number of fingers, just arranged differently."[85]

With the patent on Prilosec about to expire in 2001, the company applied for a patent for a "new" medication named Nexium. Was this a new drug? No, it was simply one of the isomers of omeprazole. Did the FDA fall for (or go along with) this rather unbelievable charade? Indeed it did. Patent law allows the practice, so the FDA probably had no alternative. As a "new" drug, Nexium had to pass a clinical trial. Although the FDA requires only that a new drug be effective, not *more* effective than the competition, AstraZeneca needed to tout Nexium as a better drug for heartburn than Prilosec. How could the clinical trials prove this? By matching up *40* milligram doses of the new Nexium against *20* milligram doses of the old Prilosec. Even then, the extra dose proved only marginally beneficial and in only two of the four trials. The FDA medical officer who evaluated the new drug application for Nexium wrote that AstraZeneca's "conclusion that [Nexium] has been shown to provide a significant clinical advance over [Prilosec] in the first-line treatment of patients with acid-related disorders is *not supported by data*." Nevertheless, the company was allowed to patent Nexium and tout it as the new and superior heartburn blockbuster. Prilosec? You can buy it relatively cheaply as the generic omeprazole, and many doctors recommend that you do.[85]

Remember Claritin, Schering-Plough's blockbuster allergy drug, which was replaced in 2001 by Clarinex? Same story, pretty much. Prozac? The original SSRI drug initially prescribed for depression and then for other conditions is now out of patent and sells for pennies as the generic fluoxetine. The me-too version, Prozac Sarafem, is a pink and lavender pill patented as a weekly dosage for severe premenstrual symptoms, and it is expensive.[1,85]

How are doctors fooled by such bogus science? The long answer is beyond my purview. The short answer is that often they do not know the specifics of the case. They accept what is written without applying the appropriate level of skepticism, which I would characterize as the same level that should be directed at any late-night TV advertisement.

* * *

Safety labels are the subject of intense negotiations between the FDA and manufacturers; as a result, the labels are often incomplete and occasionally misleading. Regarding the risk of heart attacks associated with Vioxx, after the advisory panel's conclusion, more than a year passed before the warning label was actually attached to the drug. The medical journals were full of articles touting the drug Diflucan for the treatment of ringworm in children. Doctors who read these journals would not learn that the FDA *rejected* the drug for ringworm—it was ineffective; moreover, high doses posed a risk of liver damage. Nor would the doctors have found news of the FDA's rejection in the FDA-mandated label that comes with the medicine.[86]

The FDA does not have the power to dictate the information contained in drug labels. Yes, acknowledged Dr. Sandra Kweder, acting director of the FDA's Center for Drug Enforcement and Research, the power to change labels "would be very helpful."[87] The unfettered power to write and change labels is minimal and should be granted to the agency. It is hard to believe that it does not have that power right now. Or is it? Safety has been de-funded by the FDA. *Both* the industry and the agency are in a hurry to get drugs on the market but slow to take them off. That is the basic dynamic, and it must change.

13

Daubert

Bendectin is an anti-morning-sickness medication that had been taken by more than thirty million women before its manufacturer, Merrell Dow Pharmaceuticals, was confronted in the early 1980s by hundreds of lawsuits claiming that the drug had caused birth defects. The Food and Drug Administration did *not* rescind its approval, however, and the drug was still available in Canada, but Merrell Dow voluntarily suspended sales in the United States in 1983.[1] When the first Bendectin cases began, there was little epidemiological evidence on the matter. To establish a cause-and-effect relationship between the medication and the birth defects, the plaintiffs' attorneys in these cases relied on a range of evidence, including test tube and laboratory animal studies, as well as analyses of the pharmacology of Bendectin—all requiring testimony by expert witnesses. Alone among the witnesses in any civil trial, these experts are allowed to give their informed, professional *opinion* if the judge deems it helpful to the jury. Such experts are particularly important when issues of science and causation play a role in the case. While judges and juries understand that being hit by a car can explain a broken leg, the link between a medication and a subsequent health problem must be carefully explained. The connection between exposure to a toxic chemical at a particular concentration over a given period of time and a rare cancer discovered many years later is not within the common experience of lay jurors and must be *very* carefully explained.

In order to be admissible in most courts for most of the last century, the experts' evidence had to pass the *Frye* test, which dated to a 1923 federal case that concerned the admissibility of the results of polygraph, or lie detector, tests.[2] *Frye* held that expert scientific testimony should be allowed in the courtroom only if there were, within the relevant scientific community, "general acceptance" of the theory underlying the principles involved. In *Frye* itself, the test minted on the spot disqualified the polygraph evidence. In *Daubert v. Merrell Dow Pharmaceuticals,* one of the Bendectin cases decades later, the *Frye* test was deemed to disqualify the plaintiffs' scientific evidence. So said two lower courts, but the families and their lawyers appealed, and the case eventually reached the U.S. Supreme Court.

In its ruling announced in June 1993, the Court established a new set of criteria for the admissibility of expert testimony.[3] In the federal courts, the *Frye* test was set aside. In its place we now have the "*Daubert* test." Writing for the majority, Justice Blackmun explained that henceforth scientific testimony would have to pass two tests: reliability and relevance. The "general acceptance" test from *Frye* was now just one factor to be considered. It was no longer dispositive. Reliability is judged by a number of factors, including whether the evidence derives from a scientific methodology; whether it has been published and peer-reviewed; whether it can be tested and is therefore falsifiable; and whether it has a known error rate and what the known or potential rates of error might be. This has been codified in an amended version of Federal Rule of Evidence 702.[4]

Under *Daubert,* either side in the case may file a motion that challenges the expert testimony proffered by the opposing party, thereby requiring the judge to determine whether the expert's testimony is based on an appropriate scientific methodology. Thus *Daubert* sets up the *trial judge* as the gatekeeper of the science. Because the plaintiff shoulders the burden of proof in a civil trial and must introduce scientific evidence to support the case, it is usually the defense that files the "*Daubert* challenge," as it is called. The judge can then determine the reliability and relevance of scientific evidence before a jury is even chosen and before the trial has even begun.

This new procedure has been labeled as nothing less than an "admissibility revolution."[5] Since it is the science and the accompanying expert opinion that will aid the jury in deciding whether the plaintiff's claim of a causal relationship between exposure to the defendant's product and the plaintiff's injury is "more likely than not" to be valid—the standard of proof in a civil trial—the inclusion or exclusion of this science is often crucial. If the judge excludes the evidence, there is usually nothing left to the plaintiff's case, and the judge issues a summary judgment in favor of the defendant. Alternatively, if the judge rules that the plaintiff's experts may testify, the case often settles, with both sides preferring that outcome to the high costs and the all-or-nothing stakes of a jury trial.

Simply put, in a case involving complex science, the Court's *Daubert* ruling transforms a trial by a jury—guaranteed by the Seventh Amendment to the Constitution—into a pretrial hearing decided by a single judge who addresses a single question. This is an important development with profound consequences for the increasing number of cases that necessarily turn on issues of science. In the field of "toxic torts," cases in which the plaintiff alleges that the harm done stems from exposure to a product perhaps many years in the past, the impact of *Daubert* cannot be overstated. Workplace and environmental exposure to the substances and chemicals I discuss in this book—tobacco, asbestos, beryllium, chromium, lead, vinyl chloride, and many more—has prompted litigation that often wrestles with issues rooted in complex science.[6]

The Supreme Court did not apply its new *Daubert* rule to *Daubert* itself but remanded the case to the Court of Appeals. That court applied the new rule to the science in the Bendectin case, once again excluded the expert testimony for the plaintiff, declared for the defendant, Merrell Dow Pharmaceuticals, and added a couple of new hurdles that any scientific testimony would henceforth need to clear. They added new factors for courts to consider, but the *Daubert* case made clear that the initial factors were not exhaustive and that all of the standards need not be met. These hurdles have the aim of ferreting out evidence with an inherent bias. For example, this court stated in an opinion (now dubbed *Daubert II*) that science compiled or conducted for the purposes of litigation should be inherently suspect.[7] Four years after *Daubert* the Supreme Court expounded further on the issues in *General Electric Co. v. Joiner,* a toxic torts case in which the plaintiff, a long-time smoker, alleged that his lung cancer resulted from exposure to polychlorinated biphenyls (PCBs). The judge in *Joiner* had looked at each piece of the scientific evidence individually, found each insufficient by itself, and therefore threw out the whole package.[8]

In the real world, scientists do not operate this way. They consider the strengths and weaknesses of each piece of evidence and base their conclusion on the weight of the evidence. It is entirely possible to draw a sound conclusion despite flaws or limitations in each and every test and study that constitute the evidence for that conclusion. This happens all of the time. In the PCB case, however, the district court judge threw out the plaintiff's evidence and then dismissed the case. An appellate court then ruled that the district court judge had been too restrictive in considering the admissibility of the evidence under *Daubert,* given that the exclusion of evidence would doom the plaintiff's case. The Supreme Court subsequently reversed the appellate court and set up an "abuse of discretion" standard for appellate courts to follow when judging a trial judge's *Daubert* ruling. The unanimous ruling written by Chief Justice Rehnquist stated that the appellate court couldn't simply substitute its own judgment for that of the trial court, but must defer to the lower court unless the original ruling was egregiously incorrect. In almost all instances, therefore, the decision of the single judge at the trial level will be final.[8]

Two years later, the Court issued a third ruling (in what stands now as a trilogy) when it declared in *Kumho Tire Co. v. Carmichael* that the *Daubert* test pertains not only to purely "scientific" testimony but to other types of expert testimony as well, including engineering and clinical medical testimony that relies on experience.[9]

In all, we now have three weighty Supreme Court rulings that specifically address the admissibility of expert testimony. Clearly, the Supreme Court and the legal profession as a whole understand the importance of such testimony for a wide range of litigation, including product liability and toxic tort cases. Commentators have directed a great deal of attention to the motives of the *Daubert* justices. Some of them apparently believed that standardizing admissibility issues would address the problem—or at least the perception of a problem—that expert witnesses may abandon the objectivity they presumably manifest in their professional work and, in the courtroom, become advocates for whomever signs the check (yet another manifestation of the funding effect). Other justices may have heeded the call of the "tort reform" and "junk science" movements, which, as we have seen, are funded by the corporate interests whose actions are one subject of this book. For obvious reasons, product liability and toxic torts litigation has engendered a virulent response from these interests, who would like nothing better than to shut down all such lawsuits. (As corporate defense attorneys will acknowledge, sotto voce, the main thing the corporations really fear these days is a jury.) Two antiregulation advocacy groups, the Atlantic Legal Foundation, which is committed to "redressing the bias against big business which manifests itself in favor of narrow 'consumer' or 'environmental concerns,'" and the Manhattan Institute, home to Peter Huber of *Galileo's Revenge*, have claimed credit for influencing the courts on admissibility questions.[5]

All federal courts, by definition, and more than thirty states now use *Daubert* as their standard.[10] Judges in jurisdictions that still nominally adhere to the *Frye* general acceptance test nevertheless analyze expert testimony in light of *Daubert*. On the basis of a lay judge's ruling, respected scientists have been barred from offering expert testimony, and corporate defendants have become increasingly emboldened to cavalierly accuse any adversary of practicing "junk science." Of course, when the defendant challenges the plaintiff's experts, the plaintiff responds with a *Daubert* motion against the defendant's experts as a matter of litigation tactics. Wittingly or unwittingly, therefore, the Supreme Court has created a social imbalance with far-reaching consequences for both science and justice.

Daubert has had a huge impact on our civil justice system and has been cited in hundreds of law journal articles. For all of its impact, though, this decision has received little attention outside of legal circles. *Daubert* may be the most important judicial ruling you have never heard of.

* * *

Ironically, perhaps, the main dissenting voice in the *Daubert* decision was none other than the late Chief Justice William Rehnquist. (Justice John Paul Stevens joined the chief justice's dissent.) Not doubting for a moment the capabilities of trial judges, Rehnquist nevertheless questioned the wisdom of obligating them to become "amateur scientists."[3] Seven years later, Arizona Supreme Court Chief Justice Stanley Feldman reviewed the passing parade of complicated *Daubert* rulings and wrote that *Daubert*-type tests are "more likely to produce arbitrary results than they are to produce nuanced treatment of complex issues of admissibility."[11]

Both justices are acknowledging one of my major arguments throughout this book: Absolute certainty in science is rarely an option; uncertainty is the norm, not the exception; and scientists base their judgments on the weight of the evidence because in many instances they have no other choice. Uncertainty does *not* mean the science is flawed. Disagreements do *not* mean that one of the parties is wrong or practicing junk science or just shilling for one side or outright lying. The *Daubert* decision provides no philosophical tool to help judges identify "good science," nor could it. There is not just one philosophy of science. No absolute criteria exist for assessing the validity of scientific evidence. Checklists of criteria, while appealing in their convenience, are inadequate tools for assessing many scientific issues, certainly including causation.[12–14]

When it comes to understanding the cause of disease in humans, uncertainties and complexities are a given. As I have discussed, scientists cannot feed toxic chemicals to people to find out what doses cause cancer; instead, we must harness the "natural experiments," in which exposures have already happened. In the laboratory we use animals and control the experimental conditions to learn how toxic agents affect them. Both epidemiologic and laboratory studies are characterized by many uncertainties, and scientists must extrapolate from study-specific evidence to make causal inferences. Rarely can we state that exposure to hypothetical Agent XY *unquestionably caused* the liver cancer in *a specific patient*. What we can say is that individuals who are exposed to Agent XY are statistically more likely to develop liver cancer than those not exposed. However, the epidemiologic studies that support these statements are uncommon and, for most toxic substances, nonexistent. The length and intensity of the exposure are important. The length of time between that exposure and the first onset of symptoms is also important. The presence of possible confounders is important as well. As Jerome Kassirer, former editor of the *New England Journal of Medicine,* and Joe S. Cecil of the Federal Judicial Center wrote in their evaluation of the *Daubert* ruling in the *Journal of the American Medical Association,* "In the final analysis, assessment of evidence and causal inferences depend on accumulating *all* potentially relevant evidence and making a subjective judgment about the strength of the evidence."[15]

In the *Joiner* case, in which the U.S. Supreme Court extended the original *Daubert* ruling, the trial judge had looked at every piece of the science in isolation from the others.[8] The chief justice did the same in the Supreme Court's opinion. One of those studies involved a lab experiment with baby mice. Should they have used adult mice? Under the circumstances, are animal experiments germane at all? The questions led the judge to toss that evidence, but this is not the way scientists operate. Real scientists look at the lab tests, they look at the epidemiology, they consider how similar agents are known to act—all to find the weight of the evidence. In my mind, pulling apart the evidence and judging every piece in isolation (the "corpuscular approach," as it has been dubbed[16]) was egregiously incorrect on the part of the judge. If that's what *Daubert* calls for, then *Daubert* is also egregiously incorrect. To determine whether the relationship between Mr. Joiner's lung cancer and the PCB exposure was causal, we have to look at the whole body of evidence from a scientist's (not a judge's) perspective. That is the real world, where doctors, scientists, and other experts assess the totality of the evidence and give greater or lesser importance to particular parts.

In a later case, the Supreme Court wrote that, "Since *Daubert,* moreover, parties relying on expert evidence have had notice of the exacting standards of reliability such evidence must meet."[17] This sounds excellent, but when judges who are acting as *Daubert* gatekeepers declare that isolated studies or particular experts are not reliable, they are making absolute judgments about the quality of the science, a role for which they are not qualified. It also conflicts with the nature of the scientific enterprise, which necessarily deals with "the weight of the evidence," not the "reliability" of this or that piece of the whole. In the courtroom, experts can use only their expertise to help the court *assign responsibility.* They cannot declare with unanimity what "the truth" is.[18]

The Supreme Court is looking for a magic bullet in a field that has none. If one discordant piece of scientific evidence can be used to fatally taint all the rest in civil litigation, very few juries will ever hear testimony about science in *any* case. The science will have been "*Daubert*ed," as the legal profession colloquially refers to expert testimony that a trial judge rules inadmissible. How many times will esteemed experts put themselves through such an exercise in futility? Not many. The loss will be the law's and ours.

In *Galileo's Revenge,* one of the key documents of the "tort reform" movement, Peter Huber writes, "With or without a philosophically certain demarcation between science and pseudoscience, courts are still going to issue certain judgments. *Judging is the ultimate exercise in positivism* [emphasis in original], a faith in facts strong enough to justify transferring fortunes, ruining reputations, and putting people to death. Anyone who does that for a living has a moral obligation to maintain faith in external, discoverable truth."[19]

Again, this sounds excellent, but actually it is mere sophistry because it implicitly posits a view of both science and the law that is not tenable. Interpreting *Daubert* in its light imposes on science and scientists a standard of absolute assurance and unanimity that is as unreachable in many instances as 9–0 decisions before the Supreme Court. Also note Huber's subtle implication that of course it is the *judge* who should try the facts, whereas our system has historically assigned the fact-finding duty to the *jury*—and for good reason. Both judges and jurors have limitations and biases, but *at least there is more than one juror.* Given the inherently subjective nature of the *Daubert* hearing, how do biases *not* creep into the consideration of the judge if it is a close call? Jurors can employ a deliberative process, pool their collective wisdom, discover, and account for their respective biases and limitations.

But can juries handle complex issues of science? That question is often unspoken but always in the background with *Daubert.* From the earliest days of Anglo-Saxon jurisprudence, juries have been praised by many and scorned by some. The founders of this nation viewed them as a bulwark against executive power—thus the Seventh Amendment—but in an era in which everyone assumed that the fastest a human being could ever travel would be astride a galloping horse, how could they have had any idea of today's science and technology? What would they say about juries today? Justice Blackmun addresses the question in the *Daubert* ruling. Replying to the concern of the defendant (Merrell Dow Pharmaceuticals) about a "'free-for-all' in which befuddled juries are confounded by absurd and irrational pseudoscientific absurdities," Blackmun defended "the capabilities of the jury and the adversary system generally. Vigorous cross-examination, presentation of contrary evidence, and careful instruction on the burden of proof are the traditional and appropriate means of attacking shaky but admissible evidence.... [T]he court remains free to direct a judgment... and likewise to grant summary judgment."[3]

On the other hand, Neil Vidmar, a social scientist at Duke Law School, has suggested that a 1999 appellate ruling may more tellingly express the implicit reasoning behind a great deal of subsequent *Daubert* interpretation.[20] In this decision, the court wrote that "While meticulous *Daubert* inquiries may bring judges under criticism for donning white coats and making determinations that are outside their field of expertise, the Supreme Court has obviously deemed this less objectionable than dumping a barrage of questionable scientific evidence on a jury, who would likely be even less equipped than the judge to make reliability and relevance determinations and more likely than the judge to be awestruck by the expert's mystique."[21]

As it turns out, Professor Vidmar can testify as an expert on this matter of jury competence, and he has. I quote only part of the conclusion to one of his papers on the subject: "Claims about jury incompetence, irresponsibility, and bias in responding to expert evidence [are] not consistent with a review of the many studies that have examined these issues from various methodological perspectives. . . . Critics . . . have relied exclusively on anecdote and appeals to 'common sense' rather than on systematically collected data."[20] Richard O. Lempert, a professor of law at the University of Michigan, reached a similar conclusion: "[T]he weight of the evidence indicates that juries can reach rationally defensible verdicts in complex cases, that we cannot assume that judges in complex cases will perform better than juries, and that there are changes that can be made to enhance jury performance." [22]

Brooklyn law professor Margaret Berger believes *Daubert* also raises constitutional questions. In an interview she stated the following:

> I think the Seventh Amendment could be read as not just entitling a litigant to a jury verdict, but more broadly to a jury trial when experts in different disciplines disagree. . . . Even if a plaintiff's verdict were ultimately set aside as not based on sufficient evidence of causation, a public trial means the plaintiff gets to tell his or her story and it also means that wrongdoing on the part of defendants can be exposed. Even when causation cannot be proved, that does not necessarily mean that defendants did not act in a reprehensible manner in exposing the public to risk. For example, problems often develop with drugs long after they have been approved for market. Jury trials could reveal whether corporations knowingly kept drugs or products on the market after it became clear that problems existed. If such a case ends with a *Daubert* hearing, none of this will ever become public.[23]

I concur. Moreover, the right to trial by jury under the U.S. Constitution would seem to permit the jury to consider responsible minority views within a discipline. Otherwise, why have a jury?

* * *

Scattered throughout the Court's *Daubert* trilogy are statements that appear to warn trial judges against adopting a rigid, inflexible approach to the new test. In *Kumho,* the court wrote that certain factors "do not all necessarily apply in every instance in which the reliability of scientific testimony is challenged."[9] In practice, however, many courts are adopting something close to a rigid "checklist" approach. What are these judges relying on as they judge the science? Their own experience? Common sense? Ideology?

Daubert has indirectly encouraged judges to evaluate elements of scientific evidence individually (the corpuscular approach mentioned earlier, so named by University of Texas law professor Tom McGarity).[16] This procedure ignores not only the fact that this is not how scientists search for the weight of the evidence but also the fact that many of the studies before the courts were *not conducted with the courts in mind.* It is absolutely mandatory to draw conclusions from a synthesis of these studies rather than look at each one individually.

Some judges have arbitrarily rejected scientific opinions about cancer causation based on animal studies because they simply do not accept the validity of such studies when extrapolated to human injury. These judges believe only in epidemiological studies; therefore, the animal studies, no matter how reliable under *Daubert,* fail the "relevant" standard. For many chemicals, animal studies provide virtually everything we know about their toxicity. These judges' attitude makes no scientific sense whatsoever. The entire science community could accept the methods and results of a given methodology—the criterion under the old *Frye* test—but that evidence could still be deemed unreliable by a given judge. This actually happened with a judge who refused to accept an exposure model that estimated the plaintiff's exposure to benzene simply because the judge did not think the methodology was valid and even though such modeling is standard practice in the field.[24] (Epidemiologists who work on exposure analyses often lack all of the solid data that would be desired in a perfect world, so they construct exposure models, which necessarily rely on assumptions. Disputes over the assumptions are common. One reason for the often insufficient data on employee exposures is that the employers have not gathered them. As we have seen in these pages, time after time corporations claim a "lack of evidence" as a reason for inaction, when in fact *they* are responsible for that lack of evidence.) Judges should certainly discard manifestly weak science, but should they arbitrarily reject "state of the art" science (implicitly substituting their own view of the science) and then hide behind *Daubert?* Or should a larger group of serious-minded individuals—juries—make these decisions?

I have mentioned the *Daubert II* addition to the *Daubert* checklist, which suggests that any scientific study conducted for the purposes of a trial is inherently suspect. We all know about the hired gun, a term with justifiably bad connotations. Some unethical plaintiff attorneys have their own unethical hired guns, as evidenced by the scandals in which medical experts diagnosed workers with both silicosis and asbestosis in order to be double compensated from two sets of defendants.[25,26] However, the hired gun *could be* right on target and *should be* considered along with the rest of the evidence. Besides, very little is known about the toxicity of the hundred thousand chemicals (including derivatives) that are registered for use in industry and commerce in the United States. Toxicity data are incomplete and cannot be found in the public record for the vast majority of the most commonly used chemicals.[27] According to the logic of *Daubert II*, scientific ignorance guarantees legal bliss for corporations. This is not right. This is not justice.

In the Bendectin cases that led to the original *Daubert* ruling, the defense made much of the fact that little if any of the science the plaintiffs submitted had been peer-reviewed. Well, how could it have been? Before the health problems cropped up, there had been no reason to study Bendectin. As it happens, no award has ever been paid to a Bendectin plaintiff, pre- or post-*Daubert*. So while the weight of the evidence may not have supported that litigation, do not throw out new studies simply because they have not met a standard they could never meet, almost by definition.

Meanwhile, corporations often conduct studies for litigation purposes, as internal documents that surface through legal discovery prove time and again. By and large, however, industry-commissioned studies are not painted with the brush of suspicion because they are not initially linked to any one specific case. In fact, they were probably conducted years before the case in which they are presented as evidence—sound product-defense behavior on the part of corporations that expect to be sued because they know they have some self-inflicted liability. Cases in point are the myriad of benzene analyses and reanalyses funded by the petroleum industry (described in chapter six).

Among the worst of all *Daubert* repercussions is the judges' misunderstanding of hypothesis testing and error rates, two of the *Daubert* checklist items. This was the conclusion of a recent survey of four hundred state court judges.[28] Many judges do not realize that the epidemiological studies so many seem to prefer over animal studies (because they relate directly to human beings) will be impossible to provide in the instance of a rare disease or with a product that has been taken off the market. Many fail to understand that epidemiological studies are intentionally skewed toward *rejecting* a given hypothesis, so testimony that a study failed to prove a hypothesis is not at all to say that the hypothesis is therefore disproved.

Some courts set the bar impossibly high. In *Nelson v. American Home Products Corp.*, a man who was prescribed the drug Cordarone to control ventricular arrhythmia following a heart attack began losing sight in one eye soon thereafter.[29] The plaintiff brought together six expert witnesses, including a professor of neuro-ophthalmology at the University of California–San Francisco who had diagnosed three similar cases of Cordarone-induced optic neuropathy. No matter. The judge excluded all of the plaintiff's scientific testimony and granted summary judgment in favor of American Home Products because most of the evidence was clinical evidence and case studies, not epidemiological studies. The judge declared that case reports "do not demonstrate a causal link sufficient for admission to a finder of fact in court," are not subject to peer review, and "do not advance testable scientific analysis."[29]

That statement recalls Chief Justice Rehnquist's warning in his *Daubert* dissent about judges playing scientist.[3] Regarding case reports (which, in fact, are often subjected to peer review), I would like to cite Doctors Kassirer and Cecil in their 2002 *JAMA* article: "In clinical medicine, a biologically plausible relationship, physiological studies of a drug, animal studies, or even a handful of case reports can be useful in individual cases in helping a practitioner make judgments about cause and effect relationships."[15] But should a jury be barred from hearing this testimony? Yes, according to many *Daubert* rulings.

Finally, in this brief consideration of how judges can get lost in the thickets in their attempts to comply with *Daubert*, I discuss a group of cases involving Parlodel, a drug used to stop postpartum lactation. On the basis of case reports and animal studies and the undisputed fact that Parlodel can cause a rapid rise in blood pressure in humans, the Food and Drug Administration requested in 1985 that the drug's manufacturer, Sandoz Pharmaceutical Corporation, include warnings about hypertension, seizure, and stroke on the label. It did so, but the drug remained on the market until 1994, when the FDA decided enough was enough—the reports of problems were coming in at a steady clip—and requested that Sandoz stop sales.[30]

When women sued the company, claiming that Parlodel was responsible for their strokes, seizures, and other adverse health effects, their cases were dismissed by several judges who refused to allow jurors to consider the testimony of scientists or physicians who *agreed with the FDA* that, on the basis of case reports, animal studies, and the way the drug works in the body, Parlodel could cause circulatory disorders. One of the experts was a member of the FDA's advisory committee on fertility and maternal health and had reviewed the safety of Parlodel for the government, but he was not good enough for these judges. They indicated they were looking for epidemiological studies, of which there were none either supporting or disputing the women's contention. The judges demanded a level of certainty that was virtually impossible to provide, a level of certainty far more stringent than the "preponderance of the evidence" standard in civil litigation.[15]

Then there was the judge in Alabama who thought the jury *should* hear the disputed facts about Parlodel. "It is not part of the trial judge's gatekeeping role to determine whether the proffered opinion is scientifically *correct* or *certain* in the way one might think of the law of gravity," [emphasis in original] this *Daubert* ruling reads. "[I]t is the role of the factfinder (usually a jury) to determine whether the opinion is correct or worthy of credence. For the trial court to overreach in the gatekeeping function and determine whether the opinion evidence is correct or worthy of credence is to usurp the jury's right to decide the facts of the case. All the trial judge is asked to decide is whether the proffered evidence is based on 'good grounds' tied to the scientific method."[31]

Yet another judge in a Parlodel case decided to enlist the help of a panel of independent experts. For a court to hire "impartial" authorities to judge the litigants' experts sounds like a plausible solution to the whole problem, but what happens when the impartial scientists disagree among themselves? This would often happen because the judgment of an impartial expert is no more likely to represent a scientific consensus than that of any other specialist since that consensus often does not exist. Thus it turned out in this instance, in which the judge selected three prominent scientists from different disciplines (epidemiology, clinical pharmacology, and neurology) and asked them to determine whether the plaintiff's medical experts used scientifically reliable methodologies to form their opinions about causality and to decide whether the techniques could be applied to the facts of the case. None of the three had had any relationship with plaintiffs or defendant, and they worked independently.[32]

Each report to the judge was sound, well reasoned, and effectively represented the scientific worldview of one particular expertise. Each was indubitably legitimate. They were also markedly discordant. The epidemiologist opined that the experts' testimony was not reliable because it did not include evidence from human studies (the work of epidemiologists); the clinical pharmacologist concluded that the experts' opinions were scientifically reliable because they were based on a "totality of the evidence" (clinical pharmacologists draw inferences from clinical studies and animal evidence); and the neurologist said that epidemiological evidence was not absolutely necessary, but other weaknesses in the expert's methodology made the evidence unreliable. The judge responded to the disagreement not by letting the jurors sort out the conflict—their traditional role in our system of justice—but by granting the defendant's motion for summary judgment on the ground that the plaintiff had no valid, admissible evidence.[32]

In the Parlodel cases, judges in different jurisdictions looked at similar evidence in similar cases and came to very different conclusions, just like the scientists. The court's challenge is not—and cannot be—determining "the truth" because it may not be known or even knowable. "The grand question for the law," writes Sheila Jasaonff, professor of science and technology studies at the John F. Kennedy School of Government at Harvard University, "is not how judges can best do justice to science; the more critical concern is how courts can better render justice under conditions of endemic uncertainty and ignorance."[33]

* * *

From the beginning, observers disagreed on whether *Daubert* was a victory for plaintiffs, generally speaking, or for defendants. A dozen years later, the verdict is clear: Defendants are the main beneficiaries. For the most part, big defendants have the money, and money talks in the courtroom, too. Expert testimony and *Daubert* hearings are expensive. Defendants, particularly corporations with the resources to hire teams of lawyers and scientific experts, can use the hearing or the mere threat of one to make it much more difficult for plaintiffs and their attorneys to bring or pursue a case in the first place. Long before *Daubert,* the tobacco industry had used its rather extensive resources to challenge the testimony of plaintiffs' expert witnesses, thereby driving up the costs to the attorneys. An attorney for R. J. Reynolds gloated after a particularly sweet victory: "The aggressive posture we have taken regarding depositions and discovery in general continues to make these cases extremely burdensome and expensive for plaintiffs' lawyers, particularly sole practitioners. To paraphrase General Patton, the way we won these cases was not by spending all of [RJR's] money, but by making that other son of a bitch spend all of his."[34]

I don't doubt that *Daubert* has discouraged plaintiffs with scientifically questionable claims from pursuing their claims in court, but neither do I doubt that other plaintiffs with strong claims but insufficient resources have also been prevented from having their day in court.[35] A Rand Institute study that found that judges are in fact using *Daubert* also reported that, following a spike immediately after the decision was issued, the rate of exclusion of testimony has decreased.[36] Perhaps bad cases are not being pursued, or maybe only the best, most powerful and ironclad cases are moving forward. What is the risk for an industry to leave a dangerous product on the market and take its chances in the court system, now that those chances are so much better? Could *Daubert* have an impact on corporate decision making in such cases? Of course it could.

* * *

Emboldened by their success with *Daubert* in civil litigation, industry and its coterie of trade groups and other fronting organizations now want to set up a system of *Daubert*-like hearings for the federal regulatory agencies, with the expectation that like-minded arbiters will exclude any unwanted science from the government's purview entirely. They also urge that courts that hear

174 DOUBT IS THEIR PRODUCT

appeals by regulated corporations use the stringent *Daubert* approach to judge the regulatory agency's use of science.

The push is on. At a hearing addressing OSHA's process for establishing workplace health and safety standards, a partner in the law firm Jones Day (R. J. Reynolds's firm, as noted) recommended incorporating *Daubert* into OSHA's standard setting since it "has been used successfully by the federal courts in evaluating scientific evidence for years, and provides a useful model for determining whether or not scientific evidence is, at bottom, 'reliable.'"[37] When the U.S. Chamber of Commerce adopted its official position on scientific information in federal rulemaking in 2002, *Daubert* was likewise prominently featured: "[We] believe that the same high standards of relevance and reliability that safeguard the rights of litigants in federal courts should also safeguard the public in the regulatory process. Regulations affecting business and the public should be based on scientific, not political, foundations. . . . The U.S. Chamber, therefore, advocates the adoption of an Executive Order requiring that federal agencies apply the *Daubert* standards in the administrative rule making process."[38]

Clearly, these corporate lobbyists are urging the narrowest and strictest interpretation of *Daubert*—that is, the one most divorced from the real world of science, the one most likely to lead to arbitrary exclusion of scientific evidence that any regulatory agency should consider. Judges in the courtroom often ignore or misunderstand the nuances of the Supreme Court's decision. Likewise, the legal, economic, and political obstacles that regulators already face will seem trivial compared to what they will face if *Daubert*-like criteria are applied to each piece of scientific evidence used to support a regulation.

This would be a terrible development because the rigid *Daubert* approach, methodologically questionable in civil liability cases, runs directly counter to the *precautionary* policies built into most health, safety, and environmental statutes.[39,40] When scientists evaluate scientific evidence in regulatory agencies, consensus committees, or even on the witness stand, they commonly apply a weight of the evidence approach in which *all* scientific evidence that is relevant to a causal hypothesis is taken into account. *Daubert*'s implicit demand for scientific certainty runs counter not only to the workings of science but also to the basic principle that policy decisions should be made with the best available evidence and must not wait until every piece of evidence is in and every doubt is erased.

Proponents of public health protections, especially those advanced in the face of scientific uncertainty, should be wary of calls to extend *Daubert* to the regulatory arena. Opponents of regulation have deceptively proposed the application of *Daubert* in regulatory proceedings as a plea for "sound science." In reality, these "sound science" reforms "sound like science" but have little to do with the way science and scientists work. They are simply one more tactic to delay or halt the imposition of requirements to protect the public's health and the environment.[41,42]

* * *

In the years since I since I left the government in January 2001, I have provided expert testimony in a handful of cases. In one of these my testimony was challenged under *Daubert,* providing me with personal experience in the issues I discuss here. The case involved a worker in a plastics plant who was exposed to vinyl chloride and had eventually developed brain cancer. The attorney for the worker's widow asked me to testify about the studies on vinyl chloride that had been conducted before and during the time that exposure occurred and about whether the manufacturers provided adequate warnings to purchasers of vinyl chloride so that workers could be protected from exposure to this carcinogen. As the chief safety officer for all U.S. nuclear weapons facilities and national laboratories, where workers use some of the most hazardous substances known, I felt fully qualified to testify. Before joining the federal government I designed, ran, and evaluated health and safety training programs for numerous employers and unions. Even so, the manufacturers challenged my expertise on the grounds that I am not a toxicologist and therefore am unqualified to interpret to the jury the results of an animal study. (As an epidemiologist, I would be qualified to talk only about human studies. Following this logic, only someone trained in epidemiology *and* toxicology *and* clinical medicine could make statements based on a literature that contained all three types of studies. Unfortunately, few if any people have all three degrees, while most of the literature on chemical hazards includes all three types of studies.)

My *Daubert* hearing in Trenton, New Jersey, was a day-long affair. I was questioned first by the attorney who hired me, then by an attorney for the manufacturers—each for more than two hours. Three other attorneys hired by the manufacturers attended the hearing. They did not ask questions, but I am sure they billed their client—at several hundred dollars for each hour they sat there, plus travel costs. The hearing must have cost the defendants many tens of thousands of dollars. In this case, they did not succeed. Moments after the defense attorneys completed their cross-examination, the judge rejected the *Daubert* challenge and ruled that, as a scientist, I was capable of reading studies outside my immediate discipline and was qualified to testify about warnings. (The jury found for the widow.)

These *Daubert* hurdles were unnecessary. While *Daubert* may have chased out some lawsuits based on questionable science, it serves to erect hurdles for scientific testimony and do not reflect the way science works, hurdles that may unduly protect wealthy and powerful defendants.

14

The Institutionalization of Uncertainty

Four lines of text, no more, but the brief proviso attached by Senator Richard Shelby, Republican senator from Alabama, to the 920-page omnibus appropriation bill for fiscal year 1999 turned out to be the opening salvo in a series of legislative and agency initiatives that their corporate sponsors hope will tip the balance of power in the regulatory process in their favor, once and for all.[1] The idea is to *institutionalize* the strategies I have been writing about—to construct bureaucratic mechanisms with which corporate interests can question the science underlying not just regulation but virtually any "information" disseminated by federal agencies as well. This would be the very triumph of uncertainty.

This legislation, the Data Access Act (also known as the Shelby Amendment), guarantees public access, by way of the Freedom of Information Act (FOIA), to "all data produced" by federally funded research scientists employed by nonprofit institutions.[1] Now, if any federal funds supported a scientist's study, that person is required to provide the raw research data in response to a request under the Freedom of Information Act. (This does not apply to studies paid for by corporations; we will return to that later.) According to all accounts at the time, the motive behind the action was the displeasure of corporations most responsible for air pollution, including the oil industry, diesel engine manufacturers, and coal-burning power companies, that they did not have access to the raw data at the heart of the "Six Cities Study,"[2] the massive, long-term epidemiological study by a Harvard-based research team subsequently used by the EPA as one basis for a proposed strengthening of clean air regulations.[3] For these industries, the study was dangerous; from its conclusions, the EPA has extrapolated that Americans annually suffer as many forty thousand deaths (and thousands of episodes of disease) as a result of exposure to air pollutants.[4]

The Shelby Amendment was an open invitation for *anyone* to use the Freedom of Information Act to harass scientists, question their work, muddy the waters, delay action, and perhaps even steal intellectual property. You might think that industry would be alarmed by this last threat, but industry made certain that *privately funded* research is not covered. That is, according to the logic of this legislation, industry should be free to dredge and manipulate the data of government-funded work, but federal agencies and outside groups should not be free to reanalyze industry-sponsored research submitted to the agencies during the regulatory process. Right there you have the tip-off to the hidden agenda of the Shelby Amendment.

It also should not come as a complete surprise that recent research using the documents discovered through tobacco litigation found that the true creators of the Data Access Act were *not* the coal burning electric utilities but—who else?—the cigarette manufacturers, who had realized years earlier that reanalyzing a study's raw data to change its conclusion was a particularly effective way to neutralize it. In the 1980s the tobacco companies were dragged into suits filed by asbestos-exposed workers who had developed lung cancer. The research of Dr. Irving Selikoff had shown that the combination of smoking and asbestos was a far more potent cause of lung cancer than either one alone. The asbestos industry's epidemiologists developed models that placed more blame on tobacco, and the cigarette makers had no data with which to form the basis of a counterattack. Since these studies were evidence in the lawsuits, the cigarette manufacturers subpoenaed Dr. Selikoff's raw data, with which the industry's consultants were then able to construct impressive, although dishonest, models that exonerated tobacco. As I have documented in chapter seven, when the first secondhand smoke studies were published, Big Tobacco attempted to use the same strategy but was stymied since the epidemiologists, knowing what would happen to their raw data in the reanalysis, would not give it up. In response, Philip Morris launched the "Sound Science Project," one of whose objectives was to "gain passage of federal law on criteria/standards for epidemiological studies" and "legislate public access to epidemiological data used in support of federal laws and regulations."[5] Another document adds that "our plans must emphasize all ways to develop the right criteria that will favorably evaluate and be applicable to ETS."[6] Philip Morris also recognized that its likelihood of success would be greater if its fingerprints were never seen on the data access legislation, and it appears that the power companies that were concerned about restrictions on particulates released into the atmosphere were more than willing to help.[7]

* * *

The Data Access Act was not a complete victory for industry. After receiving thousands of comments and complaints from scientists, research institutions, and public policy experts, the Clinton-era Office of Management and Budget (OMB) interpreted the famous four lines rather narrowly, "limiting requested data to published or cited research used by the federal government in developing legally binding agency actions."[8] As a result, the Data Access Act has not had the dire results first feared.

It was just an opening salvo, however, in the "sound science" campaign. The following year the tobacco industry (still behind the scenes) and its allies brought out the heavier artillery, now labeled the Information Quality Act but more widely known by the acronym of its first moniker, the Data Quality Act.[9] By any name, the DQA is a wonderful new weapon in the arsenal of all those who oppose public health and workplace regulations, as well as independent, serious science. All of two paragraphs long, its import makes the Data Access Act's four lines seem like a child's popgun.

The DQA authorized the Office of Management and Budget to develop guidelines for "ensuring and maximizing the quality, objectivity, utility, and integrity of information" and to establish procedures that allow formal challenges to information disseminated by federal agencies. (The term "information" is not defined in the act, although two parentheticals indicate that "statistical information" is subject to the law.) "Affected persons" are granted the right to challenge and request a correction of information disseminated by a federal agency that is not in compliance with those guidelines.[9]

At first, all of this sounds harmless, even beneficial. Who does not want to ensure the quality and integrity of government-disseminated information? As Dr. John Graham, former administrator of the Office of Information and Regulatory Affairs within OMB under the second Bush administration, has said, "[R]elease of governmental information that has important impacts on the private sector, is in itself in some ways, a form of regulation."[10] This viewpoint is sometimes called "regulation by information" or "regulation by publication," and it is not a trivial point. Information drives individual behavior; hence, the Food and Drug Administration's requirements for warning labels on drugs and the Securities and Exchange Commission's rules on corporate financial disclosure. Information is incredibly powerful. Of course we want "scientific due process." However, the devious conception of the DQA suggests that its creators' intentions might be devious as well.

The DQA sneaked through Congress and the White House as a rider in Section 515 of the 712-page Treasury and General Government Appropriations Act for Fiscal Year 2000, sandwiched between one provision to transfer ownership of land for the Gerald Ford Museum in Grand Rapids, Michigan, and another to settle litigation on cost-of-living allowances in nonforeign areas. There were no hearings; there was no debate; and there was no legislative history to help the courts or anyone else clarify Congress's intentions in passing the law. Representative Jo Ann Emerson, Republican from Missouri, did the deed, and she later confirmed that she acted at the request of Jim Tozzi, previously introduced as the former high-level Reagan-era White House Office of Management and Budget (OMB) official who now operates the Center for Regulatory Effectiveness (CRE), a for-profit policy shop for polluters and manufacturers of dangerous products. Since Tozzi is a veteran consultant for Big Tobacco, we should not be surprised to learn that Philip Morris was a driving force behind the DQA, one of several successes of the cigarette manufacturer's "Sound Science Project."[7]

For Philip Morris, it is all about secondhand smoke; for other industries, it is all about smoke and mirrors. Before joining the Bush administration, Dr. Graham of OMB had been director of the Harvard Center for Risk Analysis, where he was a fierce proponent of cost-benefit analyses and often produced studies that demonstrated that the costs of regulations outweighed their benefits. His nomination to his new post in Washington, D.C., was opposed by many public-interest and environmental groups, who feared he would attempt to dismantle the environmental regulatory system. Their fears were well justified. For his part, Tozzi proudly boasts about the convergence of the Data Quality Act and the "junk science" movement. From his perspective, the law would "simply stop the 'junk science' that can lead to useless and expensive regulations."[11]

"Useless and expensive" regulations? Make no mistake about it: The unstated idea here is to stop virtually *all* regulatory science and therefore virtually *all* regulation. The formal regulatory system has numerous checks and balances, and, as we have seen, regulated parties have developed over the decades an impressive array of strategies to take advantage of all of them. Their goal has always been to stall and, they hope, to stop agencies' attempts to actually issue regulations that protect the environment and public health. The DQA now gives them an official means with which to kill or alter government documents that serve as the scientific basis for action. It provides a means of challenging the supporting science "upstream"—that is, in the earliest stages of the regulatory process.[12]

We have seen how easy it is to launch an uncertainty campaign—all you really need is a lot of money—even when *the whole world* knows the truth

(I am thinking of tobacco, specifically). We have seen how easy it is for such a transparently disingenuous campaign to nevertheless buy a lot of time because, as I have said, the formal regulatory system has many checks and balances. It takes no great imagination to understand how industry can use the DQA to challenge in piecemeal fashion the quality of individual scientific studies. Their aim is to discredit and dismantle the body of evidence that an agency reviews in considering action and regulation. Jim Tozzi is right. The potential for mischief posed by the DQA is practically unlimited. For industry, it is a boon beyond calculation. William Kovacs, a vice president for the U.S. Chamber of Commerce, has predicted that the OMB's good work "will have the most profound impact on federal regulations since the Administrative Procedure Act was enacted in 1946 . . . by ensuring that [the EPA] uses better science, and *by giving industry additional grounds to sue*"[13] (my emphasis).

* * *

Passed by Congress during the Clinton administration, the Data Quality Act went into effect on October 1, 2002, during the first term of the second Bush administration. According to the advocacy group OMB Watch, ninety-eight DQA petitions were filed for fiscal year 2003, the large majority by industry. As we would expect, the industry applications are the complicated ones, those with a clear agenda. For example, on November 25, 2002, fewer than sixty days after the act went into effect, Tozzi's CRE used the DQA on behalf of a coalition of trade associations representing crop growers that rely on herbicides to challenge the EPA's dissemination of a scientific study of atrazine.[14] This research by Dr. Tyrone Hayes, professor of integrative biology at the University of California–Berkeley, concluded that atrazine, one of the most widely used weed killers, causes endocrine-disrupting effects in frogs that result in sexual abnormalities.[15] The agency cited the study in its consideration of whether to reregister the pesticide for use in this country, but the DQA petition claimed that the Hayes study violated the act's "objectivity" standard. Since the EPA had not yet established validated protocols for testing the endocrine effects of chemicals, the herbicide users argued that the study could not be considered reliable and reproducible. Therefore, the agency should change the statement that "atrazine causes endocrine effects in various organisms including frogs" to "there is no reliable evidence that atrazine causes 'endocrine effects' in the environment" and "there can be no reliable, accurate or useful information regarding atrazine's endocrine effects until and unless there are test methods for those effects that have been properly validated."[14] The EPA denied the herbicide lobby's request and asserted that using the Hayes study was appropriate and consistent with the data quality guidelines and that it was inappropriate to amend the report as suggested.[16]

In June 2002 the Competitive Enterprise Institute (CEI) filed a petition with several federal agencies to stop dissemination of the *National Assessment on Climate Change*[17] on the grounds that the assessment was based on faulty computer models and did not undergo proper peer review.[18] In fact, the National Academy of Sciences characterized these exact climate change models as "well-regarded,"[19] and they had been peer-reviewed by more than three hundred scientific and technical experts. When the White House embraced the CEI's position and posted a statement that the *National Assessment on Climate Change* had not been subjected to their Data Quality Act guidelines, the CEI claimed victory and withdrew the lawsuit, saving the administration from having to defend the report in court.[20]

In August 2003 the law firm of Morgan Lewis, working for clients unknown, filed a DQA petition with the EPA[21] that challenged the 1986 publication titled "Guidance for Preventing Asbestos Disease among Auto Mechanics."[22] This pamphlet, known as the Gold Book, is essentially a manual to help auto mechanics work safely around asbestos. (Because many automotive brake shoes contain asbestos, mechanics are at risk of exposure.) The firm claimed that the Gold Book failed to comply with the data quality standards of "objectivity" and "utility" because (1) it relies on inadequate and inappropriate data; (2) it is outdated (contradictory studies have since been published); and (3) verification of its origins, preparations, funding, review, and approval is unknown or not possible. In addition, the challenge stated that the more rigorous standard for "influential information" applies to the Gold Book since its scope and intended effect are to change the work-behavior practices of an entire industry; it relied on information derived from scientific sources; and it is routinely proffered during litigation as evidence of the EPA's current thinking on whether asbestos-containing friction products are dangerous to users.[21] This is really what the challenge was about: Plaintiffs' attorneys were using the Gold Book in court cases, and defendants wanted the book pulled.

In response, the EPA removed the booklet from its website and promised that a new brochure would be available in spring 2004.[23] It was spring 2007 when the agency finally released the revised if severely shrunken booklet. It still contained useful information, albeit with much less detail.[24]

The product defense industry has played an important supporting role in this saga.[25] Scientists at Exponent, Inc. and ChemRisk have flooded the scientific literature with analyses that conclude that auto mechanics who repair asbestos brake shoes are not exposed to much asbestos and when they are, the asbestos has been transformed into non-toxic material.[26-31] These studies do not come cheaply; between 2001 and April 2006 these two firms alone billed approximately $23 million to General Motors, Ford, and

Chrysler for their work.[32] While there is no mention of Exponent in the DQA challenge documents, the firm billed $29,000 to the big three automakers (they were splitting the costs equally) for the task labeled "Prepare Materials to Challenge 1986 EPA."[33,34] Once the revised booklet was put out for comments, two more Exponent scientists wrote to EPA complaining that, since their studies found asbestos in brake shoes to be innocuous, the brochure should be modified to "avoid introducing unnecessary concerns among current and former automotive mechanics."[35] Did the automakers also pay for these comments? We do not know; the letter to the EPA makes no mention of the financial relationship between Exponent, Inc. and auto manufacturers.

Industry representatives have challenged data from several different government agencies, and some of those agencies have stood their ground, whereas others have capitulated. In May 2003 the Salt Institute and the U.S. Chamber of Commerce jointly filed a DQA petition with the National Institute of Health's National Heart, Lung, and Blood Institute that claimed that the NIH's statement that reduced salt intake lowers blood pressure violates the DQA's standards for "objectivity," "reproducibility," and "transparency" (the higher standards applied to "influential information"). The petition sought "correction of information . . . which directly states and otherwise suggests that reduced sodium consumption will result in lower blood pressure in *all* individuals" (emphasis in original). Because these statements cannot be reproduced based on publicly-released study data, the statements are not in compliance with the Data Quality Act."[36] The petition also sought to require the Heart, Lung, and Blood Institute to make public the data from the Dietary Approaches to Stop Hypertension (DASH) clinical trial.[37] The NIH denied the request and stated that, since the petition's objective was to gain access to the DASH-Sodium study, the petitioners should pursue their request through the Freedom of Information Act.[38] After their appeal was also denied, the petitioners filed a lawsuit in which the decision not only denied the plaintiffs' claims but also ruled that the DQA is not judicially reviewable.[39–42]

The Consumer Product Safety Commission denied a challenge from the Association of Home Appliance Manufacturers to its *Final Report on Electric Clothes Dryers and Lint Ignition Characteristics*.[43,44] When the Chemical Products Corporation petitioned the EPA to replace its Integrated Risk Assessment System for barium with the industry's substitute, the EPA initially denied the request, then changed its collective mind, acknowledged the need for further consideration, and sought the industry's input.[45–47]

Enough! What toxicology experiment could *not* be challenged with a DQA petition? What epidemiological study? What analysis or report of any kind? The act is not a tool to improve the "quality sieve" that federal agencies employ. It is a strategy for raising ever more uncertainty about science in order to delay its use in decision making or to limit public awareness of an issue. In the atrazine example, the Hayes study of the endocrinology in frogs was critical to the body of scientific evidence that demonstrated that the chemical poses significant risks to the environment and public health. If the petitioners could diminish the weight of the evidence against atrazine, they would be more likely to fend off a ban or severe restriction of the pesticide. In both the salt intake guidelines and the asbestos Gold Book examples, claims against the quality of the science used in educational materials were attempts to halt their dissemination, thereby censoring the agency on the issue.

As we would expect, a lively debate has taken place within the public interest and environmental movements, as well as within the scientific community, about how to respond to the DQA. A few of these groups have filed their own petitions for correction. For the most part, however, they have heeded the advice of Tom McGarity, Rena Steinzor, and the other legal scholars associated with the Center for Progressive Reform (CPR) to acknowledge that the DQA is simply bad policy that should be repealed. McGarity, Steinzor, and I met with Dr. Graham in October 2003 and warned him that, unless the administration started to actively discourage its corporate allies from filing DQA challenges, opponents of the process would be forced to respond in kind and challenge other vulnerable government documents built on much shakier scientific foundations. We raised the specter of DQA challenges to the technical reports supporting the construction of the Yucca Mountain radioactive waste depository or the famously incompetent missile defense initiative whose interceptor missiles fail more often than they succeed. For the most part, public interest groups have held their fire; even though they may oppose these policies on other grounds, they have refrained from mounting challenges based on this ill-conceived legislation.

* * *

As good as the DQA is for using alleged uncertainty about information to jam up the works, imagine how much better it would be if industry could control information *before* it becomes an official document of the government—veto that information, in effect.

To gain this heretofore undreamed of holy grail, OMB rolled out the ultimate weapon in August 2003, a new proposal titled "Peer Review and Information Quality" which the White House claimed was authorized by that same appropriations rider as the DQA. Under this new proposal, information disseminated by the federal government (reports, websites, and even many letters and public statements) would have to undergo some form of peer review before public release. Any information that affected major regulation or that could have a "substantial impact" on public policies or private sector decisions with a possible impact of more than $100 million annually would be put through a cumbersome system in which the information would be reviewed by "experts" independent of the agency. In a step that would slow the process further, the information would first have to be published in draft form and disseminated for public comment, after which it would be sent to a peer-review panel, along with the public comments. The agency would then issue a formal response to the peer reviewers' comments before the information could be redisseminated. In contrast to the Supreme Court's decision in *Daubert*, which suggested peer review as one criterion for reliability but not a "definitive test," as I have discussed, OMB's peer-review guidelines would be compulsory.[48]

Peer review, or independent review by experts, is a pillar of modern science, a phenomenally complex enterprise in which scientists are constantly evaluating and building upon each other's work. It is invoked in at least two aspects of the process, the editorial prepublication assessment of manuscripts submitted to scientific journals (often called "refereeing") and in the decision-making processes of agencies and institutions that provide financial support for scientific research. There is significant competition for both limited journal space and scarce research funds, and peer review plays a pivotal role in the allocation of these highly valued resources.

Many federal agencies already have peer-review mechanisms for the studies and reports they produce internally or commission from outside experts. To understand the context in which OMB made its "Peer Review and Information Quality" proposal, it is instructive to look at the EPA, whose regulatory needs require research involving an extraordinarily wide range of science and technology disciplines. The agency is charged with developing environmental safeguards in areas in which there is much uncertainty and disagreement; thus, it often relies on complex mathematical models that may predict risk, exposure, emissions, and costs. The variables involved in the design and use of these models are frequently the subjects of great debate, and Congress responded to these concerns in 1978 by authorizing the EPA's Science Advisory Board, a panel of independent scientists, and charging it with "[r]eviewing the quality and relevance of the scientific and technical information being used or proposed as the basis for Agency regulations."[49]

In addition to the ongoing work of this board, both the EPA and the National Academy of Sciences have convened groups of experts to evaluate the quality of science at the agency. Since the first Bush administration, EPA policy requires that that major scientific and technical work products related to agency decisions be peer-reviewed, with independent or external peer review required for those documents that support the most important decisions. In 1992 the agency appointed a committee of independent scientists who issued a report titled "Safeguarding the Future: Credible Science, Credible Decisions."[50] In 1998 Carol Browner, EPA administrator in the Clinton administration, issued a detailed handbook to ensure uniform implementation of the peer-review policy.[51] This policy, revised and reissued in 2000, has been endorsed by several subsequent reports.[52]

No one can claim with credibility that the EPA specializes in sloppy science. On the other hand, no one can maintain that peer review is foolproof; it can be fair, or it can be stacked. Its limitations for quality control are widely recognized within the scientific community, especially by those who use it most frequently: journal editors. Richard Smith, former editor of the *British Medical Journal,* has written that "The problem with peer review is that we have good evidence on its deficiencies and poor evidence on its benefits. We know that it is expensive, slow, prone to bias, open to abuse, possibly anti-innovatory, and unable to detect fraud. We also know that the published papers that emerge from the process are often grossly deficient."[53]

The list of important scientific papers that peer-reviewed journals have rejected goes at least as far back as the rejection of Edward Jenner's report of the first vaccination against smallpox by the editor of *Philosophical Transaction.* That was in 1796.[54] One study familiar to academics includes a long list of articles by leading economists, including numerous Nobel laureates, that were initially rejected for publication.[55] In other words, peer review simply cannot be reified as the be-all and end-all of the regulatory process.

At the EPA, where the science is complex and the stakes are high for certain industries, regulated parties have historically called for more peer review, better peer review—and now *their* peer review. The process that OMB proposed would overrule the EPA's and every other agency's procedures already in place. It would be redundant, costly, wasteful of time, and, worst of all, duplicitous.

As with the fine print in the Shelby Amendment, which allowed access only to government-funded—not industry-funded—science, the fine print in the peer-review proposal tells us just about all we need to know about the real motivation of its authors and sponsors. Information related to national defense or foreign affairs was exempted, perhaps because accuracy is not so important in the matter of weapons of mass destruction and related issues. All licenses were also exempted, so when a chemical manufacturer, for example, submits its own studies to demonstrate the safety of a new pesticide that it is seeking to market, peer review is not necessary. The initial proposal excluded from participation in the peer-review process all scientists whose research has been funded by the agency involved—a move that would eliminate many, perhaps most, of the nation's leading academic experts. On the other hand, the proposal did not preclude industry-employed scientists from appointment to the panels unless they worked on the specific question the panel was to examine.

The audacity takes the breath away. Thank goodness it also got the attention of the science community. Traditionally, the organizations that represent mainstream scientists and their research institutions have focused their political efforts in Washington on research funding, thereby avoiding involvement in policy fights that might be perceived as partisan. This OMB proposal changed all that—in a hurry. The science community responded quickly and forcefully because this peer review bears only superficial similarity to traditional academic peer review. It is instead an attempt to construct a system in which regulated parties have multiple opportunities to delay or prevent the dissemination of information they simply do not like.

The opposition solidified at a remarkable workshop held in November 2003, at OMB's request, by the Science, Technology, and Law program of the National Academy of Sciences (NAS). I discuss this workshop in some detail because the meeting was so unusual, the concern of the scientists and others present so deep, and the issues so pertinent to my overall subject in this book. The day began with a talk by OMB's John Graham, who explained that the proposal was a "major priority" for the Bush administration and asserted that peer review would improve the quality of regulations and information. Au contraire, replied speaker after speaker after speaker, all invited by the NAS as experts in regulatory sciences. They warned that the proposal as drafted would mainly lead to increased costs and delays in disseminating information to the public and in promulgating health, safety, environmental, and other regulations while potentially damaging the existing system of peer review. As a former regulator in the Department of Energy, I joined many of the speakers in challenging OMB to identify *one single report* or regulation that would have been improved had the proposed peer-review system been in place.

Speakers pointed out that the proposal failed to include a cost-benefit analysis, an irony not lost on the audience. In his work at Harvard and then at OMB, Dr. Graham championed cost-benefit analyses as the fundamental standard on which regulation should be judged. Fortunately, two professors from Rutgers University—Stuart Shapiro, who had been a desk officer at OMB under Graham, and David Guston—provided the numbers they had derived after applying the methods OMB would have used if this had been a proposal sent over by an agency. Their best estimate of the cost of the proposed peer-review system was $325 million annually, the monetary value of the effects of delaying regulation that saves lives, protects the environment, or produces other societal benefits. Many observers would suggest that OMB failed to demonstrate any benefits of the proposal, but, in the comments they provided the White House, Shapiro and Guston were more charitable and asserted only that while the benefits are harder to measure, they "appear to be very unlikely to justify the considerable costs."[56]

Shapiro and Guston explained why the proposal was so problematic:

> Any individual peer reviewer will have the potential power to derail a rulemaking effort by providing a negative peer review. This is not the case in academic peer review, where editors and program managers are free to ignore negative reviews of articles or proposals. The context of regulatory peer review is very different however. It is very easy to envision a court using a negative peer review as evidence that an agency was arbitrary and capricious in promulgating a regulation. It is also very easy to envision political actors hostile to a regulation using a negative peer review to attempt to derail regulatory initiatives for purely political reasons. And such negative peer reviews need not (and indeed are likely not to) come from peer reviewers with particular anti-regulatory agendas. As discussed above, disagreement in the sciences is common. Disagreement in economics is rampant. It is unlikely that very many analyses that agencies submit for regulatory peer review will result in unanimous endorsement. Such a lack of consensus, which is useful in the academic setting may provide a death blow for regulatory efforts in the policymaking setting. This may be true even for regulations with large net benefits.[56]

These are critical points. The give-and-take at the meeting confirmed the proposal's fundamental lack of understanding of how science is used in regulation. It confirmed that the peer-review model chosen by OMB is not particularly useful or even applicable to the process through which government agencies do their work. The expert selected by the NAS to provide the "conceptual framework" for regulatory science at the workshop was Harvard professor Sheila Jasanoff, one of the nation's leading thinkers on the use of science in public policy. One fundamental flaw in the proposal, she asserted, is the apparent failure of OMB to understand that research science differs in important respects from regulatory science. The former is "investigator-initiated or curiosity-driven." It has no inherent time pressure, and no public consequences hang in the balance. On the other hand, the efficacy of regulatory science depends in part on its capacity to provide timely answers to pressing policy questions. Professor Jasanoff warned that the proposal "is likely to have significant impact on the time and cost of policy development—and, by extension, on the capacity of regulators to effectively protect public health, safety and the environment."[57]

Michael Taylor, who had served as the FDA's deputy commissioner for policy, cautioned that the centralization of authority around peer review at OMB could have the unintended consequence of constraining public health officials from reacting to a national emergency.[58] He used the hypothetical example of a food-borne disease outbreak caused by fresh produce, but if he had waited a few weeks, he could have employed the government's response to the case of mad cow disease in Washington state. Under the OMB's proposal, then Secretary of Agriculture Ann Veneman would not have been able to issue emergency guidelines without either independent peer review or a waiver from OMB (an agency without particular expertise in bovine spongiform encephalopathy or virtually any of the other technical issues that science agencies grapple with daily). In fact, it is not clear that she could have announced without OMB approval that she was serving beef to her family at Christmas.

Several speakers at the NAS workshop raised concern about the impact of the new system on already-strained federal programs that use peer reviewers. For the most part, scientists volunteer their time to provide these reviews; the huge new demand for reviewers would likely produce a new creature, the professional peer reviewer, who, by definition, would no longer be a practicing scientist and therefore not a peer. As the criticisms mounted, the invited panelists became increasingly skeptical. Then Dr. John Bailar, formerly editor in chief of the *Journal of the National Cancer Institute* and a member of the editorial board of the *New England Journal of Medicine*, said "[A]s the day has gone on, I have become more and more of a skeptic about whether this approach is appropriate. I am really concerned about the potential for mischief in it. I don't see that the added value is going to be as great as the added cost and the added hassle."[10]

The groundswell did not abate. The American Association for the Advancement of Science and the American Public Health Association passed resolutions opposing the proposal.[59,60] The Federation of American Societies for Experimental Biology, a coalition of twenty-two societies, joined the American Association of Medical Colleges in a scathing letter of opposition to the "procrustean processes" prescribed by OMB.[61] The Council on Government Relations, which represents more than 150 leading U.S. research universities, wrote a letter of opposition.[62] Perhaps most surprising is the unusually harsh language used by Dr. Bruce Alberts, then president of the National Academy of Sciences. As the nation's preeminent arbiter of science, the Academy chooses its battles carefully and rarely joins open opposition to major White House initiatives (not that there is often such open opposition from the science community). Dr. Alberts warned Dr. Graham that "the highly prescriptive type of peer review that OMB is proposing differs from accepted practices of peer review in the scientific community, and if enacted in its present form is likely to be counterproductive."[63]

The OMB proposal had the strong support of the U.S. Chamber of Commerce, the National Association of Manufacturers, the American Chemistry Council, and a host of other major trade associations, all of whom wanted the proposal to go even further and prohibit the agencies from accepting as "peer-reviewed" studies that have already been peer-reviewed in a scientific journal. Accepting traditional peer review does not do the trade associations any good and in fact defeats the whole point of their initiative because they want only *their* peer review.

The only major industry that directly opposed the OMB proposal was the pharmaceutical industry. Big Pharma, which is all too comfortable with its regulators at the FDA, appeared to fear that the proposed new peer-review system might provide an opportunity for its opponents to do some mischief. (Among those opponents might be corporations for whom lower drug prices would mean lower costs for their health insurance programs.) The drug manufacturers asserted that the proposed requirements "would contribute little value and would add to the time and expense of a gatekeeper function that has historically been criticized for obstruction and delay."[64] Not surprisingly, OMB allayed their concerns by stipulating that FDA review of new drug applications would be exempt from the new process.

Dr. Donald Kennedy, the editor of *Science* magazine, is a giant in the scientific community. A biologist who formerly served as commissioner of the FDA and president of Stanford University, he now chairs the National Academy of Sciences panel that hosted the pivotal workshop. In an editorial in *Science* he made it clear that he does not think what OMB proposed should even be called peer review. He decried the contribution of this and the Data Quality Act to the erosion of public trust in the work of scientists.[65]

In a victory for the science community, the final version of the peer-review requirements, issued in December 2004, was significantly modified to address several of the community's concerns.[66] Perhaps the most important change involved the conflict of interest provisions, which now allow scientists who have grant funding from agencies to participate in peer-review panels. OMB has also deferred to the National Academy of Sciences in stating that NAS panel reports are presumed not to require additional peer review, and OMB requires agencies to adopt the NAS policy for dealing with conflict of interest in the selection of nongovernment employee members of peer-review committees. This mollified the NAS, whose position as the ultimate framer of scientific consensus would no longer be challenged. Other modifications make the peer-review requirements somewhat less onerous for agencies; foremost among them, the level that triggers the most cumbersome and time-consuming level of peer review was raised from $100 million to $500 million. Nevertheless, the fundamental issue raised by scientists at the workshop remained: OMB failed to establish the need for a single, government-wide, peer-review policy. The final bulletin does little to allay observers' suspicion that the new requirements are a poorly camouflaged attempt to introduce delays into already slow regulatory processes and to further hamper government activities aimed at protecting the public health and the environment.[67]

* * *

All in all, Big Tobacco's efforts over the past several years have paid off. The antiregulatory zealots at OMB and the political leadership of the agencies have embraced the DQA as a way to control career science staff who are bent on fulfilling the agencies' public health responsibilities. The roadblocks have successfully slowed agency activities by pulling scarce staff and resources from useful projects. Senior management at the regulatory agencies have been warned repeatedly by the White House that anything the least bit controversial will not be permitted though OMB review unless it has undergone internal and often external peer review as well.

These "sound science" administrative controls have delayed numerous documents and regulations, from OSHA's proposed update of the workplace silica exposure standard to new designations of Superfund sites. If no regulatory action is proposed, the "sound science" controls are silent—there is no opportunity for peer review or a data quality challenge when an agency decides not to act, no matter how compelling the evidence. These controls are invoked only to impede regulation. Oliver Houck of Tulane Law School aptly describes these controls, which are implemented only when regulation is under consideration, as "a knife that cuts only one way: against environmental protection."[68]

In virtually every instance in which a federal regulatory agency proposes protecting the public's health by reducing the allowable exposure to a toxic product, the regulated industry hires scientists to dispute the science on which the proposal is based. They have had some success, but they have not been able to *utterly* thwart the will of the people. Every reputable poll still demonstrates widespread support in the United States (and elsewhere) for a broad range of environmental and public health regulations and protection. Now, however, the new tactics embodied in the Shelby Amendment, the Data Quality Act, and the OMB peer-review rules take industry's guerilla war against science to frightening new levels of deception and perhaps effectiveness.

Industry's motive is transparent. The politics is transparent. The dogged work of the think tanks and the product defense industry is transparent.

(The involvement of Big Tobacco with the birth of the DQA was not so apparent at first, but it is now well recognized.) Industry's goal is to maximize its ability to manufacture, magnify, and institutionalize the uncertainty inherent in the scientific enterprise. The hard work of recent decades is in jeopardy. Contrary to the old adage, it *is* possible to roll back some clocks, and that is exactly what this coalition of industry and politicians is striving to do.

15

The Bush Administration's Political Science

In 1991, on the basis of evidence reported in chapter four, the Centers for Disease Control and Prevention (CDC) lowered the definition of what was considered an elevated blood level of lead, a highly toxic metal, in children from 30 to 10 μg/dl (micrograms per deciliter of blood).[1] Today the CDC's best estimate is that more than 300,000 under the age of six have exposures exceeding that target level, and new studies indicate that even lower exposure levels may affect children's learning.[2] When Senator Jean Carnahan (D-MO) asked the CDC in 2001 to lower the threshold to 5 μg, the head of the CDC division in charge indicated that the agency would probably make the change.[3] Soon after, however, the CDC's advisory committee on childhood lead poisoning prevention had some new members.

Among those disqualified from serving were Bruce Lanphear of the Cincinnati Children's Hospital Medical Center, whose research supported the suspicion that levels below 10 μg could be harmful, and Michael Weitzman of the University of Rochester, who had been on the committee for five years.[3] Among those nominated to replace them were Joyce Tsuji, whose work at the product defense firm Exponent, Inc. was paid for by Asarco, a leading metals smelter facing large clean-up costs that would be reduced substantially if lead were deemed to be less hazardous.[4,5] (Citing scheduling conflicts, Dr. Tsuji asked to have her nomination withdrawn after reports of her corporate ties surfaced.) Also nominated were Sergio Piomelli of Columbia Presbyterian Medical Center in New York, who labeled the members of the 1991 advisory committee "well-meaning fanatics";

and William Banner, a pediatric toxicologist at the University of Oklahoma Health Sciences Center, who is on record in a court deposition as believing that levels below 70 µg do not pose a threat to children and who dismisses all conclusions to the contrary.[6]

Federal advisory panels are the most important means by which the government harnesses the expertise of the scientific community. The committees that advise agencies on the kinds of public health and environmental issues discussed in this book have a particularly difficult job because the science is complex, certainty is not in the cards, and conflicts about economic impact are a given. In previous administrations, a wide range of views for the members has been the norm. For example, the EPA's Science Advisory Board, as important and high profile as any of the committees, has long had as members scientists employed by Exxon, Monsanto, DuPont, and General Motors, as well as the World Wildlife Fund and the American Lung Association.

With this second Bush administration, that ecumenical approach has changed. The story of the lead committee is not an aberration. This White House has stacked advisory panels with individuals chosen for their commitment to the administration's allies and ideas rather than to the best and latest science. In 2002 fifteen of the eighteen members of the committee advising the director of the National Center for Environmental Health were replaced, for the most part with representatives of regulated industries, product defense specialists (including ChemRisk's Dr. Dennis Paustenbach), and organizations ideologically opposed to federal regulation.[7] The initial choice to head the FDA's Reproductive Health Drugs Advisory Committee was Dr. W. David Hager, a physician who reportedly refuses to discuss contraception with unwed female patients; only after much opposition was he demoted to panel member.[8,9] Not surprisingly, Dr. Hager was one of the four (out of twenty-seven) members who voted against recommending that the FDA permit over-the-counter sales of the "Plan B" morning-after pill to prevent unwanted pregnancies.[10]

When I first learned about this committee stacking, I contacted Dr. Donald Kennedy, editor of *Science* magazine, and proposed an editorial on the issue. This editorial, coauthored by members of the Project on Scientific Knowledge and Public Policy (SKAPP) planning committee and titled "Advice without Dissent," concluded with this observation:

> Instead of grappling with scientific ambiguity and shaping public policy using the best available evidence (the fundamental principle underlying public health and environmental regulation), we can now expect these committees to emphasize the uncertainties of health and environmental risks, supporting the administration's antiregulatory

views. And in those areas where there are deeply held conflicts in values, we can expect only silence. Regulatory paralysis appears to be the goal here, rather than the application of honest balanced science.[11]

Shortly after publication, I received a call from Dr. William E. Howard III, a consultant to the Army Science Board (ASB) who had recently been nominated to become a full member. This board is not one of the public health or environmental advisory boards that I wrote about in *Science;* its mission is to advise the U.S. Army on technical matters, many of which are related to weapons development. The ASB's members are scientists, engineers, and retired flag-rank military. Dr. Howard told me—and later wrote to *Science* magazine—that his nomination was one of several killed by the White House Liaison Office in the Office of the Secretary of Defense. He had learned from an ASB colleague that political appointees checked the names of the nominees on a website that lists donors to political campaigns, on which a man with a similar name (William S. Howard), who lived in a different but nearby town in Virginia, was listed as a contributor to the presidential campaign of Senator John McCain. Thinking this simple mistake could be rectified (after all, as a consultant he was already doing the work of a panel member and contributing in this capacity to the nation's defense), he requested that the ASB appeal the decision. The ASB refused. The career staff told him they "did not want to upset" the apparatchiks in the White House liaison office.[12]

Our editorial also spurred other scientists around the country to reveal their own experiences with the advisory committees in the new era of the second Bush administration. Perhaps the most chilling was the report by Dr. Dana Loomis, a University of North Carolina School of Public Health epidemiologist who was chair of the "study section" that reviewed research proposals for NIOSH. Study sections are advisory committees that review research proposals. That's it. They do not consider public policy. They do not even advise agencies about what topics to research. They simply examine and rate the proposals presented to them. This work is mostly drudgery, and we scientists serve on these panels (I served on the NIOSH study section some years earlier) as part of our commitment to advancing scientific research. Chairpersons and staff also work hard to recruit a balanced committee—not politically balanced but balanced by expertise, in this case, epidemiology, toxicology, industrial hygiene, ergonomics, and other disciplines.

But now, Dr. Loomis reported, Health and Human Services Secretary Tommy Thompson refused to appoint candidates that Dr. Loomis nominated. No one could remember such a veto in the past. The problem with two of the rejected nominees was straightforward: They were ergonomics researchers, one of whom had been an advisor to OSHA in the development of the ill-fated ergonomics standard. In the replacement process, different experts were called and asked their opinions on the OSHA ergonomics standard.[13] To many of the scientists who have served on these study sections, this interference threatened the system that has worked well to ensure that the best studies are chosen for federal support. If appointment was now contingent on political viewpoint, membership would be seen as a political payoff. Some scientists would no longer be asked to serve, and others would no longer be willing to serve.

All of these developments prompted a groundswell of interest in public policy circles. Two members of the House of Representatives requested an investigation by the General Accounting Office.[14] Resolutions condemning the stacking of advisory committees were passed by the American Association for the Advancement of Science[15] and the American Public Health Association.[16] The National Academy of Sciences began a study of ways to ensure the government gets the best scientific advice.[17] Dr. Donald Kennedy penned two more pertinent editorials in *Science* magazine.[18,19]

In his January 31, 2003, *Science* editorial, Dr. Kennedy expressed his deep disappointment with such politicization of science and added a couple of remarkable stories to the growing list. A nominee for the Muscular Dystrophy Research Coordinating Committee at the NIH was asked by a White House staffer whether she supported President Bush's stem cell policy. A professor of psychology and psychiatry nominated to serve on the National Council on Drug Abuse was told by the vetting staffer who called him that the purpose was to "determine whether he held any views that might be embarrassing to the president." The staffer kept a running score. After the nominee answered incorrectly regarding needle exchange programs, he was two out of three; when he answered incorrectly about his vote in the presidential election, he was two out of four. The staffer asked, "Why didn't you support the president?"

"This stuff would be prime material for a Robin Williams comedy shtick, but it really isn't funny," Dr. Kennedy wrote. He cited the federal statute about inappropriate influence and concluded that "It would be a good idea for HHS Secretary Tommy Thompson and the White House Personnel Office to read the law, and then follow it."[18]

Defending against these protests, a spokesperson for Secretary Thompson bluntly stated that the secretary has the prerogative to solicit only advice he would want to hear.[7] Can such selective executive ignorance serve the national interest over the long run? I do not think so, regardless of the political viewpoint behind it. Moreover, the claim for such an executive privilege is not even correct. The Federal Advisory Committee Act requires that committees be "fairly balanced in terms of the points of view represented and...not be inappropriately influenced by the appointing authority or by any special interest."[20]

I wish I could now report that this second Bush administration was chastened by the criticism, that it recognized the need for using the best science, and that it started to respect the integrity of the federal science advisory system. Unfortunately, this has not been the case. New reports continued to surface. After he left federal employment, Dr. Gerald Keusch, the director of NIH's Fogarty International Center, divulged that Secretary Thompson rejected almost 75 percent of the experts Dr. Keusch had nominated to serve on the center's advisory committee (including several internationally known figures, one a Nobel laureate). They were replaced by several individuals Keusch deemed inappropriate.[21] In a better-known case, Elizabeth Blackburn, a renowned cell biologist who dissented from the administration's position on stem cell research, was dropped from the President's Council on Bioethics. She and another member were replaced by three scientists whose views are much more in line with those of the religious right, for whom the White House was apparently vetting all candidates.[22] Amazingly, Dr. Leon Kass, the chair of the committee, claimed to have no idea of the views of any of the three new appointees.[23]

In its second term, the Bush White House *has* gotten a little more subtle and added a new trick to the system. Instead of simply stacking committees, a high-profile action that allows scientists and the press to focus on rejected nominees and their replacements, it may simply disband a panel that is not giving the right advice. That is what happened to the Secretary of Energy Advisory Board (SEAB), a panel that I know provided valuable advice to the Department of Energy when I was assistant secretary. According to press reports, however, the SEAB serving this Bush administration recommended an unpopular restructuring of the nuclear weapons labs.[24] The members were all thanked and politely asked not to return. Other committees, like the EPA's Clean Air Scientific Advisory Committee (CASAC), cannot be axed because Congress requires them, but they can be devalued or ignored, and that is what happened with CASAC. After taking the unprecedented step of publicly criticizing the EPA about its unwillingness to issue a sufficiently protective air pollution standard, the board was told it would no longer be asked for advice in shaping policy (its entire raison d'être). Along with everyone else in the country, it can comment on EPA policies after they have been formally proposed.[25]

* * *

From the moment George W. Bush took the oath of office in January 2001, his political appointees, working at the bidding of the corporate polluters who in many cases were their former and subsequent employers, have gutted, evaded, and opposed environmental regulations. I doubt they would even bother to deny that a main agenda of this administration is to ensure that certain industries face no additional regulatory burden, no matter how toxic or dangerous their products. The manipulations of the scientific advisory panels are indicative of this policy and quite significant, I believe, but they have not created a major stir outside the scientific community and the federal agencies. That is precisely why I have featured them in the beginning of this chapter. The story needs to be out there. The next subject—the denials and distortions of the Bush administration on global warming—is more widely known, but it is too important to pass over entirely. On the other hand, the deniers' argument is rooted in the classic "Uncertainty!" attack we have seen played out in industry after industry, so this section can be a short one. We know this drill.

Is the greenhouse effect—global warming caused by the burning of fossil fuels—fact or fiction? Neither, yet. It is the best hypothesis of the best scientists who have studied these very complex issues over the course of decades. As Dr. James Baker, former head of the National Oceanic and Atmospheric Administration (NOAA), has said, "There's a better scientific consensus on this than on any issue I know—except maybe Newton's second law of [thermo]dynamics."[26] The climate scientists and the policy makers around the world who accept this consensus believe a precautionary approach is the only responsible one. We should act to control fossil fuel emissions. If the global warming hypothesis is correct, we may be able to prevent potentially catastrophic consequences. If it is incorrect, the consolation prize is not too bad: a more energy-efficient global economy and a cleaner environment. Isn't this a no-brainer? Win-win? A slam dunk? Such is the worldwide consensus, and isn't it interesting that essentially the only voices challenging it are the industries that would be affected by immediate action?

To see the specific tactics that foes of environmental regulation use, it is instructive to return to the operative strategy paper prepared by Frank Luntz, a famous consultant to conservative causes worldwide. He specializes in words—that is, convincing his clients that simple code words and phrases are everything in political debate today, when most Americans are paying very little attention and, when we do, are inundated by a flood of conflicting information. Thus, we get "sound science" and "junk science" and "uncertainty."

The title of this particular Luntz document is "The Environment: A Cleaner, Safer, Healthier America," and it is dedicated to challenging the presumed orthodoxy that "**'Washington regulations'** represent the best way to preserve the environment"[27] [emphasis in the original]. Of course, the ability of free markets to protect the commons has yet to be proved; the numerous disasters that birthed the regulatory system lead us to believe otherwise. The legal obligation of corporations to serve the interests of shareholders above all else might also lead us to believe otherwise, but it has not been my purpose to get into a grand debate on the attributes and limits of corporations and markets. My purpose has been to get into a grand debate on the nature of science, its role in public policy, and its susceptibility to craven manipulation.

"Winning the Global Warming Debate—An Overview" reads the title at the top of page 137 of Luntz's document. Item number one is this: "**The scientific debate remains open.** Voters believe that there is *no consensus* about global warming within the scientific community. Should the public come to believe that the scientific issues are settled, their views on global warming will change accordingly. Therefore, *you need to continue to make the lack of scientific certainty a primary issue in the debate*, and defer to scientists and other experts in the field". On the following page is this paragraph: "*The most important principle in any discussion of global warming is your commitment to sound science.* Americans unanimously believe all environmental rules and regulations should be based on sound science and common sense. Similarly, our confidence in the ability of science and technology to solve our ills is second to none. Both perceptions will work in your favor if properly cultivated." And below that paragraph is this boxed statement: "**LANGUAGE THAT WORKS**[:] *'We must not rush to judgment before all the facts are in. We need to ask more questions. We deserve more answers. And until we learn more, we should not commit America to any international document that handcuffs us either now or into the future'*"[27] [emphasis in the original].

There are thousands of scientists on our side of the debate and a mere handful on the other, but uncertainty can reign in the mass media and the public mind if that handful has a large enough megaphone—and they do because they are underwritten by ExxonMobil, by all analyses the hands-down largest funder of the warming deniers.[28] According to the authors of the internal ExxonMobil memo titled "Global Climate Science Communications Action Plan," "[v]ictory will be achieved when ... average citizens 'understand' (recognize) uncertainties in climate science; recognition of uncertainties becomes part of the conventional wisdom."[29]

The consequences of global warming could dwarf those of all the other issues discussed in this book put together, and the movement to delay and subvert action now has a powerful ally in Washington, D.C.: the second Bush White House. In February 2001—within a month of George W. Bush's inauguration—ExxonMobil faxed a memo to the White House that asked, "Can Watson be replaced now at the request of the [United States]?"[30] "Watson" was Dr. Robert Watson, esteemed climate scientist, chief scientist at the World Bank, and chairman of the UN Intergovernmental Panel on Climate Change (IPCC). This panel had been studying the issue for a decade (since the first Bush administration, when it was created by the World Meteorological Organization and the UN Environmental Programme). Its most recent assessment had concluded, "[M]ost of the observed warming over the last 50 years is likely to have been due to the increase in greenhouse gas concentrations."[31]

The answer from the White House was "sorry, no" because Dr. Watson still had one more year in his five-year term. When his time was up, the White House refused to support him for a second term and pushed for and got Rajendra Pachauri, an Indian engineer. Perhaps Pachauri has surprised the White House with the outspoken approach he has taken on global warming issues since his term began because administration officials still seemed unwilling to accept the IPCC's findings. In May 2001 the White House asked the National Academy of Sciences to look yet again at the work of the IPCC.[32] The ensuing report stated, "The changes observed over the last several decades are likely mostly due to human activities, but we cannot rule out that some significant part of these changes is also a reflection of natural variability."[33] That second clause is what the administration was after all along. Ignore the first clause, emphasize the second, call for more research, and buy more time. Uncertainty!

Within two months of taking office, the president stepped back from his campaign promise to lower carbon dioxide emissions from coal-burning power plants. Among other points, the White House argued that CO_2 was not a pollutant under the Clean Air Act,[34] a specious assertion reminiscent of Ronald Reagan's famous observation that trees cause more pollution than do automobiles.

Every two years, the United States has to report to a UN body on its greenhouse emissions, efforts to reduce them, and consequences of action and inaction. As we have seen, one of the first petitions filed under the Data Quality Act challenged the dissemination of this report, the *National Assessment on Climate Change,* on the grounds that it is based on faulty computer models and did not undergo proper peer review—charges that are simply false. The EPA did deny the petition under the DQA, but when that agency's six-hundred-page draft report for 2003 included all of six paragraphs on global warming, the White House deleted five of them. The one that made the cut contained no reference to repercussions from global warming.[35] The White House also instructed the agency to insert a reference to a study disputing the global warming hypothesis (and not just human activity as the major factor, but the warming itself), written by scientists associated with the Center for the Study of Carbon Dioxide and Global Change, one of the "think-tanks" funded by ExxonMobil.[36]

When the Bush administration pulled out of the Kyoto Accords, it offered a specious sop to the world by establishing a voluntary goal to reduce

200 DOUBT IS THEIR PRODUCT

emissions intensity by 18 percent by 2012. "Intensity"? That's output *per economic unit*. With robust economic growth, therefore, we could achieve such a reduction in "intensity" while contributing *more* greenhouse gases to the environment—and would, in fact. When it comes to global warming, actual emissions are the only ones that count. Moreover, the Government Accountability Office had already estimated that the United States would achieve a reduction of 14 percent in intensity over the next decade, thanks to already-planned improvements in efficiency.[37]

After Dr. James Hansen, chief of the NASA Institute for Space Studies and one of the nation's leading climate scientists, called for limiting greenhouse gas emissions, White House appointees threatened him with "dire consequences." NASA scientists, many of whom worked on global climate issues, were a particular target. *New York Times* reporter Andrew C. Revkin documented NASA's almost comedic attempt to spin the agency's science. In the months leading up to the 2004 election, Revkin reported, the White House told NASA's public affairs directors to highlight the president's "vision" for space travel to Mars in NASA news releases, even if the subject at hand was earth science. This manipulation initiative was transparent: A December 2004 news release describing research on the relationship between wind patterns and recent warming of the Indian Ocean included a statement that the analytical tools used in the study "may someday prove useful in studying climate systems on other planets." The term "climate systems" by itself must have been a red flag for the political apparatchik who reviewed it because NASA scientists were subsequently not allowed to talk about new satellite data on ozone and air pollution until after the 2004 elections. Meanwhile, news releases were compiled by political appointees who held little regard for the science. George Deutsch, a NASA public affairs political appointee with little technical background (who left the agency after his resume was alleged to contain false statements), considered it his assignment to insert the word "theory" after every reference to the Big Bang. In an email later leaked to the press, Deutsch explained, "It is not NASA's place, nor should it be[,] to make a declaration such as this about the existence of the universe that discounts intelligent design by a creator."[38–41]

Scientists at NOAA were also targets for manipulation and censorship. Following the devastating 2005 hurricane season, the agency put out a statement that there was a consensus among its experts that natural, rather than man-made, factors were to blame. Several scientists within the agency (as well as many outside it) disagreed with this statement—and some reported that they had been censored in conversations with the media on this topic.[42] In the end, the attempted silencing of James Hansen and the other scientists at NASA and NOAA backfired to some extent. Formerly well known only among scientists, Hansen was interviewed on CBS's *Sixty Minutes* and became a media star. The administrators at both NASA and NOAA have issued policy statements that declare their dedication to "scientific debate and transparency,"[43,44] although it is not clear that this affirmative policy has trickled down to the rank and file in those agencies that are not working on the high-profile issue of global warming.

In June 2005 we learned from the front page of the *New York Times* and elsewhere that one Philip Cooney, chief of staff for the White House Council on Environmental Quality, edited a federal report on climate change to magnify the level of uncertainty. Suddenly the word "uncertainties" was preceded by "significant and fundamental." Or consider the following sentence: "The attribution of the causes of biological and ecological changes to climate change or variability is extremely difficult." Cooney added the "extremely."[45] Well, so what, we might ask. These are not really substantive changes. No, they are not, and this document is not going to make or break any policy on climate change, but it is all of a piece with this administration. Before his appointment by the president, Cooney was a lobbyist with the American Petroleum Institute, one of the nation's leading manufacturers of scientific uncertainty, and immediately following the *New York Times* report he left the White House for a post at ExxonMobil.[46] His job title may have changed, but his job description did not.

As late as June 2006 President Bush was still claiming it wasn't certain whether humans had any role in global warming.[47] A few weeks later, when the U.S. Supreme Court was hearing arguments on a suit that was attempting to compel the EPA to regulate carbon dioxide as a pollutant, the Bush administration said, "Let's debate the science." Referring to a legal brief written by a familiar group of global warming deniers whose work the oil industry supports and promotes, the administration argued that the EPA's inaction was justified by the differences among scientists (specifically between those paid by the industry and everyone else). "I think one thing that we ought to be able to agree on," asserted the deputy solicitor general, "is that there is uncertainty surrounding the phenomenon of global climate change."[48]

Such uncertainty is just what ExxonMobil, the coal industry, and the other carbon polluters want and are paying for because it avoids discussion of the much tougher set of policy choices necessary to reduce carbon levels in the atmosphere. Rest assured, we will eventually be forced into that discussion.

Almost inevitably, the global warming deniers will go the way of the tobacco lung cancer deniers. It is happening already, overcoming the rear-guard efforts by the Bush administration, which continued to follow Luntz's advice. Even the oil companies, whose products make a substantial contribution to the atmospheric accumulation of the greenhouse gas carbon dioxide, are coming around. In October 2006 John Hofmeister, president of Shell Oil Company, said, "We have to deal with greenhouse gases. From Shell's point of view, the debate is over. When 90-plus percent of the world's leading figures believe that greenhouse gases have impacted the climate of the Earth, who is Shell to say, 'Let's debate the science'?"[49]

Let us just hope we overcome the obstruction before we reach the tipping point for the Greenland glaciers, when their melting cannot be stopped; before dramatic increases in insect-borne diseases like malaria further afflict poor populations throughout the tropics; and before lower crop yields devastate regions where much of the world's population is already hungry. If we get to this point, billions of tons of carbon dioxide later (along with billions of dollars of corporate profits), how many lives and opportunities will have been squandered? How much harder will it be to work our way out of these problems?

* * *

Near the end of the Clinton administration, the EPA issued regulations aimed at reducing the allowable drinking-water level of arsenic, a known human carcinogen, from 50 parts per billion (ppb) to 10 ppb, the level recommended by the World Health Organization and already in effect in Europe.[50] "Junk science!" cried the antiregulatory crowd, and its cronies within the new Bush administration immediately froze that recommendation and made plans to kill it. They probably did not expect the public outcry (which was loud) or the vehement response from the scientific community. In fact, I will bet that Karl Rove, President Bush's political guru, did not even know about this decision because he would have understood the potent symbolism: Here was a new group in Washington, D.C., so beholden to industry that it balked at removing from our drinking water a chemical whose name is almost synonymous with poison. Requested by the EPA to review the proposed standard, a panel of the National Academy of Sciences stated that, if anything, the proposed standard should be lowered to 3 ppb, since 10 ppb represented a risk of 30 excess cancer deaths for every ten thousand people exposed.[51] The EPA did not go that far, but in October 2001, eight months into the new administration, it embraced the previously derided 10 ppb standard.[52]

This did not stop the "Republican war on science," as journalist Chris Mooney has called it.[53] And why should it have? No one knows better how to play the regulatory game in Washington. I have described in some detail how OSHA has surrendered to special interests and used the scientific uncertainty subterfuge to stall or weaken protections for workers in a host of industries. An even longer list of polluters has been able to weaken or eliminate regulations of the Environmental Protection Agency during this second Bush administration. Portions of the agency's proposed regulations to control mercury emissions from power plants were written by industry lobbyists and simply inserted verbatim into the rules. Congress's Government Accountability Office has determined that the EPA's mandatory cost-benefit calculations in 2004 had skewed the numbers to make the administration's "cap and trade" approach seem more cost effective than simply capping pollution at every power plant.[54] This was nothing new; the political appointees in the agency have wanted to weaken the Clean Air Act since they took power in 2001. They doctored the cost-benefit analysis presented to Congress to promote the administration's proposed "Clear Skies" legislation over the alternative that environmentalists backed. "Clear Skies"? Pure Orwell. The Congressional Research Service determined that the agency's analysis exaggerated the costs and underestimated the benefits of enacting more protective legislation.[55]

In 2004 the EPA issued rules exempting much of the U.S. plywood industry from controlling emissions of formaldehyde. It justified the new, less stringent rules by using a risk assessment conducted by the Chemical Industry Institute of Toxicology (CIIT), a laboratory, as its name suggests, run by the chemical industry.[56] The agency ignored two studies published in the months before the rule change, one by scientists at the National Cancer Institute,[57] the other from the National Institute for Occupational Safety and Health,[58] both of which found increased risk of leukemia among workers exposed to the chemical. Using the same data as CIIT, a scientific advisory committee in California unanimously rejected the formaldehyde industry's request to reconsider the state's risk assessment.[56] A few weeks later the International Agency for Research on Cancer designated formaldehyde as a human carcinogen.[59]

The list of similar stories is too long for me to chronicle here. Some involve lying about or manipulating science, others issuing bad or no regulations. Each would also require me to emphasize that what is going on within the agency is not the fault of most of the career employees, many of whom are heartsick that their work has been so undermined, to put it mildly, and that their once-proud agency has become just another enabler for the polluters and the poisoners. I could also devote dozens of pages to stories about every other agency involved in regulation and some that are not, but I will settle for a brief selection that demonstrates the range of the issues at stake, both at home and abroad.

I begin with rare wildlife species. It is difficult if not impossible to attack the position that these creatures merit special protection from development that threatens the destruction of their habitats. On this question at least, the American public is close to united. We understand that while the snail darters and spotted owls and sea turtles may not be vital to the ecology, the *principle* is vital because this really is a slippery slope. So, save the spotted owls and the old-growth forests in which they live. Corporate interests understand that public opinion is adamant, so they have tried a clever end run by going after the *science* that estimates the population of a species—in effect, its degree of endangerment. For decades, wildlife biologists have employed statistical models to estimate the size of animal populations because the methods are as good as or better than counting and because the time and money involved in trying to count all animals would be prohibitive. This is standard practice, and it is never challenged within the scientific community.

Starting in 2003, Republican opponents of the Endangered Species Act introduced several bills that would limit regulators' ability to use statistical models to estimate species populations.[60] Instead they want us to count every bird instead—an onerous and unnecessary obligation. If the tree-huggers cannot prove with an actual head count that an elusive creature is endangered, they cannot stop development in order to protect it—a new wrinkle in the same old uncertainty game. At a hearing on the bill before a committee of the House of Representatives, I testified that legislators dictating the scientific methods a policymaker may or may employ is antithetical (and probably damaging) to the science enterprise itself. I compared the proposal to Lysenkoism, the label given the Soviet Politburo's campaign to dictate methodologies to Soviet scientists.[61] Actually, the name of the proposed legislation tells anyone who is paying attention all they really need to know about its provenance and its purposes: The Sound Science for Endangered Species Act Planning Act of 2003.[62] In September 2005, when the Republican-controlled House of Representatives passed another version of the bill, it was misnamed the Threatened and Endangered Species Recovery Act.[63] Fortunately, the Senate failed to act on this misguided legislation and, with the 2006 election of a Democratic-controlled Congress, this initiative appears to be doomed.

In June 2005 two retired scientists—a biologist and a hydrologist—from the Bureau of Land Management, a division of the Department of the Interior, charged that their analysis of the impact of cattle grazing on public lands had been changed in order to smooth the way for new regulations that would relax grazing restrictions. The initial statement that the new regulations would have "significant adverse impact" on wildlife was replaced by the statement that the rules would be "beneficial to animals." *That* is a substantive change. Missing entirely from the final rules was their statement: "The Proposed Action will have a slow, long-term adverse impact on wildlife and biological diversity in general." The biologist called the promulgated rules a "whitewash." The bureau called the changes to the original study "standard editing."[64]

Jump from rare species and grazing animals to family planning. The Bush administration has been manipulating the science on issues related to sex from the beginning. Foremost is the Plan B debacle, in which the FDA—for the first time in anyone's memory—ignored the recommendation of its advisory panel and refused to license a postcoital contraceptive for sale without prescription. The rationale it gave was that easier access to Plan B might increase sexual activity among teenage girls. The agency had no data on this question, and it did not look for any. That was beside the point. The morality commissars seem to believe that fear of pregnancy—and only fear of pregnancy—will stop teenagers (and adults, too) from having sex. (The FDA eventually jettisoned the rationale. In July 2006, when the agency gave in to political pressure and announced that it would accept an application from the manufacturer of the Plan B contraceptive and increase the minimum age for purchase from sixteen to eighteen, the FDA did not even attempt to claim that new data on teenage sexual behavior led to the change since no new studies had been done.[65])

Early in the Bush administration, the Centers for Disease Control pulled a fact sheet from its website that provided information on proper condom use. It replaced the fact sheet in October 2002 with one that stressed condom failure rates and promoted abstinence, even though abstinence generally has a far higher failure rate than condom use, as many studies have confirmed.[66,67] In fact, misinformation about the effectiveness of abstinence has been widely distributed through several new programs. In 2005 the federal government spent $170 million on abstinence programs, more than twice what it spent in 2001 (although $100 million less than the president had requested). Representative Henry Waxman, one of Congress's public health watchdogs, issued a report that demonstrated that more than 80 percent of this abstinence-only curriculum presents false, misleading, or distorted information about reproductive health.[68]

Forget the science. This administration pushes abstinence, period. Either it has deluded itself and the public about the most effective means to prevent pregnancy and sexually transmitted diseases (STDs), or it feels no compunctions about deceiving the public in order to advance the agenda of one of its vital political constituencies. After Representative Mark Souter (R-IN) complained to the CDC about the "obvious anti-abstinence objective" of the 2006 National STD Prevention Conference, the public health agency changed the name of the panel from "Are Abstinence-Only-Until-Marriage Programs a Threat to Public Health?" to "Public Health Strategies of Abstinence Programs for Youth." It removed one of the speakers and added two others who were not reviewed by the meeting's organizers. The session's convener, Dr. Bruce Trigg, who is medical director of New

Mexico's STD prevention program, said, "It is unprecedented that this type of interference takes place at a scientific meeting."[69]

The likely outcome of these lies is more sexually transmitted diseases and, ironically for an administration that opposes abortion rights, more unwanted pregnancies and resulting abortions. This has been pointed out time and again. The American Medical Association, hardly a hotbed of secular advocacy, believes that the Plan B pill could prevent 1.7 million unintended pregnancies and eight hundred thousand abortions.[70] It doesn't matter.

Scientific data related directly to abortion have not been immune to manipulation, either. In 2002 the National Cancer Institute posted information on its website that promoted the totally unsupported theory that abortions increase the risk of breast cancer. There is no credible evidence for this canard, and the NCI did not get away with it. After much public outrage, the institute convened a meeting of leading scientists, who easily rejected the new claims, and the agency pulled the erroneous information.[71] The abortion opponents would not be swayed. In 2006 Representative Waxman released a study that found that more than a third of the federally funded pregnancy resource centers in the survey told female investigators who posed as pregnant seventeen-year-olds that having an abortion would increase their risk of breast cancer. This is a shameful deception. In all, twenty of the twenty-three centers provided false or misleading information about the health effects of abortion.[72]

Traditionally, the National Institutes of Health (of which the NCI is one component) have been more insulated from politicization than, say, OSHA and the EPA. However, in this Bush administration, the NIH generously provided a conservative Christian group that calls itself the "Traditional Values Coalition" with a hit list of agency grantees who were studying prostitution, substance abuse, homosexuality, or sexually transmitted diseases. Research in these areas could decrease the incidence and impact of sexually transmitted diseases, including HIV, but the coalition still opposed it. The House of Representatives came within two votes of defunding five research programs that had been selected for financial support through the NIH's peer-review system.[73] No doubt the agency got the message and is avoiding areas that will invoke the displeasure of Congress and certain constituencies to which it answers. Now, researchers who focus on areas like sexual behavior and drug abuse know that if they want to obtain federal funding (and who else would fund them?), they have to avoid the wrong research questions. They will be forced to abandon certain areas of investigation that hold great promise for public health.

To be completely fair, anything having to do with sex and drugs is going to be controversial in this country. During the Clinton administration, the same types of issues and controversies arose, but they were handled in a different way, one much more aligned with the facts—the way the world is, not the way we might like it to be. Concerned that needle exchange programs would promote intravenous drug use without reducing rates of HIV transmission, Congress instituted restrictions upon federal funding for these programs in the 1980s.[74] In 1992, the CDC commissioned the School of Public Health of the University of California–Berkeley and the Institute for Health Policy Studies, University of California–San Francisco, to examine those important questions. Chosen as principal investigator was Dr. Peter Lurie, who later was my collaborator on chromium 6. The results, released just after Clinton took office in 1993, concluded that needle exchange is a cost-effective strategy for reducing HIV drug risk behavior that increases neither the numbers of intravenous drug users nor the quantity of drugs injected. The study's straightforward recommendations called for "federal, state, and local governments to remove the legal and administrative barriers to increased needle availability and to facilitate the expansion of needle exchange programs."[75]

What would the administration do with this controversial recommendation? Donna Shalala, Secretary of Health and Human Services (HHS), clearly wanted this entire issue to disappear, but it was too incendiary, so she first tried what the Bush administration has become so expert at: misinterpreting the data. She pretended that the experts were expressing scientific uncertainty and disagreement. However, the science could not really be disputed, at least not by honest scientists, and after scientists and AIDS activists around the country berated her for selling out,[76] she and the Clinton administration eventually gave in. In April 1988, Secretary Shalala finally certified that needle exchange programs indeed decrease HIV risk behavior without increasing drug use.[77] She did not, however, remove the restriction upon federal funding for needle exchange programs, arguing that the decision to implement the programs involved more than the public health part of the equation. Community values, she posited, needed to be considered. At least she acknowledged the science. The Bush administration refuses to do that.

Now consider the fate of Richard Foster, Medicare's chief actuary, whose job was to estimate the cost of President Bush's Medicare Prescription Drug proposal in 2003. The White House announced the bill would cost $400 billion over ten years. When Foster's estimates for the same period came in at 25–50 percent higher—numbers that could kill the bill's chances among fiscal conservatives—Foster testified that he was warned by Tom Scully, Medicare's administrator and his boss, that he would be fired if he revealed his estimate to Congress. Foster kept his mouth shut. With only the White House estimate at hand, the House of Representatives passed the legislation on a close vote: 220 to 215. Five months after the bill was passed, Foster's dangerous estimates surfaced in the press. Why then? The buzz in Washington held that his pension had just fully vested, and so he had become immune to the administration's threats. Perhaps, but Scully did better than that. He jumped ship and took a lucrative job with a law firm that represented many clients who stand to profit substantially from the program. (Incredibly, he had been authorized to negotiate a job with his future employer while negotiating with Congress on the bill.)[78] By the way, the White House later estimated the real cost to the taxpayers at something like $720 billion over ten years, almost double the prediction it made when it was selling Congress the program.[79]

It necessarily follows that an administration that specializes in uncertainty and censorship at home will not want to provide straight answers overseas. It is leading the charge against a European Union initiative named REACH (for registration, evaluation, and authorization of chemicals), which would require chemical manufacturers to perform basic toxicity testing on chemicals in common use and to find substitutes for particularly hazardous ones. As we have seen, U.S. manufacturers have resisted acquiring such basic information for decades, and they will not capitulate in Europe without an all-out fight. In this shrewdly disingenuous sentence C. Boyden Gray, U.S. ambassador to the European Union, expressed the stance of the United States: "We should not regulate if there is no harm to address and there is no benefit of safety to confer."[80] The bottom-line message was this: What we do not know can hurt you, but it cannot hurt us, and we are the ones who count. (Gray served as counsel to former president George H. W. Bush and has been involved in numerous antiregulatory activities, including serving as cochair of the Air Quality Standards Coalition, an organization of polluters that attempts to minimize EPA standards on air quality.[81])

This administration keeps a close watch on all international initiatives. There is no telling how dangerous they might be. In April 2003 the World Health Organization (WHO) and the UN Food and Agriculture Organization issued a report titled *Diet, Nutrition, and the Prevention of Chronic Diseases*, which recommended that added sugar should constitute no more than 10 percent of the calories in a healthy diet and that governments should attempt to limit children's exposure to the advertising of junk food.[82] At the behest of what might be called the junk food lobby (including the extravagantly subsidized sugar industry and its big purchasers, who make up the National Soft Drink Association), a high-level official with Health and Human Services wrote to the head of the World Health Organization and questioned the science behind the report's "linking of fruit and vegetable consumption to decreased risk of obesity and diabetes." While claiming that the U.S. government is committed to addressing "the growing challenges of obesity and chronic diseases through evidence-based policies," he complained about the report's "unsubstantiated focus on 'good' and 'bad' foods" and about its "assertion that heavy marketing of energy-dense foods or fast food outlets increases the risk of obesity."[83,84] When WHO's executive board debated these questions in January 2004, HHS Secretary Tommy Thompson emphasized the administration's commitment to the junk food lobby by including in the U.S. delegation lobbyists from the Grocery Manufacturers of America.[85]

* * *

What's truly scary about this administration's manipulation of science is that some of the consequences will linger long, long after these people are gone. Some of their policies and procedures can be reversed and potentially terrible impacts averted—global warming, most notably—if we are fortunate. Others stand to inflict longer-term structural damage to the government's ability to address issues that involve science.

For starters, good people are leaving the federal agencies. They have had it. I have mentioned the plummeting morale at the EPA. The same holds for the FDA, perhaps the most important of our public health regulatory agencies. It regulates 25 percent of the economy, in effect. It is charged with ensuring the safety of our food, medicines, and medical devices. For decades it was the model that public health authorities emulated throughout the world. Hundreds of scientists who were employed as inspectors and compliance officers with extensive technical training looked on their work with pride because they knew the importance of their contribution to public health. On this topic, Dr. Jerry Avorn, professor of medicine at the Harvard Medical School and chief of the Division of Pharmacoepidemiology and Pharmacoeconomics at Brigham and Women's Hospital in Boston, has written that the FDA was "once the most vigilant drug regulatory body in the world."[86] *Once.* In the past. When the Bush administration took office, the number of FDA "standards violations" identified by the staff remained steady, while the number of enforcement actions taken by the agency dropped by half. A 2006 report by the ever-vigilant Representative Waxman documents how attempts by inspectors to enforce the FDA's regulations are regularly overridden by central office bureaucrats (that is, the political appointees up above), who refuse to even issue warning letters.[87] As previously noted, no one can recall a situation like Plan B, where an advisory committee's overwhelming vote was arbitrarily overturned by a political appointee serving one narrow constituency. If scientists want to meet with international counterparts, including visits to the Washington, D.C., offices of the World Health Organization or the World Bank, they must clear it with the appropriate political apparatchiks weeks in advance.

Simply put, daily life for senior federal scientists has become more un-pleasant. As a result of all of this, morale is plummeting.

Adding insult to injury, the Bush administration is reducing the agency's budget. Forget Vioxx and the increasingly difficult issues of drug safety. Forget mad cow disease and the challenges of ensuring a safe food supply. Instead, starve the beast that regulates our food and our medicine. To meet these cuts, senior employees are being offered incentives to retire early.[88] Not surprisingly, many dedicated scientists who are fed up with political interference take these offers, leaving gaps that will be difficult to fill.

The problem is not confined to the FDA, however. The Union of Concerned Scientists and Public Employees for Environmental Responsibility (PEER) carried out a survey of biologists, ecologists, botanists, and other professionals who work for the U.S. Fish and Wildlife Service and found that most of the respondents were aware of political interference with scientific work. Half of the respondents rated morale as either poor or extremely poor.[89] Similar results were found in a survey of scientists at NOAA fisheries.[90]

A second long-term danger is the selective ignorance this administration practices. Much as they love uncertainty, they prefer complete ignorance—why complicate things by collecting potentially troublesome data? Corporations have played this angle for decades, but I believe this administration is the first to play it with such a vengeance in the regulatory process. Even if such policies are overturned by a future administration, what research and opportunities have been lost forever? What hazards have not been prevented? A shining example is the EPA's Toxics Release Inventory, or TRI, authorized in 1986 by the Emergency Planning and Community Right-to-Know Act.[91] As it has with so many important pieces of safety and health regulation, Congress passed this legislation in response to a disaster, specifically, the 1984 chemical release at Union Carbide's plant in Bhopal, India, that killed untold thousands, and was soon followed by a leak at a Union Carbide sister plant in West Virginia that hospitalized one hundred neighbors. The law requires facilities in certain industries that manufacture, process, or use significant amounts of toxic chemicals to report annually on their releases of these chemicals. These reports are made public through TRI for use by neighbors, community organizations, local politicians, and the news media.

Credit the TRI program with encouraging companies to markedly reduce the production and therefore the possible accidental release of toxic waste—a tremendous achievement that cost taxpayers very little.[92] Since the program kicked off in 1988, reported releases of the original 299 chemicals tracked by the TRI have dropped almost 60 percent.[93] The TRI now requires reporting on an additional three hundred chemicals—and the program continues to encourage reductions, especially in some of the newer chemicals added to the list.[94] The TRI remains a popular program with local government entities, and it has *not* proved costly to the industry, which is doing just fine despite its knee-jerk predictions to the contrary. It is not well liked by the trade associations that represent most of the major polluting industries.[95-98] In late 2006, over the opposition of a bipartisan coalition of legislators, the EPA dramatically reduced TRI reporting requirements.[99]

There is no shortage of examples of Bush administration decisions to withhold or simply not collect information that reveals policy failures. For example, on Christmas Eve 2003, the Bureau of Labor Statistics announced it would stop publishing statistics on the impact of factory closings; in the final issue of the Mass Layoff Statistics monthly report, BLS had reported that in the previous month 240,000 workers lost their jobs in 2,150 mass layoffs.[100] Similarly, when a Department of Education study found that charter schools were not superior to public schools in increasing students' academic performance,[101] the administration announced it would simply collect less data on charter schools in the future.[102]

The less-information-the-better policy has been applied to many aspects of federal policy. In their first year in office, Bush administration appointees at the Treasury Department decided to end production of reports showing how the benefits of tax cuts were distributed by income class.[103] The country may be engaged in a "global war on terror," but in 2005, following an increase in the number of terror attacks reported around the world, the State Department stopped including statistics in its annual report on international terrorism.[104]

Measures that demonstrate lack of progress in the Iraq war are particular targets, even those that had long been openly available. To ensure that the public is not given the complete picture, the Bush administration has suppressed access to previously available data on a range of measures, from the number of attacks on U.S. forces[105] to the number of hours electricity is delivered to Baghdad residents.[106]

Here is one last example of our inalienable right not to know the truth: Two networks of climate research stations that provide much of the data essential to resolving uncertainties about the role of greenhouse gas emissions and climate change received devastating budget cuts in 2005. In the following year NOAA dropped several key climate instruments from a team of satellites originally designed to monitor earth's changing climate from space.[107] Kevin Trenberth, head of the climate analysis section at the National Center for Atmospheric Research in Boulder, speaking in *Science* for many members of the scientific community, said, "It's almost as if some people don't want to know how the climate is changing. Maybe they prefer uncertainty, so that they can avoid taking action."[100]

16

Making Peace with the Past

In 1939 the great physicists of the day were thinking deeply about the military implications of Albert Einstein's famous equation, $E = mc^2$. Could the Allies use the unimaginable energy revealed by this simplest of equations to produce a new weapon of unimaginable power? Could the Nazis? The consensus among the physicists was, yes, in theory—but in theory *only*, thought Niels Bohr, the Nobel Prize winner from Denmark, "unless you turn the United States into one huge factory." Years later, Bohr said to Edward Teller, "I told you it couldn't be done without turning the whole country into a factory. You have done just that."[1]

Indeed. The speed with which America's vast nuclear weapons complex was conceived, engineered, and built was among the most notable engineering achievements of the twentieth century. Beginning in 1942, the U.S. Army constructed vast complexes in New Mexico, Tennessee, and Washington State. These were soon supplemented by dozens of other production facilities, laboratories, and nuclear test sites scattered around the country from Florida to Alaska. Unfortunately, one legacy of this remarkable effort was a level of environmental degradation never previously seen in the United States. Another, less well-known legacy is the adverse health effects among the nuclear weapons workers, who were exposed to some of the deadliest substances ever used.

As a former Assistant Secretary of Energy for Environment, Safety, and Health, I know the health story firsthand. It demonstrates that it is possible to do the right thing by sick workers in this country. Granted, the circumstances were unique, but it nonetheless holds lessons for the development of public policy that acknowledges the existence of real (rather than manufactured) scientific uncertainty without being paralyzed by it.

In the beginning, the purpose of the three primary facilities—Los Alamos, New Mexico: weapons design and final assembly; Oak Ridge, Tennessee: production of enriched uranium-235; Hanford, Washington: production of plutonium—was kept secret from the construction workers, many employees, and the public. Originally chosen because of their isolation from population centers and for the availability (in Tennessee and Washington) of massive amounts of cheap hydroelectric power, the facilities needed a massive influx of workers to operate.[2] In the spring of 1944 the construction workforce reached 60,000 at Hanford and 47,000 at Oak Ridge. The overall Oak Ridge workforce reached 82,000, half of whom were employed in operating the Tennessee facilities at the time of the victory over Japan.[3,4] Other work (primarily uranium processing) was contracted out to private facilities in Buffalo, St. Louis, Cleveland, and elsewhere across the swatch of the Northeast and the Midwest we now think of as the Rust Belt.

This original cost of this Manhattan Project was huge—about $27 billion in 2005 dollars.[5] But it was minor compared with what was to come. Following the war, the weapons complex was placed under the direction of the Atomic Energy Commission (AEC), a newly formed civilian agency that controlled the massive expansion of the weapons complex during the conflict in Korea and the Cold War. Each of the three seminal facilities doubled in size, and the prospect of a Soviet nuclear attack that could destroy any one of them dictated a policy of redundancy. As a result, far-removed sister facilities with the same capabilities as the Oak Ridge uranium enrichment plant were rushed into service in Portsmouth, Ohio, and Paducah, Kentucky. A new plutonium production facility was constructed on a twenty-four-thousand-acre reservation on the Savannah River in South Carolina to duplicate the capability of Hanford. Two new weapons laboratories, Sandia and Livermore, were built to expand the activities formerly conducted only at Los Alamos.

The scale of the secret nuclear weapons complex was breathtaking. In 1956 the weapons plants consumed 12 percent of the nation's electricity production; the three uranium-enrichment plants that separated uranium-235 from uranium-238 consumed more electricity than the daily power production of the entire Tennessee Valley Authority and the Hoover, Grand Coulee, and Bonneville dams *combined*.[6,7] Building the facilities consumed more than 11 percent of the nation's annual nickel production and one-third of its stainless steel. From 1947 to the mid-1950s the capital investment in the weapons complex exceeded the combined capital investment of DuPont, General Motors, U.S. Steel, Bethlehem Steel, Alcoa, and

Goodyear. The weapons complex expansion employed 65,000 construction workers, or five percent of all construction workers in the United States.[6] With the second wave of construction under way, the weapons plants employed almost 150,000 highly paid workers in 1953.[8] From 1945 through 1997 these men and women manufactured more than seventy thousand nuclear warheads, along with enough surplus highly enriched uranium (250 tons) and plutonium (26 tons) to make many thousands more.[9,10]

Without a doubt this was an engineering triumph—and an environmental and public health nightmare. The production of plutonium and enriched uranium are fundamentally chemical processes that require and produce enormous quantities of toxic chemicals. All in all, it is safe to say that America's nuclear weapons program and the corresponding scorched-earth campaign in the Soviet Union created what are probably the two most toxic industrial environments on earth, exposed their workers to some of the most dangerous materials known to humankind, and produced almost unimaginable quantities of insidious waste you would not wish on your worst enemies.

From the beginning, the scientists and engineers who constructed and ran the weapons complex knew of these almost unique dangers, but the army and then the AEC were much more concerned with winning World War II and the Cold War than in addressing safety and public health concerns. The exception was exposure to high levels of radiation. Protection against this threat was a high priority and was disguised as "health physics," a euphemism coined by scientists at the University of Chicago for purposes of security since it conveyed less information and would presumably draw less interest than "radiation protection."[11] Otherwise, an early (1947) memo from Oak Ridge supervisors to AEC headquarters highlights the institutional attitude:

> Papers referring to levels of soil and water contamination surrounding Atomic Energy Commission installations, idle speculation on the future genetic effects of radiation and papers dealing with potential process hazards to employees are definitely prejudicial to the best interests of the Government. Every such release is reflected in an increase in insurance claims, increased difficulty in labor relations and adverse public sentiment.[12]

When the Department of Energy (DOE) was created in 1977, it absorbed not only the weapons facilities of the Atomic Energy Commission but also that agency's disregard for public health concerns. Understandably, much of the weapons work was and still is shrouded in secrecy, and this secrecy insulated the program from the scrutiny of its own workers, the growing communities surrounding the facilities, and even other government agencies with health or environmental responsibilities. And then it got worse in the 1980s, when President Ronald Reagan ratcheted up the nuclear arms race with the Soviets, who could ill afford the enormous expense but would try to keep up with the United States anyway. There is little doubt that the enormous economic cost of that arms race substantially contributed to the collapse of that communist empire.

In this country, victory in the Cold War came with its own price. After the initial splurge in the rapid expansion of the program, capital investment had languished for several decades; the primary Oak Ridge weapons facility did not even meet local electrical codes. Nevertheless, to overwhelm the Soviets, the aging plants were operated at full throttle twenty-four hours a day, seven days a week. In short order, the significant environmental pollution problems of the 1950s, 1960s, and 1970s became *massive* environmental pollution problems that we will be paying to clean up for many years to come.

The accounts of the mismanagement of the weapons complex that surfaced in the 1980s and 1990s, which identified the enormous quantities of radioactive waste dumped in the 1950s and 1960s, were staggering:

- Among the by-products of plutonium production are highly radioactive liquid chemical mixtures; the nuclear plants produced more than 100 million gallons of this waste, the equivalent of ten thousand tanker trucks. Much of this waste has been stored in underground tanks, many of which are long past their prime and leak. The tanks had never been seen as a complete solution, though, and contained only a portion of the waste. At Hanford alone, more than 120 million gallons of liquid waste were intentionally dumped from the tanks into the ground between 1946 and 1966.[7]
- The Y-12 plant in Oak Ridge, Tennessee, used 20 million pounds of mercury to enrich lithium for hydrogen bombs from 1950 to 1963, at which point we had more than enough lithium. During those years, it is estimated that that facility alone released 550,000 pounds of the metal into the local air and water.[13] By comparison, a national debate is currently raging over the 40 tons of mercury put into the environment annually by *all* of the coal-burning power plants power in the United States.[14]
- Many of these horrors were revealed for the first time to the U.S. public in *Time* magazine's October 31, 1988, cover story, headlined "The Nuclear Scandal" and "They Lied to Us." The piece focused on

the uranium-processing plant in Fernald, Ohio, where three hundred thousand pounds of uranium had gone up the stacks. Neighbors said they had no idea this was a uranium plant. The water tower had a red-and-white checkerboard design, so some of the local people assumed it produced cattle feed or pet food.[15]

Responding to the growing pubic relations crisis—one that might have threatened the entire nuclear weapons program—President Reagan's successor, President George H. W. Bush, appointed Admiral James Watkins as the secretary of energy. Watkins sent "Tiger Teams" into all of the major and many of the minor weapons facilities, where they documented thousands of environmental, safety, and health violations. Some of the facilities were shut down pending resolution of these problems. Several facilities never reopened; all were subjected to real environmental scrutiny, some for the first time.

The tasks ahead for the weapons complex dwarf most other environmental cleanup programs. Two examples give a sense of the enormous scale of the problem. Depleted uranium hexafluoride is the primary by-product of the uranium-enrichment process. The Department of Energy is currently storing more than 700,000 metric tons (1.5 billion pounds) of this unstable, toxic material in fifty-eight thousand cylinders, a sizable portion of which are decades old and leaking.[16] Here is another staggering statistic: DOE is storing 150,000 tons of radioactive scrap metal.[17] The metal cannot easily be recycled because few scrap metal processors want to risk mixing radioactive metals into their product, so much of it will have to be buried. DOE currently estimates, probably with unwarranted optimism, that cleaning up the pollution created while manufacturing and testing our nuclear weapons will cost more than $300 billion and take most of the twenty-first century to complete.[18]

The legendary lack of concern the AEC and then DOE had for the environment was captured for me in an encounter with Representative Harold Rogers (R-KY) in 2000. I was testifying at an appropriations hearing about the planned disposal of a huge pile of radioactive scrap metal at the Paducah, Kentucky, site. The pile had been given the name "Drum Mountain" because it was primarily 55-gallon drums that had contained uranium. Representative Rogers asked me to tell him when DOE first learned of Drum Mountain. I replied that, while I had joined the department only in 1998, federal officials had been on the site since the collection of scrap began there in the 1950s. Since the pile had reached thirty-five feet in height and contained eighty-five thousand rusty, crushed metal drums (along with some residual uranium), DOE had undoubtedly known about it for many years. Representative Rogers had expected me to testify that DOE had just discovered the problem. After the hearing, he thanked me for not lying to him.

* * *

As for the workers in the weapons project, protection from the highest levels of radiation exposure was the primary focus of the government's concern. Many of the workers were not told the names or the hazardous nature of the other materials with which they worked; if they were told, they were prohibited from sharing this information with their spouses and physicians. (To this day, many workers are *still* not told this information.) If they subsequently became ill, that was just too bad. First the Atomic Energy Commission and then DOE, hand in hand with their private-sector contractors, *systematically* denied that working with some of the most hazardous materials ever known had made any workers sick. This was an utterly indefensible position, but boundless resources were expended on its behalf.

There is no danger. Therefore you are not sick. Now go back to work.

I have cited one telltale Oak Ridge memo from 1947. Here is another, dated 1948, from the AEC's Insurance Branch to its Declassification Branch, which calls for "very careful study" before releasing a Los Alamos report that found health effects from radiation exposure at levels previously thought to be safe: "We can see the possibility of a shattering effect on the morale of the employees if they became aware that there was substantial reason to question the standards of safety under which they are working. In the hands of labor unions the result of this study would add substance to demands for extra-hazardous pay. . . . [K]nowledge of the results of this study might increase the number of claims of occupational injury due to radiation and place a powerful weapon in the hands of a plaintiff's attorney."[19]

That was the prevailing attitude of the federal government—a position further revealed in the outrageous treatment afforded Dr. Tom Mancuso, one of the giants in occupational epidemiology, previously introduced in these pages through his landmark work with chromium and beryllium. In 1962, after leaving the Ohio Department of Health and joining the faculty of the School of Public Health at the University of Pittsburgh, Dr. Mancuso was awarded a contract by the AEC to conduct the largest occupational epidemiologic study to that date: the health effects of radiation among half a million workers in the nuclear weapons complex.[20] (The fact that the agency commissioned this study does reveal some concern for the workers. It was also an opportunity to look closely at the relationship of radiation and health in a huge population with significant radiation exposure, although far, far less than the survivors of Hiroshima and Nagasaki had received.)

In 1974 the AEC pressured Dr. Mancuso to repudiate findings by the Washington State epidemiologist who detected increased cancer risk among workers at the plutonium production facility in Hanford, Washington. Although his own preliminary findings did not support the other researcher's conclusion, Mancuso refused to endorse an AEC press release that disputed the study because his own findings were only preliminary. This was the responsible position, but no matter: Mancuso's AEC funding for the comprehensive study was terminated.

When the AEC chose one of its own contractors to continue the investigation, Mancuso, not trusting the independence of the new group, refused to cooperate. The AEC had to re-collect the data that he had gathered to that point while he continued with his analysis of the data he had collected.[20] He eventually published several papers that documented an elevated risk of cancer risk among the workers at Hanford.[21-24] As a result, first the AEC and then the DOE hounded him relentlessly and questioned his results with a ruthlessness that would have made the tobacco and asbestos industries proud. I believe this campaign of character assassination cut short Dr. Mancuso's career.

In the 1980s the bill for the government's cavalier attitude toward people finally came due, just about when it did for environmental degradation. Veterans of the armed forces were the first to step forward in force and demand justice when it was no longer possible to dismiss the excess cancers afflicting the group that, as uniformed soldiers, had been marched onto the Nevada Test Site three decades earlier and stationed, unprotected, near atomic tests for experimental purposes. (During the Cold War, military planners envisioned battles with Soviet troops in Europe, with conventional and nuclear weapons exploding simultaneously on all sides. Our soldiers would have to be prepared for such battlefield conditions, so the guinea pig soldiers in Nevada were given no protection other than instructions to look the other way.) These "atomic veterans," as they styled themselves to good effect, lobbied for fair compensation for the cancer cases now cropping up with disturbing regularity.[25] With the justice of the cause beyond doubt, Congress responded with the Radiation-exposed Veterans Compensation Act of 1988, which provided benefits for veterans with certain cancers who had been exposed to radiation not just from the detonations in Nevada and in the Marshall islands but also in Japan (if they had been stationed in Hiroshima or Nagasaki) and even at weapons-production facilities like Hanford, where tremendous quantities of radioactive material were released into the environment, intentionally and unintentionally.[26]

A difficult question was, what was fair compensation for the atomic veterans? Cancer caused by radiation looks the same as cancer caused otherwise. Doctors cannot tell the difference. Congress therefore linked compensation to the *likelihood* of radiation-related disease by stipulating two points. First, certain types of radiation-sensitive cancers (e.g., leukemia, multiple myeloma) were presumed to be service related and would yield automatic compensation to any soldier with radiation exposure. Second, the National Cancer Institute (NCI) was directed to develop a system to calculate the "probability of causation" for other cancers that may have additional causes.[27] Taking into account the soldier's age, dates of exposure, and the intervening time period, what is the likelihood that the radiation caused the cancer? As it happened, the survivors of the bombing of Hiroshima and Nagasaki helped the scientists at NCI develop the answers. Epidemiologic studies of these survivors provided the best available dose-effect curve. They could not identify which specific cases in Japan were caused by radiation, only that a particular exposure increased the risk by a certain amount. (Leukemia cases and other cancers of the blood and lymph system began to appear most quickly after the bombings—a few years—followed by other cancers, especially those of solid organs like the lung.)

In the end, the NCI produced what we came to call the "radio-epidemiologic tables."[28] If the probability of radiation causation was "as likely as not" (compared with the standard threshold in our civil justice system, "*more* likely than not"), the American veteran was compensated. The studies out of Japan were the best available, but there were tremendous uncertainties in exposure assessment and in the overall epidemiology, so the Veterans Administration was told to err on the side of the veteran.

Following the passage of that legislation, other individuals suffering diseases related to nuclear weapons production and testing demanded equivalent recognition and compensation. The most famous were the "downwinders," a name that hardly needed explanation. One of the key reasons the testing program had selected the U.S. Air Force base north of the then sleepy town of Las Vegas as the prime new test site in 1951 was the relative dearth of nearby human settlement. Neighboring residents were assured that little risk was associated with the radiation released in these gigantic fireballs, and such radiation as there was would certainly not affect them, even downwind. In fact, however, the AEC had known the full extent of the unique danger from the very first nuclear test, called "Trinity," detonated in the New Mexico desert a month before Hiroshima and Nagasaki. The photographic film industry understood the problem of radioactive fallout because radioactive dust from Trinity fell on an Iowa cornfield and contaminated the shucks that were used by Eastman Kodak to manufacture the paper used to separate sheets of X-ray films. The paper had enough radioactivity to cause black spots on the X-rays.[29] Years after the Nevada desert tests (finally halted in 1992), excess cancer cases were reported among the downwinders in the desert, most notably in St. George, Utah.[30]

The uranium miners in the West, many of whom were Navajo, were another group that was decimated by the weapons program. The AEC knew that these miners on the Colorado Plateau received some of the highest doses of radon (a radioactive gas that comes from the natural breakdown of uranium in rock and soil) ever recorded. I heard the story of the complicity of the U.S. government from Stewart Udall, who had served as Secretary of the Interior during the administrations of Presidents Kennedy and Johnson. On one of my many visits to the Los Alamos Laboratory, I was sent to investigate an incident in which a group of workers had been dosed with plutonium. While there, Representative Tom Udall asked me if I would like to meet his father, Stewart. I had read his father's history of the Cold War, *The Myths of August*,[31] and jumped at the chance. That night the congressman drove me to his father's adobe house in the hills. I sat riveted as Secretary Udall told me how the AEC knew that the radiation would probably kill many of these men, but the agency did and said nothing other than to silence its critics and successfully oppose every case in the courtroom.

Stewart Udall had grown up on the edge of the Navajo reservation in Arizona. When he returned west after his government service, he took up the cause of these uranium miners and brought suit against the government. The former Interior secretary told me about the visits he and Tom, just out of law school, had paid their clients, the Navajo uranium miners and their widows, to learn about what these workers had endured while mining uranium for nuclear weapons. He documented the complicity of the AEC and the U.S. Public Health Service in allowing thousands of miners to work in an environment so full of radon that a sizable proportion would inevitably develop lung cancer. The government scientists provided regular medical examinations but were required to say nothing that might alarm the miners. As a result, physicians from the federal health agency did nothing to prevent the ensuing lung cancer epidemic but watch it unfold.[31]

The Navajos and the Udalls did not prevail. The court ruled for the government, which had successfully asserted its "sovereign immunity" in cases where the national security could be invoked.

In 1990, two years after passing the legislation that compensated the atomic veterans, Congress responded to public demand and passed the Radiation Exposure Compensation Act (RECA), which covered the downwinders and the uranium miners, as well as civilian test site workers.[32] The sponsors of the legislation had wanted to use the science-based solution— the "probability of causation" tables—for this new compensation program as well, but the residents of southern Utah, by this point profoundly distrustful of the government, insisted on "presumptions" only.[33] If a downwinder or a test-site civilian lived in a certain county or were on a test site at the time of detonation and developed one of the common "radiogenic" cancers, compensation would be automatic. The government adopted this presumption approach and extended it to the uranium miners. Lung cancer or noncancerous lung disease would be presumed to be work related and therefore compensable if the individual had worked a certain number of months in a mine with high radiation levels. The payment schedule eventually determined was the result of political compromise: $100,000 for a uranium miner, $75,000 for a test-site participant, and $50,000 for a downwinder.

The immediate problem was that the RECA program was given to the Department of Justice (DOJ) to administer, and it has always been a stepchild in that agency. The compensation payments were not funded as entitlements like the veterans' benefits, always and automatically payable. Compensation was simply a part of the DOJ's budget and thus competed for funding with law enforcement and justice activities. The department never asked for enough money for RECA, and Congress never allocated enough. In 2000 RECA actually ran out of money. Widows of uranium miners who had died of lung cancer received an IOU letter from the U.S. government.[34]

* * *

This is where matters stood in 1998, when President Bill Clinton appointed me as the Assistant Secretary of Energy for Environment, Safety, and Health. The compensation program for the atomic veterans worked fairly well, and the program for miners and test-site civilians and downwinders was in place, although underfunded. Only the civilian employees at the many weapons facilities around the country had been left completely out in the cold—workers who had been exposed in some cases to toxic peril, including exposure to beryllium, plutonium, and uranium, just as injurious as that faced by the other groups.

The legend around DOE was that not a single worker in the weapons program had ever successfully filed a worker's compensation claim—never, over a span of fifty years. I can report that this was a *slight* exaggeration. I was able to identify a small number of cases that successfully went through the state "workers' comp" systems, but there is no question that most workers did not even bother to file claims. They knew that the AEC, then the DOE, threw powerful resources at any worker who dared to file a claim. The government could have acted responsibly, but instead it reimbursed contractors for any expenses incurred in their efforts to deny compensation to the workers, whether in the workers' compensation system or in litigation.[35] Word of this policy spread among the employees, and most of them took the path of least resistance: *Do not even bother filing.*

Moreover, many workers were trapped by the time limits the states imposed to file a claim. In Pennsylvania, for example, where a number of beryllium factories had been located, any workers' comp claim had to be filed within three hundred weeks (less than six years) after the last exposure.

However, as we learned in a previous chapter, chronic beryllium disease (CBD) is progressive and may not be recognized or even manifest itself for years after the final exposure, and then it might not be correctly diagnosed. These workers' factories, owned by private manufacturers who sold beryllium products to the AEC, had closed years earlier. The workers with CBD were simply out of luck.

Even when sick workers' employers have not disappeared, getting compensated for occupational illness is a rare event. Most workers in the weapons complex are considered private sector workers since they are employed by the contractor the government hired to run the facility. As a result, they are covered under antiquated state workers' compensation laws, which were first enacted in the early twentieth century to provide monetary benefits to workers who are injured or the families of workers killed on the job. Most states (Texas is an exception) require employers to carry workers' compensation insurance to cover medical expenses, wage-loss payments, and rehabilitation and death benefits.

Historically, the principal function of the system was to provide benefits to injured workers, who exchanged their right to sue their employer for guaranteed, if modest, benefits. Previously, injured workers had no option for compensation other than litigation against their employers. The legal arguments used by employers who were defending these suits often prevented injured workers and their families from receiving any compensation whatsoever, although a small proportion of injured workers were victorious in court.

Several features characterize all state-based workers' compensation insurance systems. They provide a portion of lost wages (although, as we will see, not a very large portion) along with "first-dollar" coverage of medical expenses, so there are no deductibles or copayments for the covered service. With very few exceptions, the workers' compensation system is the injured workers' exclusive remedy for compensation; every state system precludes workers from suing their employer, no matter who is at fault for the injury. Moreover, having been constructed in an era before the environmental causation of chronic disease was recognized, the systems are almost incapable of dealing with most occupational diseases that first appear years after exposure.

By the mid 1990s hundreds of cases of beryllium disease among the weapons workers had been diagnosed, and more were appearing each month. The Oil, Chemical, and Atomic Workers Union (now part of the United Steelworkers of America), which represented the largest number of DOE workers, was raising the workers' compensation issue in Washington but getting little traction. For the most part, the agency stuck to the position that no evidence existed that workers had been sickened by such hazardous exposures in the weapons complex; it had spent millions of dollars defending this position against the claims of sick workers. In early 1998 an acting secretary had issued an order to stop fighting all CBD claims, but the mandate had not worked. Dozens of CBD sufferers from the Rocky Flats weapons plant were still in "comp courts" in Colorado, and it was a legal debacle. Different insurance companies who had provided coverage to the contractor at different times each insisted that some other carrier was responsible for the problem, and, because of the way the contracts were written, the U.S. government was paying for the legal costs of *all* parties—except those borne by the sick workers. Some of the workers tried to get out of the workers' compensation system's exclusive remedy and sue the U.S. government since it was not the official employer. While these cases were very expensive for the government to contest, they never produced the desired results for the workers (sovereign immunity, again), even though there was and still is little question that the DOE's beryllium had caused their CBD. It was truly a lose-lose situation.

The Department of Energy faced a serious problem with its "deny and defend" policy. I had just been sworn in and had not even organized my desk when my boss, Secretary of Energy Bill Richardson, who had taken office only a few months earlier himself, called me into his office for my first big assignment. Some weeks before, a group of sick workers in Oak Ridge, Tennessee, had made their anger known to the secretary in very explicit terms. Richardson did not know the long history of stonewalling within the weapons program. He was caught off guard. "Go to Oak Ridge immediately," he said to me. "Give them a message. Tell them I want to help."

That was on a Friday. On Monday I flew to Oak Ridge, my first visit to this famed, federally planned community where the three main facilities were coded-named Y-12, K-25, and X-10. (The first two kept their code names; X-10 was eventually renamed Oak Ridge National Laboratory, although the old-timers still call it X-10.) Until 1955 residents could not even own their own homes at Oak Ridge. In the early years black residents were segregated by federal decree in one neighborhood and then resettled in another immediately adjacent to Y-12.

That evening I had a private meeting with about two dozen of the sick workers. At their insistence, no local DOE officials attended; quite simply, the workers did not trust their bosses. At the meeting I did something no DOE national official had done with these brave men and women in years: I listened. One by one, they described in detail how the government refused to acknowledge that their claim for compensation might have any validity whatsoever. Asking for their medical records to show to their doctors, they received photocopies with whole sections blacked out—"classified" information. If they complained about their treatment, they felt, and with plenty of justification, that their security clearances would be pulled and their jobs endangered. Lawsuits were not going anywhere. Beryllium suits, specifically, had been dismissed under the government's same claims of sovereign immunity that had stymied the uranium miners' quest for justice. The meeting finally broke up after midnight.

Based only on the descriptions I heard that night, I felt that some of the illnesses described were probably caused by toxic exposure at Oak Ridge, some pretty clearly were not so caused, and about others I just was not sure. Crystal clear, however, were two facts: These civilian workers had put themselves in harm's way while producing the nuclear weapons on which this nation had relied for its defense for half a century, and they had not been informed of the dangers, for the most part, much less provided with adequate protection. Their government owed them a fair hearing. It was that simple.

Secretary Richardson agreed with me—and gave me sixty days to come up with a plan. Two decisions were easy: The various states' workers' compensation programs would never do justice here, and the eventual claims process, in whatever form, should be removed from the DOE, which had lost all credibility with these workers and their communities—and for good reason. These cases were relegated to the state workers' compensation systems because these workers were all classified as private sector workers, but that seemed to me to be not much more than a convenient fiction that protected both the government and the contractors. The workers were employed by a private contractor, but they worked for the U.S. government. After all, when the management of Oak Ridge was transferred from Union Carbide to Martin Marietta (later Lockheed Martin) in 1984, the top dozen or so managers changed, but every one of the workers punched the same clock on Monday morning. Nothing changed. They were de facto federal workers, and they needed a *federal* workers' compensation program comparable to the Federal Employees' Compensation Act (FECA) program, which covers millions of other federal employees from office custodians to cabinet secretaries.

Administered by the Department of Labor, FECA is not a perfect system, but it is far better than any state system. In the first place, it is not adversarial by nature. The "employer" (that is, the federal agency at which the injured party works) has no role other than to supply information; the agency cannot fight a worker's claim, as many employers and insurance carriers do in the private sector, almost as a matter of course. The federal benefits are not ridiculously insufficient and unfair, as are those of every state system. In most states, lost wage compensation payments to higher-paid private-sector workers, like those employed in the nuclear weapons complex, are capped at two-thirds of the state's median wage. Injured federal workers get two-thirds of their lost wages tax free, no matter what the wage; if they have dependants, they get 75 percent.

I proposed a new federal compensation program based in the Department of Labor, one that would have a benefit structure the same as that of all federal agencies. This seemed eminently fair. The White House—specifically, the Office of Management and Budget—agreed with our assessment *in part*. Officials at OMB gave the okay to move forward on cases of chronic beryllium disease and to set up a new program that would apply the FECA principles. However, OMB asked for an interagency process to determine whether other illnesses were occurring and whether the state compensation systems were indeed inadequate for compensating those workers.

Once the Department of Energy announced this change in policy—this change in *attitude*—the floodgates opened. *You mean our government is going to stop fighting us and start helping us instead?* Workers could hardly believe their ears. Those who had felt they could not talk out of fear of reprisal came forward to tell their stories. Whistleblowers and others who had raised health and safety concerns and who had been shunned if not discriminated against felt vindicated. At my first meeting in Oak Ridge a few months earlier, I had learned the power of simply listening to these workers tell their stories, and I believed this power could be magnified with a series of such meetings. We subsequently organized a listening tour among communities across the nation. In this way we could address, to some extent, OMB's concerns, start the healing process, and make a measure of peace with the past.

Coincidentally or otherwise, our listening tour had not even begun when a scandal at the Paducah, Kentucky, uranium enrichment plant broke on the front page of the *Washington Post*.[36] A lawsuit had been filed in secret alleging that Lockheed Martin and Union Carbide, the first two contractors to operate the Paducah plant, had cheated the federal government by collecting million-dollar fees for operating the plant while concealing evidence of environmental contamination by plutonium and other radioactive materials (charges which the contractors have denied). This was what lawyers call a *qui tam* lawsuit, one that is filed in secret in order to give the Justice Department a chance to investigate the charges and perhaps join the action on behalf of the original plaintiffs. That decision is supposed to be made within six months. After three *years* the government finally decided to join the lawsuit.[37]

The scene in Paducah was bad. Our oversight team had to search through documents that had been stored in barrels contaminated with radioactive waste. Once retrieved, however, the documents presented a damning case, a decades-long legacy of poor safety and health practices.[38]

Workers were never warned that the uranium with which they were working was contaminated with plutonium and neptunium. Management did not evaluate the exposure because, if it had, the workers' union would have demanded hazard pay.[39] Shameless, but not surprising. As we have seen, this was standard operating procedure in many industries. If an employer did not officially investigate a hazardous condition and put peril to paper, and if it could then pretend not to know about that danger, how could it be held responsible later?

The Paducah scandal made us wonder whether the uranium at the uranium-enrichment plants in Oak Ridge and Portsmouth might also have been contaminated with plutonium. The investigators headed to those two sites, and no one was surprised to learn that the work at the plants had been integrated to such an extent that uranium contaminated with plutonium contaminated all three facilities.[40,41] The situation that all of these workers faced resembled that of the downwinders and civilian test-site workers in Utah and Nevada, as well as the uranium miners. The government was complicit in their exposure, but it would be difficult to assess that exposure precisely because the government and its contractor had not kept good records. We decided these workers must be covered in new RECA-like legislation.

In town after town around the country—beginning in Paducah—everyone was invited to the DOE town hall meeting, and many of them showed up: workers, former workers, spouses, children, grandchildren, friends, neighbors, and businesspeople. Anyone could testify; some of the evening meetings went well past midnight. Taking our listening tour to most of the major sites, we held nine public meetings in ten months. Generally, the story led the local evening news broadcast and was on the front page in the local newspaper the following morning.

For our meeting with workers at the Portsmouth uranium-enrichment plant in Ohio, we rented the largest conference room available in Piketon, the town nearest the plant. This was the poorest area in Ohio, and the plant provided the only well-paid jobs for miles around. We were concerned that the workers, afraid they might lose their jobs or that the plant might even close following their revelations, would not talk openly about the working conditions. But talk they did, and listening were their two senators, George Voinovich and Mike DeWine, and Representative Ted Strickland.[42] Members of Congress have tremendously busy schedules. When I saw all three of these men sitting in this packed room, I understood how important this issue had become. As a result of their experience listening to these workers, all three of these legislators became powerful advocates for the program.

At Los Alamos, New Mexico, the iconic cradle of the entire nuclear weapons program, we set up a separate area in the meeting room for people who did not want to be seen or videotaped. Such was the culture of fear and paternalism that permeated the place. I had raised this concern with representatives of the University of California, the institution that had operated the Los Alamos National Laboratory since its inception, and they issued a strong statement assuring workers they could participate without fear of reprisals. Still, the seating area that ensured anonymity filled up quickly. Senator Jeff Bingaman and Representative Tom Udall issued stern warnings to the University of California not to take reprisals against these workers. They pledged their best efforts to make a fair compensation program a reality.[43]

In Iowa we set up shop in the Mississippi River town of Burlington, the home of the Iowa Army Ammunition Plant, which many years earlier had been an AEC-run nuclear weapons assembly plant until that function was moved to the newer Pantex facility in Amarillo, Texas. We had not planned to visit Burlington since it was no longer a DOE facility and therefore did not have any current safety and health concerns, but Senator Tom Harkin asked us to add this venue. He had been contacted by Robert Anderson, a constituent who had served as a security officer at Burlington decades earlier, now had lymphoma, and thought it might be related to radiation.

Senator Harkin and Secretary Richardson hosted that meeting. One man told us that he had honored his pledge of secrecy—not saying a word about his work for twenty-five years after the plant had closed—because the AEC had never released these workers from their pledge. Loyal Americans, they had never said a word. There were many wet eyes in the audience that night. Secretary Richardson apologized to this man and the other workers and released them from their pledge of secrecy.

At the Pantex plant in Amarillo, we were reminded that the bad old days were not over yet. A Pantex machinist, Pete López, explained to us that he had been screened for beryllium disease and confirmed as "sensitized"; that is, his immune system was reacting to the metal, and he was likely on his way to beryllium disease. López needed to be removed from any beryllium exposure and to get regular medical follow-up. With the assistance of the plant physician, he had applied for state workers' compensation benefits. This should have been an easy case. The agency itself had diagnosed the disease, and it was agency policy not to contest beryllium disease claims. There was not even an insurance carrier to fight, and DOE was going to pay the costs of the claim. Nevertheless, the company that DOE hired to process claims did what it always did and what it had been instructed to do: deny the claim while providing the standard ludicrous explanation that beryllium disease "is an ordinary disease of life" and therefore not work related. This was not 1950 or 1960 or even 1990. The date stamped on the denial was May 31, 2000, almost two months *after* Secretary Richardson announced our intention to compensate all valid work-related claims. In Amarillo we got a better understanding that our efforts to make peace with the past could run up against an institutional commitment to *defend* that past.[44]

In Las Vegas press coverage was dominated by interviews with Wayne Cates, whose lungs had been destroyed by silicosis and who was now hoping a lung would become available through the transplant network. Silicosis is an ancient, now *completely preventable* disease. Nevada senator Harry Reid had a special understanding of silicosis; his own father was a miner who had suffered from the disease. The senator made it quite clear that the government had failed to protect these workers from silica dust, that they had the standard difficulties gaining compensation through the workers' compensation system, and that he wanted the federal program to cover the workers who were afflicted with silicosis.

Agency staffers in our nation's capital are often disparaged as "bureaucrats," but our interagency team with staff from Labor, HHS, and other agencies did a remarkable job designing a program that would be fair to both the sick workers and the taxpayers, who were footing the bill. Once we completed our public meetings and the data gathering phase of our work, we received permission from the White House to expand the compensation program beyond the previously authorized beryllium component to the other illnesses caused by toxic exposures at the plants. Accompanied by eleven members of Congress, Secretary Richardson made the historic announcement. With the backing of the Clinton White House and a groundswell of local support from the affected communities (often organized by the tireless Richard Miller, the union policy analyst who was a walking encyclopedia on the DOE system), momentum for the legislation grew. Legislators from all ends and angles of the political spectrum, from Senator Ted Kennedy of Massachusetts to Senator Strom Thurmond of South Carolina, cosponsored our bill. Lobbied hard by their increasingly vocal constituents, other members of Congress, both Republicans and Democrats, introduced *their own,* more generous versions of the compensation legislation.

However, the measure met outright opposition from other precincts within the government, including the Nuclear Regulatory Commission (NRC), the agency charged with ensuring the safe use of nuclear materials, especially at commercial nuclear reactors. The NRC seemed to believe that radiation at levels other than the highest is not particularly hazardous to human beings. I always presumed this stance was simply a means of defending the nuclear power industry, which feared having to compensate *its own* workers if DOE started a radiation disease compensation program. (The NRC is overly sympathetic to the commercial reactor operators. This is not surprising; government agencies are often advocates for certain commercial interests.)

So the NRC pushed back, but the NRC carries little weight in Washington. The real problem was the heaviest hitter of them all, the Department of Defense, which faced many of the same problems DOE faced—civilian workers who had been exposed to beryllium, radiation, nerve gas, rocket fuel, munitions, and asbestos—and had never addressed any of them. The Pentagon could not even tell us how many of its people were exposed to beryllium. It had never run *any* sort of CBD medical surveillance program. It was opposed to the whole idea of a federal program compensating private-contractor workers. From its blinkered perspective, this would be a terrible, dangerous precedent, given the tens of thousands of naval shipyard workers who had developed lung disease as a result of exposure to asbestos (widely used as an insulating material aboard ships). These shipyards were government owned but operated by private contractors, analogous to DOE's nuclear weapons facilities. The industry had tried to shift the blame to the federal government by claiming that the asbestos suppliers were only following government procurement specifications. Many workers had successfully sued the asbestos manufacturers, but the Department of Justice had always been successful in shielding the government from liability in these claims. Now the Pentagon was concerned that a new program to compensate nuclear weapons workers would open the floodgates for the shipyard workers.

We argued that DOE's situation was unique, primarily because it had always taken full responsibility for protecting exposed workers by developing standards for exposure to radiation and beryllium long before OSHA. The AEC would even shut down facilities from which they purchased beryllium products if they failed to meet the standards. (As it turns out, the standards were not fully protective, but at least there were standards.) Caught in the middle of this internecine bureaucratic battle was the Justice Department, whose very capable and caring attorneys were supportive of our objectives but who were also charged with protecting the government from liability claims, particularly asbestos litigation. So we crafted a compromise. Stipulating that nuclear weapons production was fundamentally different from other government work, we proposed splitting the compensation program into two parts. One would be a new federal program for workers who were made sick by exposure to beryllium or radiation, hazards considered unique to nuclear weapons. The second part of the program would assist those who were sick from exposures *other than* beryllium or radiation (including asbestos) to receive compensation through the state workers' compensation systems. In this new Worker Advocacy Program, the DOE was supposed to serve as the workers' advocate rather than opponent.

One cliché in Washington holds that the perfect is the enemy of the good. It is true, and this part of the program was explicitly designed to mollify the Pentagon and the Justice Department—a political compromise we swallowed because it was a great start. If we could not help all of the sick workers for which the government was at least partially responsible, at least we would help some of them. Another cliché holds that a camel is a horse designed by a committee. In the nation's capital, how true it is. Historians who look back on this legislation will shake their heads in wonder at the strange beast with all the weird appendages. The final compromise provided $150,000 for each sick worker or the survivors, plus full reimbursement for those medical costs incurred after applying for compensation. To bring them to parity, Representative Henry Hyde (R-IL) insisted that the widows of the uranium miners who had received $100,000 under RECA would receive another $50,000, plus medical benefits.[45] The final act was twenty-one pages, and it has already been amended twice; I would need a page or more to outline the simplest explanation of its provisions, but suffice it to say that passage of the Energy Employees Occupational Illness Compensation Program Act (EEOICPA) was a huge victory for the workers of the nuclear weapons complex.

The hard work of actually implementing much of the compensation program fell to the Department of Labor, which has performed admirably by quickly staffing up, writing regulations, and cutting the first checks in less than a year after the legislation passed (many were written to the widows of workers who had died decades earlier).

Would that the same could be said of the Department of Energy. Its implementation was farcically incompetent at best and intentionally subversive at worst. (Within that agency, the job fell to the Worker Advocacy Program, which had also been charged with helping employees with their work-related disease claims before the state workers' compensation programs.) After four years and more than $90 million, the agency had managed to compensate thirty-one workers.[46,47] Fortunately, the program never lost its strong, bipartisan congressional support; after an ugly hearing in which she was berated by a group of Republican senators for neglecting the program, the individual President Bush appointed to succeed me as Assistant Secretary of Energy for Environment, Safety and Health resigned to "spend more time with her family." Congress then fired the DOE and turned the rest of the implementation job over to the Department of Labor.

Since our program was set up as an entitlement, with mandatory payment made without the need for congressional appropriations, the Justice Department sheepishly approached the White House and asked permission to introduce legislation that would make the always underfunded RECA program an equivalent entitlement so that the surviving wives of uranium miners would not receive an IOU from the government if their program ran out of funds again. In 2004 Congress finally passed this legislation, thereby ensuring that these recipients would be fully paid out through the new Department of Labor program.[48]

My greatest regret regarding the program? That name! I had proposed the Energy-related Occupational Illness Compensation Act because it yielded a sweet acronym, EROICA. Like Beethoven's *Third Symphony*, whose dedication referred to heroism (after the composer had ripped up a dedication to his former hero, Napoleon), this acronym for the new program would signify that these civilian workers, having put themselves in harm's way defending their country, were also heroes. But the Pentagon objected fiercely: EROICA—EROTICA—too close for comfort and an invitation for ridicule and sarcasm, they claimed. I think they just did not want to venerate a program they fundamentally opposed. I gave in, and now this program, which has disbursed more than $3 billion to sick workers and their survivors, is saddled with the meaningless, unpronounceable acronym EEOICPA.

17

Four Ways to Make the Courts Count

In the public mind, the regulation of the corporations—good and bad—is the job of the EPA, OSHA, FDA, and other agencies in the executive branch that perform their duties as authorized by Congress. These agencies are seen as the mechanism through which the government attempts to compel corporations to act responsibly, and to not damage our health and the environment. In fact, however, the third branch of the government—the judicial system—also plays a crucial role in this effort. If the tide has turned against the entire tobacco industry—and I believe it has—it is not due to actions by the FDA or the EPA, although the pioneering work of both of these agencies raised public consciousness and helped reveal the workings of the tobacco industry. Rather, it is because the cigarette manufacturers have lost legal battles waged by the widows and widowers of deceased smokers and by the states attempting to recoup the taxpayers' money spent providing medical care for smoking-related diseases. As strong as it was and still is, the strength of the science did not convince Philip Morris to admit that tobacco causes lung cancer. Only after being pummeled by much detrimental and expensive litigation has the cigarette maker come up with a new strategy that involves telling at least the partial truth. Similarly, the asbestos industry was tamed neither by OSHA and EPA nor by a frank acknowledgment of the science but by lawsuits brought against Johns Manville and other producers filed by victims of mesothelioma, lung cancer, and asbestosis.

Tobacco and asbestos are the best-known examples, but in industry after industry it has been litigation that has uncovered and published the damning

232

facts about hazards and toxicity. I have referred to many such lawsuits, and the courts have heard many, many more. The manufacturer of the infamous Dalkon Shield contraceptive device, A. H. Robins, did little safety testing on its product and concealed the unfavorable results it had at hand.[1,2] This device would have damaged the reproductive capabilities of many more women had not lawsuits revealed the truth. The manufacturer of the diet-drug combination Fen-Phen concealed numerous reports of pulmonary hypertension that were brought to light thanks only to legal discovery.[3] Moreover, with the pharmaceutical companies, the revolt of the medical journal editors was an important turning point for the reform movement, as we have seen, but I believe the intervention of New York attorney general (later governor) Eliot Spitzer may have made the biggest difference. In June 2004 Spitzer filed suit against GlaxoSmithKline (GSK), charging that the pharmaceutical company had concealed unfavorable scientific studies on the efficacy and safety of the antidepressant Paxil for children. Specifically, he alleged that GSK had withheld data that adolescents who were taking Paxil were at increased risk of suicidal thoughts and acts.[4] Less than a month later GSK announced it would release the clinical data on the safety and effectiveness of Paxil, as well as of other drugs it manufactures.

Spitzer's efforts have already paid out additional public health dividends. Cleveland Clinic cardiologist Steven Nissen suspected that GSK's Avandia (rosiglitazone), one of the nation's largest selling diabetes drugs, might also cause heart disease. Dr. Nissen accessed GSK's now public clinical trial data base and, combining data from 42 studies, confirmed what he had feared (but what the FDA's system to detect drug-related adverse events could never detect): that diabetics taking Avandia were at significantly increased risk of heart attacks.[5,6]

Litigation works, and it will need to work overtime in the years ahead. Unless the regulatory system is radically restructured and strengthened, it will never have both the carrots and the sticks necessary to ensure responsible corporate behavior. Even then, the agencies still need the willpower and the political support to use them. Given the all-out assault on the very idea of regulation by the corporations and their allies in the Republican Party and this second Bush administration, what will prevent the federal regulatory agencies from getting weaker and weaker? The way things are going, litigation could end up being just about all we have.

The Ford-Firestone tire debacle is an excellent case in point. Soon after Ford began marketing the Explorer SUV equipped with the ATX Bridgestone/Firestone tires in the early 1990s, both manufacturers received the first reports of accidents involving tire tread separations. So many problems cropped up in Arizona that the state procurement office asked Firestone to replace all ATX tires that had been bought under state contracts.

That was in 1996. Ford dealers in tropical countries (where the heat led to more separations) also took note of the tread separations and in Saudi Arabia, Thailand, and Malaysia offered to replace the dangerous tires. Nevertheless, neither company notified the National Highway Traffic Safety Administration (NHTSA) of the problem or their actions taken overseas. This agency, charged with preventing vehicle-related deaths and injuries, was apparently not a regulator that needed to be taken seriously. It was aware of at least some of the tire tread separations, however, because State Farm Insurance filed notices of twenty-one specific cases with NHTSA. That was in 1998. Yet NHTSA did nothing. The next year State Farm sent in thirty more reports, but each was greeted with more inaction. The *next* year a TV station in Houston aired the first widely publicized investigation. Firestone denied the veracity of the report, but the damage was done, and NHTSA was shamed into opening an investigation.[7]

Now compare the paralysis of NHTSA with the activity in the courts. The first lawsuits that alleged personal injury due to the tire defects were filed in 1995, shortly after the tires were introduced, and continued to accumulate at a steady pace. In fact, much of the information that made headlines following the television report was originally unearthed by these lawsuits. In theory, the mission of public health regulatory agencies is to identify serious risks and take preventive actions that minimize the number of people hurt. NHTSA's actions came after the pressure of litigation had already compelled the industry to improve tire safety. No evidence suggests that NHTSA, without the litigation and the ensuing media coverage, would ever have acted at all. On November 1, 2000, Congress provided the agency with more authority to require recalls and to increase penalties for failure to report defects.[8] By then, tread separations had already resulted in accidents that killed more than one hundred people, while hundreds more suffered nonfatal injuries. Massive recalls and tire replacements were under way, all necessitated by the spotlight directed on this scandal by lawsuits.[7,9]

Bronchiolitis obliterans caused by diacetyl, the artificial butter flavor ingredient, is a similar story. As we have already seen, OSHA would not and, short of an act of Congress, will not issue standards to protect the workers in microwave popcorn plants from the deadly vapors that have destroyed so many lungs. No doubt the more than $100 million awarded to sick workers will encourage the flavor manufacturers to prevent more cases and protect their employees.

Lawsuits also work as an engine that powers technological progress. A study by the Rand Corporation concluded that potential liability was the single most important factor in shaping decisions on product design.[7] The chemical industry acknowledges that litigation avoidance plays a central role in promoting responsible corporate behavior.[10] Everyone in the business world would agree, and this is why industry lobbyists and the Bush administration are working hard to convince Congress, state legislatures, and the American people to limit the ability of injured individuals to receive compensation through the judicial system. They call this "tort reform." Like their efforts to cripple our environmental health protection system by clamoring for "sound science," this campaign is designed to let corporations off the hook when they endanger our lives and health. It is profoundly cynical and profoundly dangerous because in many industries the courts are just about the only check we still have on the unlimited resources of corporations. Instead of making it ever harder for cases involving toxic exposures and product defects to be heard in court, we should acknowledge the courts as a critical component of the public health system and develop policies that promote this role. To this end I put forward four proposals.

1. No More Court-Sanctioned Secrecy

Courts are a repository of large amounts of information that is potentially important in public health protection. Every chapter of this book contains material that was uncovered during the discovery process in a legal proceeding: documents that prove industry campaigns to manufacture uncertainty; others that prove corporate knowledge of significant health hazards years, if not decades, before they were acknowledged; and vital scientific studies that should have been in the literature but were hidden by their corporate sponsors. It is almost always in the public's interest to place these documents in the public domain, but defendants, who want to avoid bad publicity and the encouragement of additional lawsuits, are often willing to offer the plaintiff a more generous settlement in return for secrecy. Seduced by the larger settlements, plaintiffs and their attorneys have little incentive to oppose the practice, and judges benefit by clearing their dockets of complex, time-consuming litigation. So the deal is done, and the documents are sealed from public view, sequestered forever. The loser is society. Secrecy diminishes our ability to both identify public health and safety hazards and prevent further harm.

Protective orders and secrecy agreements have hidden critical evidence of hazards associated with dozens of materials, products, and processes: automobiles, medicines, child car seats, BB guns, toys, cigarette lighters, school lunch tables, water slides, and many more.[11,12] No price is paid by the parties involved—to the contrary, it is a win-win deal for them—while the public and regulators are left in the dark. Secrecy agreements are a nefarious practice, and the courts have the means of limiting if not eradicating them. Some do so. The judges of the U.S. District Court for the District of

South Carolina have issued rules "disfavoring court-ordered secrecy in cases affecting public safety,"[13] but they appear to be in the minority on the federal bench. Judges in toxic tort cases may consider this issue in approving secrecy agreements, but such consideration does not carry the day often enough.

How could the courts put some teeth into rules to discourage the sealing of important documents? Dan Givelber, former dean of the Northeastern University School of Law, and Tony Robbins, former head of NIOSH, the U.S. National Vaccine Program, and two state health departments, have coauthored an intriguing proposal. They suggest that, if harm has been caused by a hazard that was the subject of previously sealed documents, a jury could use that earlier secrecy agreement as good cause for assessing punitive damages in this later case. With such a rule in place, secrecy agreements would not be a risk-free default position; for hiding the truth, the corporation could pay a steep price the next time around.[11]

Ending this practice will come down to the judges and the rules established for them. It is their responsibility to protect the public. They should do so.

2. Allow Injured Workers to Sue Their Employers

Injured workers are generally barred from suing their employers, no matter how negligent those employers may have been with regard to conditions in the workplace. Instead, the employees must rely on limited benefits provided through dysfunctional state workers' compensation systems. No other recourse is allowed. This feature of the workers' compensation system (called the "exclusive remedy") has contributed to numerous outrages over the decades, including the abysmal failure of the compensation system in a dozen different states where nuclear weapons workers developed beryllium and radiation-related diseases. The federal government finally did the right thing and developed its own system for compensating sick employees in that industry. Similarly, the federal black lung program was set up because the compensation systems in the coal-producing states failed to prevent pauperization of sick miners and their families. On the other hand, some states have made exceptions to the exclusive remedy rule in egregious cases in which the employer willfully failed to take preventive actions that were obviously necessary to mitigate workplace hazards. As a result, the large monetary awards in a small number of the lawsuits are probably much more effective than fear of an OSHA inspection in encouraging employers to control hazards.

A case in point is window washing. Clearly, workers in this inherently dangerous trade must be provided with adequate training and equipment, but Kansas City window washer Les James received no training from his employer, Quality Window Cleaning, before starting work one morning in July 2000. Less than an hour later, this twenty-five-year-old father of three fell to his death. The investigation revealed similar fatalities of Quality employees four years earlier. On that occasion OSHA had issued no penalty; with this second death it hit Quality with a fine of $2,700 (no missing zeroes: two thousand seven hundred dollars). Because of the prior fatality and the company's clear obligation to provide training, the James family was able to overcome the exclusive remedy bar and sue Quality Window Cleaning. The judge awarded the family $7.2 million as compensation for the company's negligence.[14-16]

It is reasonable to assume that such awards send a stronger message to window-washing firms across the nation than did the single OSHA fine for $2,700. (In 2002 yet another Quality Window Cleaning worker fell to his death, and again OSHA issued no penalty.) With the dramatic weakening of OSHA, the state legislatures should eliminate the workers' compensation "exclusive remedy" in cases in which the employer is guilty of what OSHA itself terms "willful" violations of safety and health regulations.

3. Develop Better Compensation Systems

The blanket preemption of lawsuits by injured parties is generally bad policy, but several times Congress has established reasonable-alternative compensation programs for victims who under normal circumstances might have sued manufacturers. From the public health perspective, the most important of these programs is the National Vaccine Injury Compensation Program, which is designed to ensure that anyone injured by a vaccine will be fairly compensated and that vaccine manufacturers will remain in the market. In this program, families cannot file a lawsuit until they have finished pursuing a claim for compensation through the VICP, but such a preemption of lawsuits is not necessary in order for these programs to work. When we in the Department of Energy were designing the Energy Employees Occupational Illness Compensation Program (EEOICPA) for the compensation of the nuclear weapons workers, the beryllium industry lobbied hard for a clause that would preempt all suits against it. I felt this would be bad policy and a bad principle. Instead, I recommended to the Clinton White House that we structure our program as a *nonexclusive* compensation scheme. Workers could either accept this no-hassle, fair compensation in return for dropping action against the federal government and its contractors or opt out and pursue their lawsuits in the courts. The nonexclusive approach was adopted, and it has been an unqualified success. To my knowledge, every single lawsuit brought by a nuclear weapons worker or family member has been dropped, and the victims and their families have received compensation.

The same approach is now becoming standard in alternative compensation programs. Less than a year after Congress acted on behalf of the weapons workers, the World Trade Center and the Pentagon were attacked on September 11, 2001. Congress immediately moved to protect the airline industry from what the industry viewed as possibly ruinous litigation by the surviving families. With amazing and bipartisan dispatch, Congress adopted the approach we used for the weapons workers: The 9/11 families were assured of generous compensation from the federal government in exchange for an agreement not to sue it or the airlines. With a handful of exceptions, the widows and widowers of 9/11 accepted this offer.

The rationale of these programs is straightforward: Federal intervention is necessary to ensure that victims receive fair compensation without damaging an industry or group of corporations whose work is important to the national good. In addition, the federal government fulfills its important regulatory role in each of these industries because the incentive for responsible corporate behavior—fear of future litigation stemming from *new* occurrences—is retained.

Similarly, the rescue and recovery workers who inhaled clouds of toxic dust at Ground Zero in the weeks after 9/11 should not be forced to navigate the byzantine New York State workers' compensation system if they believe their lung disease is associated with exposure at the World Trade Center site. Congress is likely to consider a federal compensation program for these heroes, just as it did for other workers who put themselves in harm's way in other national defense and homeland security efforts, and for those killed in the 9/11 terrorist attack.

Asbestos-related disease is another area ripe for an alternative compensation program. In 2006 Congress considered but did not adopt Senator Arlen Specter's proposal to create a national compensation fund. The initiative was unsatisfactory to representatives of large numbers of the victims and to some of the manufacturers and their insurers who would be funding the multibillion-dollar program, but the basic approach is a good one, assuming the details can be worked out.

4. End "Preemption by Preamble": Bad Public Policy and Bad for Public Health

Since the beginning of the regulatory era in the 1970s, the corporations have argued that compliance with all pertinent regulations should inoculate them against litigation. To the naïve and the uninitiated, this seems fair enough; to those who understand the influence the corporations exert over the writing of these same regulations and therefore know how pathetically weak many of the regulations are, it is patent nonsense. My colleague David Vladeck, a professor at the Georgetown Law School, uses the tragedy of the *Titanic* to illustrate the point. When the cruise ship sank in the early morning hours of April 15, 1912, there were 2,227 passengers and crew on board. More than 1,500 perished in the icy waters of the North Atlantic, mostly because of a shortage of lifeboats; the *Titanic* had only sixteen in all, with a total carrying capacity of 980 people. However, these sixteen lifeboats actually exceeded the required number because the regulation had been established almost thirty years earlier, when cruise ships were much smaller than the awesome *Titanic*. Lifeboat capacity was designed to meet the inadequate standard, not to provide protection for the number of people the ship was designed to carry.[17] That was outrageous negligence, but under the rule of "preemption," the cruise ship company and its insurers walked away from that tragedy without a scratch.

The Bush administration issued several sets of regulations that likewise preemptively override state laws governing lawsuits and thereby eliminate an important incentive for good corporate behavior. To illustrate the issue here, let's consider specific cases. Vehicle rollover crashes kill more than ten thousand people each year in this country, which is about one-third of all vehicle occupant deaths, and injure another sixteen thousand.[18] In 2005 NHTSA issued a rule on vehicle roof strength that is so weak it could have been written by the auto industry lobbyists: Almost 70 percent of existing vehicles already meet this proposed standard, and the agency itself estimates the new rule will prevent between thirteen and forty-four deaths each year, less than one-half of one percent of the annual total.[19] Additionally, buried in this almost worthless rule was an even worse provision that preempts all state laws, including those that permit product-defect lawsuits if vehicle manufacturers meet these minimal new standards.

Here is another case in point: The Consumer Product Safety Commission has included a similar preemption in a rule that addresses mattress flammability. And yet another, the most dangerous of them all, in terms of public health: In January 2006 the FDA added a provision to its rule on prescription drug labels that states that FDA approval of a drug label "preempts conflicting or contrary State law."[19] We have already seen how this drug label is not a document the FDA *even controls*. It is subject to extensive, closed-door negotiation with the manufacturer and is primarily based on data that the manufacturer generates and supplies to the regulator. If the manufacturer does not provide complete information on a drug's toxicity or neglects to conduct the long-term follow-up necessary to determine that toxicity—and we have seen Big Pharma's track record in this regard—the label will be hopelessly inadequate. Yet the FDA wants this label to protect the manufacturers from liability.

There is that word again: Orwellian. Fortunately, many judges are rightly skeptical of the Bush administration's preemption philosophy. "The FDA's current view on the question of immunity for prescription drug manufacturers is entirely unpersuasive," was the ruling in 2007 of a Federal judge in New Orleans. Merck had asked Federal District Court Judge Eldon E. Fallon to dismiss the case of two people who began taking the drug after the FDA approved the label warning that Vioxx might increase heart attack risk. The drug manufacturer had argued that the FDA's approval of the label exempted the company from claims its warnings were inadequate. Judge Fallon wrote that "[b]ecause there are no federal remedies for individuals harmed by prescription drugs, a finding of implied preemption in these cases would abolish state-law remedies and would, in effect, render legally impotent those who sustain injuries from defective prescription drugs."[20] On the other hand, some state judges have embraced preemption by preamble. In April 2007, a Texas judge threw out 1,000 Vioxx lawsuits, asserting that the label Merck negotiated with the FDA could be considered adequate warning of the drug's risks.[21]

Preemption by preamble is particularly bad public policy because these preemptions have implications far beyond the compensation of actual victims. If widely upheld, what incentive would the automakers, for example, have to improve the safety of their products? None whatsoever, and no one can doubt they would not work to improve their products because the U.S. car industry has fought numerous life-saving safety improvements. According to the industry, mandatory seat belts would be the end of their world. With antiregulatory zealots running the health and safety agencies, issuing weak standards, or simply ignoring hazards and refusing to issue any standards at all, lawsuit preemption would be catastrophic to the public's health.

18

Sarbanes-Oxley for Science

A DOZEN WAYS TO IMPROVE OUR

REGULATORY SYSTEM

If a camel is a horse designed by a committee, what in the world is the U.S. regulatory system, which was designed by a host of congressional committees over a number of years? If it were not so sad and frustrating, the anarchic and overlapping division of responsibilities between the agencies would be funny. To wit, a dozen federal agencies regulate food safety, while at least six different agencies are responsible for ensuring the safety of a frozen pepperoni pizza. This total does not count the workplace and transportation safety agencies, whose inspectors are often on the same premises as the food inspectors.[1]

The lack of a consistent philosophy shared by the agencies is just as dispiriting. The EPA's mandate attempts to protect the entire population from risks that might harm a relatively small number of persons, whereas OSHA will not consider regulating a chemical hazard in the workplace unless it stands to hurt at least one in a thousand individuals exposed. Some statutes, like the Safe Drinking Water Act of 1974, require agencies to conduct cost-benefit analyses, whereas others (Clean Air Act of 1970) prohibit them from doing so.

Naturally enough, the opponents of strong environmental and public health regulations are quick to point out every inconsistency, every foible, and every bureaucratic foul-up in the system. This campaign is analogous to the one used to undermine the legal system; some of the anecdotes in circulation are valid, while others are not. In any event, the regulatory system is an easy target for political attack, and the concerted campaign to undermine it has been successful in one way. While the antiregulatory forces have been unable, for the most part, to convince Congress to pass legislation that would slash the agencies' power, they have used the administrative powers of the executive branch to accomplish the same goal. As a direct result, some agencies have virtually abandoned their efforts to fulfill their public health responsibilities. For example, OSHA, as we have seen, has stopped issuing new standards and has severely cut back on workplace inspections. Other agencies are functioning but under great strain. At the EPA, public health regulations are being written by corporate lobbyists instead of career staff. Key scientists are fleeing the agency. There is widespread recognition that the FDA's current approach to evaluating the safety (as compared with the efficacy) of drugs is simply not working. For the first time in anyone's memory, political meddling has occurred in purely scientific areas that had been considered off-limits to politicians. Morale among the career staff is abysmal, and public confidence in the agency has dropped precipitously.[2] These developments have put those of us who believe the government must take a central role in protecting public health in the uncomfortable position of defending legislation and regulatory approaches that we have to concede are working poorly. We can only hope that the agencies can be strengthened under different political leadership.

When crises happen, such as the twelve deaths at a West Virginia coal mine in January 2006, the news media and the public respond with outrage. Legislators react by proposing more and stricter regulation, not less. The public supports a strong role for government in protecting their health and their environment. They know at gut level that no one else can do the job, but they are not aware that powerful forces working behind the scenes are determined to moot this broad support. After all, the system still provides great benefits. The Cuyahoga River no longer catches fire. In most localities, the air is cleaner than it was decades ago. We have made real gains, but most people cannot see how much remains to be done. Pollution and toxic chemicals may still be major killers, but they do their work silently. For the most part, the epidemics are invisible: The World Health Organization estimates that three million people die each year because of air pollution.[3] Nevertheless, who associates a single death with the invisible particles we know to be responsible?

The public is also largely ignorant of the depth and reach of corporate deception. For decades, the cigarette manufacturers took advantage of the rules on attorney-client privilege and attorney work products in order to sequester data. Who knows what portion of the worldwide epidemic of asbestos-caused disease, currently estimated at one hundred thousand deaths a year, might have been prevented had the manufacturers reported the results of inhalation studies in the 1940s that linked asbestos with lung cancer?

But looking back, why should we have expected them to behave differently? Time after time we have seen the same scenario played out in different industries. When a study suggests a corporation's product may be hazardous, rare is the CEO who announces that the firm will examine the evidence carefully and honestly. Instead, the professional spokesperson immediately denies that the study could be accurate, often before the company's own scientists could possibly have examined the work. The company hires product defense specialists to refute and reanalyze the original study with the sole purpose of manufacturing and magnifying uncertainty.

I draw an analogy between what has happened to science, especially the science on which our public health and environmental regulatory systems are based, and what happened to accounting in the go-go 1990s. The best-known example is the respected accounting firm Arthur Andersen, which assisted not just Enron but also WorldCom and Waste Management, in allegedly hoodwinking stockholders and the SEC through what are now recognized as questionable accounting practices. Several of the other giant accounting firms have been implicated in similar schemes. This behavior was so common at major accounting firms that it was apparently seen not as deviant but rather as a means to make more money for their clients. Just as Enron and WorldCom used the accountants at Arthur Andersen, so do the manufacturers of chromium, beryllium, and other notoriously toxic but underregulated hazards employ the scientists at product defense firms. Instead of concocting misleading balance sheets, product defense scientists specialize in producing scientific data or interpreting them in ways that all too often make hazards appear benign, thereby helping their grateful clients avoid victim compensation and costly environmental regulation.

To be sure, science is not accounting; there are limits to the analogy. While there are conventions and guidelines for the application of certain scientific methods and techniques, science is overall less amenable to practicing and reporting standards than is accounting. The scientific enterprise requires interpretation of results and often the synthesis of the results of many studies. It looks for the weight of the evidence, so the policies science shapes are driven by interpretations and syntheses rather than by the data directly.

However, science is also becoming more like accounting in that it is increasingly and inextricably linked to commerce. The separation between academic science and the business world is disappearing. As a result, the whole culture of science is changing rapidly. One hundred years ago Marie and Pierre Curie and Wilhelm Roentgen (discoverer of X-rays) refused to patent their remarkable discoveries. Nowadays scientists patent everything they can get their hands on: seeds, hormones, and risk assessment models. Universities and university scientists have enrolled in joint ventures and profit-sharing arrangements with chemical and pharmaceutical manufacturers that would have been unimaginable to scientists just a few decades ago. As a result, the model of the disinterested scientist searching for truth with no financial interest in the outcome, proposed by Robert Merton a half-century ago, is no longer held up as an ideal, not even by scientists.[4] This concept is no longer operative. Laughable is more like it. Instead, the most valued scientist is the one whose work contributes most to the bottom line.

The social and economic impact of the big accounting scandals was devastating: Thousands of workers lost their jobs and/or their pensions, and billions of dollars of shareholder assets disappeared virtually overnight. In response, Congress enacted the American Competitiveness and Corporate Accountability Act of 2002, commonly known as Sarbanes-Oxley.[5] This law, named for its primary sponsors, Senator Paul Sarbanes and Representative Michael Oxley, makes corporate executives responsible for ensuring the accuracy of the information their firms provide to the public and to the financial regulatory system.

We need an equivalent Sarbanes-Oxley for Science, tough federal legislation that parallels the reforms in the accounting trade. Science is the basis for our public health and environmental regulatory system. Each year thousands of studies are conducted for the purpose of influencing this system, most of them by the corporations who are the subjects of regulation. Drug manufacturers, not the FDA, conduct the clinical trials for new medicines. For the most part, chemical manufacturers, not the EPA, test the toxicity of new, and sometimes older, chemicals. Since science is now almost inextricably meshed with corporate sponsorship and commerce, the regulatory controls now applied to the accounting of this commerce (thanks to Sarbanes-Oxley) must be applied to the science that underpins the commerce and has profound effects on our public health and environmental protection systems.

We also need to make changes in our regulatory system. I am under no illusion that a wholesale restructuring is in the offing anytime soon, but incremental changes are possible and definitely feasible with a different administration. We must make these changes and be poised and ready for the next disaster—the next mine explosion, oil spill, or E. coli outbreak—that spurs the public to pay attention, pick up the phone, and send emails. This attitude may seem calculating and callous, but it simply reflects political reality. The public supports regulation, but it also requires a strong incentive to demand major changes.

I conclude this book with a dozen recommendations for "Restoring Scientific Integrity in Policymaking," the title of a statement from the Union of Concerned Scientists that I helped formulate in 2003 and that has since been signed by more than ten thousand scientists. Here is the key passage: "The distortion of scientific knowledge for partisan political ends must cease if the public is to be properly informed about issues central to its well being, and the nation is to benefit fully from its heavy investment in scientific research and education. To elevate the ethic that governs the relationship between science and government, Congress and the Executive should establish legislation and regulations that would . . ."[6]

In that statement we presented a set of broad initiatives. Now I elaborate with twelve specifically targeted recommendations. I think of the first five as Sarbanes-Oxley for Science, a set of initiatives that regulate the behavior of corporations regarding the science they generate to influence the regulatory arena. These proposals address the key principles of scientific completeness, full disclosure, and accountability and responsibility. The last seven recommendations are directed at the regulatory agencies, which must change both the way they deal with the corporations and the way they use science. Some of the twelve could be implemented immediately by an executive branch committed to responsible regulation. Others are bolder and more radical and thus require far more debate and analysis since they would entail a restructuring of the major components of the regulatory system.

1. Require Full Disclosure of Any and All Sponsor Involvement in Scientific Studies

Money changes everything. Financial conflict of interest inevitably shapes judgment—the funding effect—and this correlation must be factored into the consideration of the analyses and opinions of scientists employed by industry. During the late 1990s there was a series of alarming instances in which corporations blocked the publication of research that was detrimental to the companies but important for protecting the public's health. Outraged, the editors of thirteen of the world's leading biomedical journals, including the *New England Journal of Medicine* and the *Journal of the American Medical Association*, declared in 2001 that they will publish only studies done under contracts in which the investigators are "free of commercial interest." The editors would no longer accept papers about studies performed under contracts that allowed the sponsor to control the results. In a joint statement, the editors asserted that contractual arrangements that allow sponsor control of publication "not only erode the fabric of intellectual inquiry that has fostered so much high-quality clinical research, but also make medical journals party to potential misrepresentation, since the published manuscript may not reveal the extent to which the authors were powerless to control the conduct of a study that bears their names."[7]

Federal regulatory agencies, charged with protecting the public's health, must make life-and-death decisions based largely on scientific evidence submitted by the regulated parties themselves. Yet the policies of the federal regulatory agencies to ensure the honesty of the reporting of this research have not kept pace with developments in the academic and biomedical communities. In many ways, the FDA is somewhat more insulated from corporate data manipulation than the other agencies. When a manufacturing company applies for approval to market a new drug, it must supply the FDA with all of the raw data from its clinical trials and safety studies. Granted, the manufacturer's scientists may also publish the study results in a medical journal, where they may apply whatever spin they want. However, the FDA's scientists will generally ignore those papers and perform their own analyses of the raw data. Even with this system, the world of pharmaceutical research continues to be filled with scandals. No wonder the other federal agencies, which have fewer resources and no legislative authority to demand raw data, have such problems coping with the corporations. They are condemned to rely on the work of the hired guns in the product defense industry—studies bought and paid for by the regulated parties.

As a regulator in the Department of Energy, I thought I knew the provenance of the studies submitted to my agency, but I could never be sure. The EPA, OSHA, MSHA (Mine Safety and Health Administration), and most other regulatory agencies have no formal mechanisms to identify potential conflicts of interest, and their regulations do not provide any incentives for sponsors to ensure that research is free of sponsor control. When studies are submitted to EPA or OSHA, for example, these agencies do not have the authority to inquire who has paid for the studies or whether they were performed under the types of contracts the medical journals have banned. I do not believe that regulators should use conflict disclosures to exclude research (we have an obligation to consider all of the evidence and to accord greater importance to those studies that are of higher quality and relevance), although we should certainly be informed about those conflicts.

Recognizing that sponsors with clear conflicts of interest have no incentive to reveal them or to relinquish control over sponsored research, University of Texas law professor Wendy Wagner and I developed a series of recommendations that would *begin* to improve the situation. Writing in the journal *Science*, we proposed that federal agencies should adopt, at a minimum, requirements for "research integrity" comparable to those used by biomedical journals. Corporations, trade associations, unions, public interest groups, and others who submit studies for consideration should be required to disclose the financial and other conflicts of interest of the investigating scientists, and they should also divulge whether the scientists had the contractual right to publish their findings without influence and without obtaining consent of the sponsor.[8]

Disclosure is a necessary reform, but it is not a panacea. The pressures on scientists who receive corporate money are too great. Even with contracts that forbid the sponsor's control of full disclosure, the fear of losing the next contract will limit true scientific independence. I prefer a system in which research and testing are carried out with true independence. Any study desired by (or required of) industry would be paid for by the industry but conducted by independent researchers, under federal auspices. Subsequent publication would be completely independent of the sponsoring corporations.

I am not the first to propose this model, of course. The approach is regularly proposed for the pharmaceutical industry, perhaps first by Senator Gaylord Nelson in 1971,[9] and more recently by Sheldon Krimsky in his important book *Science in the Private Interest.*[10] Is this a pipe dream? Not *completely*—because editorials in some of the leading biomedical journals— all of which have been so burned in the past by bogus articles—have endorsed the idea. Those who oppose regulation would doubtless view such a system as a nightmare. But regulation that protects the public's health and the environment must be based on the best available science, and the best science is science done by independent investigators.

2. Is This Stuff Safe? Manufacturers Must Test Chemicals before Exposing Workers and the Public

I find it remarkable that in this day and age one of the primary ways by which the toxic effects of chemicals are discovered is *still* the "body in the morgue" method. An industrial worker dies from some very unusual condition, and we ask why. Well, some of us ask. Often enough, the manufacturer would rather not know. As we have seen, before the epidemic of lung disease cases in popcorn factories, the U.S. flavor manufacturers did not attempt to learn whether breathing diacetyl, the primary component of artificial butter flavor, was dangerous to workers or to consumers who prepare microwave popcorn; the product had been tested only as a food, and it came up clean. Only after dozens of workers in the manufacturing plants developed lung disease did federal scientists expose lab animals to the diacetyl vapors and learn how quickly high levels destroy the lungs.

Why was diacetyl, a widely used chemical to which thousands of workers and countless consumers are exposed, not properly evaluated? The answer is simple and absurd: For the most part, U.S. chemical manufacturers have no legal obligation to test the chemicals they produce. Under the Toxic

Substances Control Act (TSCA, pronounced "Tosca," like the opera), the EPA theoretically has the power to regulate the entire life cycle of chemicals from their production and distribution to their use and disposal. The agency can require a manufacturer to conduct toxicity testing and to list potential hazards on their products' labels. In theory, the EPA can even prohibit the use of spectacularly dangerous chemicals; however, in the thirty-plus years since the TSCA legislation was enacted, the agency has limited the use of only five chemicals or groups of chemicals (polychlorinated biphenyls or PCBs, chlorofluorocarbons, dioxin, asbestos, and hexavalent chromium—but only when it is used as a water treatment chemical), and its attempted ban on asbestos was slapped down by a federal court.[11] The EPA has lost so many legal and political battles that it no longer even attempts to act with authority. This timidity extends well beyond the outright banning of chemicals. Of the sixty-two thousand chemicals that were already in commerce when the EPA began reviewing chemicals under the auspices of TSCA in 1979, it has invoked its authority to require the testing of fewer than two hundred.[12]

What do we know about the toxic effects of the other 61,800 chemicals? Surprisingly little. There are large gaps in our knowledge of the toxicity of the majority of the almost 3,000 high-production volume (HPV) chemicals (that is, more than one million pounds produced or imported per year). In 1997 the advocacy group Environmental Defense examined existing toxicity data on a sample of the HPV chemicals that had also been subject to regulatory attention under major environmental laws—in short, chemicals with a high-priority need for hazard identification. The group found that 71 percent of the sampled chemicals did not meet an internationally accepted minimum health hazard screening data requirement.[13] Embarrassed, the EPA followed up on this report and determined that 93 percent of the HPV chemicals were missing at least one basic toxicity screening test and that 43 percent were missing *all* of the tests. The agency estimated that it would cost the industry about $400 million to fill all of the basic data gaps for the HPV chemicals. That sum amounts to about 0.2 percent of the annual sales of the top one hundred U.S. chemical manufacturers.[14]

To start to fill this immense data gap, the EPA set up the "HPV Challenge Program" in 1998. In this *voluntary* initiative, the chemical companies would commit to generate basic toxicity information on these most commonly used chemicals. This is an important start, but the limits of the well-meaning program are clear. Tens of thousands of the more minor chemicals, including many that we know are likely to be toxic based on their chemical structure, are not included. And there are more than 250 HPV "orphans"—common chemicals that no manufacturer has agreed to test.[15]

That is the situation with "older" chemicals. To deal with new chemicals, TSCA provides the EPA with a little more firepower. The agency does not require preproduction testing of chemicals, but manufacturers are required to notify the agency of their intent to manufacture a new one. The EPA then attempts to predict the toxicity of these chemicals by using computer models that compare the new chemicals with substances that have similar molecular structures and about which toxicity information is known. Using these models is not the same as testing, of course, and if limited or no toxicity information is available on the class of chemicals, then the model is not much help at all. Still, EPA's reviews have resulted in action being taken to reduce the risks associated with exposure to more than thirty-six hundred new chemicals.[12]

It is time for the EPA to *require* manufacturers to conduct basic toxicity testing of heavily used chemicals, as well as substances that are likely to be especially toxic. The European Union is trying to move in exactly this direction with legislation called REACH, which stands for Registration, Evaluation, and Authorization of Chemicals. Once implemented, this will require manufacturers to provide basic toxicity information on all chemicals of which one ton or more is marketed annually.[16] While REACH has been fiercely opposed by the U.S. industry, our manufacturers will likely adapt to it in order to sell their products in Europe. They will come up with the data and live to tell the tale. It is always the same story, as we have seen throughout this book: balk, obfuscate, delay, complain, go to favored senators, go to the White House, go to friendly media—and then, if finally forced to comply with this or that terribly onerous, perhaps even fatal, regulation, do so with little or no loss of profitability.

Why should the United States wait for the Europeans to act? We should require manufacturers and vendors to generate basic information about the toxicity of chemicals to which workers, neighbors, and consumers are exposed.

3. No More Secret Science: Manufacturers Must Disclose What They Know about the Toxicity of Their Products

Too few toxicity studies are ever conducted by the manufacturers. That is one problem. Just as bad (or worse) for public health is the hiding of much of the information that is generated. On the subject of science and research, the corporations have developed their own "Don't ask, don't tell" policy. We have seen how this dynamic has played out with the pharmaceutical companies: the systematic burying of unwanted results from clinical trials; the selective, misleading publication of positive results in the medical journals and the belated revolt of the editors of those journals; the justified rejection by the medical community of Big Pharma's voluntary registration scheme; and the movement in Congress to require mandatory public registration of all clinical trials.

The TSCA legislation requires corporations to inform the EPA each time they learn about an adverse effect of a chemical exposure, but the agency rarely goes after manufacturers who fail to report. Much of the information about toxic exposures that is provided, especially the toxicity studies of new substances, is forwarded in sealed envelopes marked "confidential business information" (CBI) and as such cannot be released to the public. The CBI loophole ostensibly protects the companies against the unwarranted circulation of trade secrets—proprietary formulas and manufacturing processes—but it is widely abused. The CBI claim is now the rule rather than the exception: Chemical manufacturers seal the envelope in 95 percent of their premanufacture notifications, and the EPA says okay.[12]

Manufacturers are given wide latitude to classify *any* type of information with the CBI claim, often without even having to specify the nature of the trade-secret concerns. Toxicity studies are often sequestered, even though TSCA specifically states that such health and safety information cannot be classified as a trade secret and thereby hidden from the public.[17] The burden of disputing the thousands of CBI claims falls on the resource-poor EPA, which rarely if ever does so. Challenges by consumers or watchdog groups are also rare—and not just because they are difficult and expensive. Since CBI information is secret, few people know that the research exists and has even been filed with EPA. No corporate official is required to take responsibility for the CBI claim, and no penalties are levied for asserting a claim that is later proven wrong or inappropriately made. Given all this, no wonder filing a CBI claim is now standard operating procedure for corporations, not only in matters dealing with toxic chemicals. In 2006 the special inspector general for Iraq reconstruction issued a blistering report that criticized a Halliburton subsidiary that abused the proprietary information label in its filings, thereby inhibiting transparency and impeding government oversight of its work.[18]

I am not suggesting that there are never reasons for corporate confidentiality. Secrecy serves many functions, including protecting national security, investment value, and individual confidentiality, but excessive secrecy will damage the scientific enterprise itself—it already has. The tremendous societal costs of that excessive secrecy have been the subject of this book. Sheila Jasanoff of Harvard University's John F. Kennedy School of Government has described the contours of the debate over data secrecy: "Openness and transparency in science...cannot be treated as absolute goods. Rather, the degree of openness is context-specific and needs to be traded off against other important social values. The problem for contemporary law and policy is to develop principled approaches to maintaining the desired balance."[19]

Right now, the balance is out of whack, and confidentiality, not transparency, is the default position. The reverse should be the case, and we have the legislative means to at least begin to address the problem as it concerns toxic chemicals: Enforce TSCA as Congress meant it to be enforced. Give EPA sufficient resources to validate CBI confidentiality claims. If necessary, revise the enabling legislation to give it more teeth.

4. Put an End to Rigged Data Reanalysis

For the most part, only government studies and government-funded studies are reanalyzed. Studies funded by private industry are reexamined only if the corporate sponsor is unhappy with the original results and brings in a product defense reanalyzing specialist to get things right. This reanalysis asymmetry stems from several basic inequalities. Foremost is the unequal treatment of public and private science: Corporate researchers have access to government-supported studies, but privately funded science has no comparable public access (the subject of the following recommendation).[20] A related issue is money: Corporations and trade associations that need to attack a government study generally have adequate resources to do so—reanalysis can be expensive, but it is far cheaper than doing a study from scratch. Finally, industry studies are often set up to find nothing (for example, by having too few study subjects or too short a follow-up), so even if the government or public health advocates had access to the data and the budget with which to reanalyze it, no amount of reanalysis could find a positive result.

As we have seen, the objective of industry and product-defense reanalysis is to force regulators to consider studies that appear to be equal but come to differing conclusions. Uncertainty. That's a recipe for regulatory paralysis. Epidemiologists understand that data analyses that use methods and comparisons selected post hoc—after studying the distribution of the data—do not have the same validity as those that test prior hypotheses. Many regulators understand this, too, but industry sponsors hope that even if they cannot convince the regulators, their machinations may not be as clear to a federal judge reviewing a regulatory action. Moreover, once the reanalysis is done, that is where it usually ends. Federal support for occupational and environmental epidemiology is limited and shrinking as we speak. The government agencies and institutes that fund scientific research are generally unwilling to spend more public money to conduct additional studies to clarify the confusion and uncertainty caused by the reanalysis. As a result, the validity of the criticisms raised in the reanalysis is rarely tested.

252 DOUBT IS THEIR PRODUCT

I am not saying reanalyses are necessarily corrupt; there are important and positive reasons for such studies. When honest scientists conduct them in an objective and transparent manner, they can make a useful contribution to the scientific literature. However, for reanalyses to be recognized as valid, the sponsors and investigators must afford honest and deliberate consideration of the complex issues involved. It can be done. It has been done. In chapter fourteen I wrote about the attack by legislators doing the bidding of polluting industries on air pollution studies conducted by epidemiologists at Harvard University and the American Cancer Society. No doubt fearing rigged reanalyses, the scientists refused to give up their raw data. A compromise was reached: The Health Effects Institute (HEI), a research group originally set up by the EPA and the automobile industry, agreed to organize a truly independent reanalysis of the studies. The HEI developed procedures specifically designed to preserve objectivity and transparency. The resulting reanalysis reached the same conclusions as the original work and thus strengthened the evidence that air pollution is an important cause of premature mortality in the United States.[21]

This is the quality of reanalysis we need. In 2004 I gave a plenary lecture at the annual meeting of the International Society for Environmental Epidemiology (ISEE), in which I decried rigged reanalyses and other methodological tricks that product defense consultants use to manufacture uncertainty. My lecture triggered a year-long discussion that culminated in a proposal by the ISEE ethics committee to create guidelines for ethical reanalysis of another scientist's research. The guidelines call for scientists who want to reanalyze another's data to agree *beforehand* which hypotheses will be explored (no more Texas sharpshooting) and the extent to which different patterns of evidence would support or cast doubt on each of the different hypotheses. There should also be assurances that the results of the reanalysis and reinterpretation will be made available regardless of the result.[22]

5. The Lessons of Enron: Hold Real People Accountable

Enron and WorldCom executives claimed they had been out of the loop and totally unaware of the accounting misrepresentations in which their companies were engaged; juries, however, believed they were lying and brought in guilty verdicts. Sarbanes-Oxley aims to put an end to that "strategic ignorance" across the board by holding most senior managers responsible for their companies' false or misleading financial data. They cannot hide behind their ignorance. They are in charge, and they are paid enormous sums, so they are also responsible, and real-world consequences will result for cheating and lying about the books.

The exact same responsibility should apply to required disclosures of scientific information. As I described in the chapter on chromium, executives of that industry filed hundreds of pages of documents and sat through eleven days of public hearings but never once informed OSHA that they had commissioned a study that demonstrated high risk of lung cancer at low levels of exposure to this toxic metal. A manufacturer of diacetyl, a toxic component of artificial butter flavor, did not reveal a study that showed that one day's exposure to diacetyl would destroy the lungs of rats. We can put a stop to these lies of omission. Corporate officers who participate in regulatory processes should be required to certify that their submissions are accurate and complete, under the threat of civil and criminal penalties. We cannot rely on old-fashioned notions of conscience because they do not seem to operate when people can hide behind the shield of a faceless corporation.

6. Level the Playing Field: Require Equal Treatment for Public and Private Science

Corporations that face expensive and burdensome regulation have a strong financial incentive to produce scientific evidence useful in opposing that regulation. As long as sponsors retain control, studies can be designed and reported in ways that support the sponsor's objectives. Furthermore, dissemination of unfavorable results can easily be suppressed or limited. Many studies that chemical companies perform, for example, are never given to public health agencies. If they are, the confidential business information label hides them from public viewing.

By contrast, I believe that publicly funded research is much less likely to be distorted by the financial incentives that shape studies to meet a sponsor's needs. In addition, publicly funded studies are more likely to be published since unpublished research does not advance the careers of independent investigators. Yet the raw data from the more trustworthy government-funded studies are generally available to private parties for scrutiny and reanalysis, while industry is under no obligation to release comparable raw data from its own inherently suspect studies. These remain largely insulated from outside review and meaningful agency oversight.[8,20]

This imbalance is ridiculous on its face and should be corrected. "Sound science" reforms like the Data Access Act (also known as the Shelby Amendment) and the Data Quality Act get the problem precisely backward (but on purpose, of course). Privately sponsored research conducted to influence public regulatory proceedings should be subject to the same access and reporting provisions as those applied to publicly funded science. In the absence of equal treatment of public and private science, what incentive will the regulated parties ever have to produce private research of high quality? We need to better scrutinize privately produced data, and these data should be made available to interested scientists and regulators. The public good cannot possibly be served by the unequal treatment of public and private science, especially since the regulatory agencies depend to a great extent on this private research in setting protective standards.

The laws that govern the workings of federal agencies, especially the Administrative Procedures Act, require the agencies to consider and respond to questions and comments made by the public. This good government reform has been turned on its head by opponents of regulation and used to make sure the government does nothing good. Corporations and trade associations have multiple opportunities to challenge and delay any proposed regulation or even a report they do not like. Industry has the resources to hire the best scientists money can buy (that is not to say the best scientists, period; the qualifier is an important one). And they do. Faced with strengthened environmental regulation or potential litigation, corporations will spend huge amounts of money creating uncertainty. They hire mercenary scientists to fill captured journals with studies that create no new knowledge and whose only purpose is to gum up the works.

The objective is to paralyze the regulatory process. The goal has been achieved, for the most part, because the playing field is so decidedly lopsided. Occasionally an environmental organization or union will challenge the work of the product defense scientists or try to influence a government agency to take a stronger position, but these groups have relatively few resources at their disposal. University scientists are generally uninformed about the regulatory process and rarely participate; their work is published in academic journals and used in the regulatory arena only when advocates translate it and inject it into the regulatory discussions.

We also have the Small Business Regulatory Enforcement Fairness Act (SBREFA), which established a Small Business Administration Office of Advocacy to promote the needs of small businesses to the EPA and OSHA. SBREFA, a remnant of Newt Gingrich's Contract with America, establishes a formal mechanism in which these two public health agencies must present regulations still in the planning stage to panels of small business representatives and advocates and invite their input.[23] This is yet another opportunity for polluters to demand that concern about public health and the environment be balanced against economic impact on small businesses. The EPA and OSHA already consider the economic impact of their regulations, and if they did not, the White House and Congress would remind them of their need to do so. Every proposed regulation goes through extensive interagency review. However, the Small Business Advocate gives antiregulatory forces another bite of the apple by pushing EPA and OSHA to weaken standards.

To help level the playing field, the system needs an equal and opposite advocate—this one for public health and the environment, a well-funded office with the power to review *all* of the science used by the regulators, including privately funded science, and to advocate for standards that would truly protect the public.

7. Protect the Independence of Federal Scientists and the Science Advisory Committees

The Bush administration has turned too many scientists into either whistleblowers or refugees. Many of the best scientists have left government service. Their replacements—if they are replaced—are less experienced and, in many cases, less talented because the best young scientists do not want to join a demoralized agency where their work will be scrutinized and perhaps censored by political appointees who care little about the public's health or the environment. Congress can ameliorate this problem by passing laws that provide stronger protection for federal whistleblowers and by conducting oversight into the muzzling of scientists across the agencies. A bit of progress has occurred on this front. The National Academy of Sciences has denounced the practice of asking potential appointees to federal advisory panels for whom they voted and to whose campaigns they donated money.[24] In 2005 Congress passed an appropriations rider that prohibits the government from spending federal funds on political litmus tests for scientific panel appointments, but only for a one-year period.[25] Congress needs to make this permanent and remind future administrations that the U.S. government wants the advice of our best scientists, not our most compliant ones. In the end, however, no legislation can change work environments made toxic by political appointees who tell scientists what to think and what to say, so the best solution is leaders who respect science and scientists.

Drug companies hire the best and the brightest scientists to design and test new medicines; chemical manufacturers employ fine toxicologists and epidemiologists, along with chemists who develop new products. The work of these scientists is often of the highest quality, but for all their exceptional work we cannot assume that they provide an unbiased interpretation of the literature. The Vioxx debacle is a powerful example: Scientists working for Merck, including academic scientists who were only consultants, interpreted (or presented) the initial studies incorrectly—and helped convince the FDA to do the same. Tens of thousands of preventable heart attacks later, the correct interpretation of the early studies is now clear.

If it is dangerous to rely on scientists with financial conflicts of interest to interpret raw data, why should we depend on these scientists to provide advice to the regulatory agencies? It makes no sense, and the law reflects this view: Scientists with financial conflicts of interest cannot now serve on advisory panels unless they receive a waiver. However, this stipulation has so little currency today that waivers are routinely granted, no matter how glaring the conflict. "Conflict of interest can be managed" is the current mantra. Well-meaning administrators of these committees believe they desperately need the leading researchers in their fields, regardless of how conflicted they may be. In some areas of medicine, it is difficult to find experts completely unaffiliated with the drug companies because so many physicians, especially the most respected academic ones, have received money from them. Even after the tsunami of publicity about Vioxx as a cause of heart attacks, ten of the thirty-two scientists the FDA named to the panel that considered whether the COX-2 inhibitors should be allowed on the market had financial ties to COX-2 manufacturers. Nine of the ten scientists voted in favor of permitting Vioxx to be marketed. Had their votes been eliminated, Vioxx would have lost that vote instead of receiving narrow support.[26] After much bad publicity, the FDA relented, and has proposed a change in policy that will restrict the service of scientists with financial conflicts on the agency's advisory panels.[27]

A common response from scientists with financial conflicts is that their judgment is not influenced by their employment relationships. To give them the benefit of the doubt, most of these scientists honestly believe this, but the evidence strongly suggests otherwise: Financial ties cloud judgment. If we cannot predict which scientists will be influenced (and all evidence is that we cannot), we need to limit the use of all conflicted scientists. Moreover, the headlines about these conflicts look bad; the public is justifiably skeptical about the panels' objectivity, and that skepticism threatens the value of their work. When a major committee appointed by the NIH issued a recommendation that Americans with lower cholesterol levels than previously recommended should go on cholesterol-lowering statin medications, the conclusion was immediately questioned because eight of the nine panel members had financial ties to companies that sell these drugs.[28]

I am convinced that conflict of interest cannot be "managed." It must be eliminated. Too much is at stake. Data interpretation requires independent judgment; the public needs assurance that the opinions expressed in these settings are unbiased by commercial interest. The cholesterol question impacts the daily lives and wallets of millions of Americans, and it has a multibillion-dollar impact on the companies and the economy. For a decision this important, the NIH could have convened a panel of very smart scientists who had never received money from a drug manufacturer. If these scientists were not sufficiently knowledgeable about the drugs under study, the NIH could have paid them adequately to study the literature and become sufficiently expert. I think the U.S. government and our twelve-trillion-dollar economy could afford this.

The recognition that conflict of interest must be avoided rather than managed is gaining some traction. In 2005, after a period in which the integrity of the agency's work was questioned, the International Agency for Research on Cancer (IARC) announced a major policy shift, which stated that scientists with "real or apparent conflicts of interests" could no longer serve on the panels that produce IARC's famous monographs on the causes of cancer. Instead, the agency has invented a category of participants known as "invited specialists"—experts with critical knowledge and experience who are recused from certain activities because of a conflicting interest. They contribute their wisdom but do not draft text or vote on the monograph's content.[29]

The policy has worked with great success and has disposed of the argument that certain experts are so important that they must be included on panels no matter how conflicted. Could the policy work for federal agencies? It would be very simple—no additional legislation would be required—to conduct an experiment. Convene some panels with only unconflicted experts and see how they do. I do not have any doubts. They would produce quality results, while ensuring the impartiality and integrity of the product.

8. Regulation by Shaming: Increase Public Disclosure of Hazards

"Sunlight is said to be the best of disinfectants; electric light the most efficient policeman," wrote Supreme Court Justice Louis Brandeis.[30] Fear of public disclosure of hazards can be a powerful motivation to clean them up. Public disclosure encourages the responsible parties to control the hazards rather than suffer the public embarrassment and political pressure that often follows disclosure. No disclosure, no embarrassment, no pressure. Thus the Bush administration's attempt to dramatically roll back the reporting requirements of the EPA's Toxics Release Inventory (TRI), as discussed in the chapter on this administration. The TRI effect is sometimes called regulation by information. I prefer the term given it by Mary Graham, of Harvard's Kennedy School of Government: "regulation by shaming."[31]

I am a big fan of shaming. I know its power in the regulatory world from personal experience. By an act of Congress, the Department of Energy's nuclear safety enforcement program could not issue fines to the nonprofit organizations that run DOE facilities. When safety violations occurred at the Los Alamos nuclear weapons laboratory—some that were pretty severe and resulted in dangerous radiation doses to the workers involved—I of course could not issue fines against the University of California, which ran the lab. But I *could* issue a press release, and I did. The announcement declared that I would have fined the acclaimed university $220,000 if it were a private employer.[32] While big fines are probably more effective, fear of future public embarrassment helped improve safety performance at Los Alamos and elsewhere in the weapons system.

I imagine cynics will suggest that a public university in a progressive state is hardly typical, and that many corporations are beyond shaming. There is good reason for this supposition. Certainly the tobacco industry seems immune to shame, but many of the other industries discussed here may seem beyond shaming *only because their actions remain out of view.* That is, they have never been publicly shamed. Throw a spotlight on their behavior, and let's see what happens. It can only be for the good.

9. Require Corporations to Make a Plan and Stick to It

The well-meaning legislators who wrote the idealistic legislation that created the EPA, OSHA, and the other regulatory agencies envisioned departments that would use the best available science to set standards that would protect the public. As scientists learned more about toxic chemicals, the relevant regulatory agency would issue the appropriate standard. That was the vision, but the past few decades have served as a sobering lesson about how good intentions can go astray. The prime example is OSHA. When Congress enacted the OSHA law in 1970, it believed the new agency would adopt private industry consensus standards as a stopgap measure *only* and then issue new standards based on current research. But in the late 1980s, when the agency tried to update several hundred workplace exposure standards en masse, it generally selected industry's own newer, voluntary standards that were not necessarily as protective as a strong public health agency might require. Even so, dozens of corporations and trade associations took OSHA to federal court and demanded that OSHA address each change in separate chemical-by-chemical efforts. The court agreed and in 1992 ruled that health standards had to be issued one chemical at a time; OSHA announced that the outdated standards would remain unchanged.[33]

Chemical-by-chemical standard setting would be a painfully time- and resource-intensive process for any agency, much less this beleaguered one. Since that landmark ruling, OSHA has issued three new standards that cover toxic substances (one of which was required by a federal court ruling), plus its ergonomic standard, which Congress repealed in 2001. Unless things change radically, only a handful of the thousands of chemicals in daily use in American workplaces will ever be the subject of an OSHA standard. As I discussed in the chapter on diacetyl (the artificial butter flavor that obliterates workers' lungs), OSHA does not need a new standard if a hazard is serious and recognized measures are available to mitigate the hazard. It can invoke the "general duty clause," but the agency has refused to do so. As things stand now, no standard, no responsibility. This works out nicely for the employers. Absurd examples abound. In September 2004, for instance, a zoo employee was severely mauled by a black bear who escaped after its den was left unlocked. The OSHA inspectors concluded that no citation could be issued since the agency has never issued a regulation saying that bears should be prevented from escaping their dens.[34,35]

Then again, the idea that OSHA might *ever* issue a citation is not relevant at most workplaces in the United States. Given OSHA's current staffing numbers, the average workplace can expect the inspector once every 133 years. In 1975 there was one OSHA employee for every 27,845 U.S. workers; by 2005 that ratio had fallen to one for every 59,589.[36]

With OSHA barely functioning and the EPA hamstrung and able to regulate only a small proportion of the chemicals to which Americans are exposed, we need a different approach (or several different ones) to reducing environmental and safety hazards. And one is right at hand: Require corporations to develop and follow a hazard reduction plan. I have had first-hand experience with this sort of requirement. In DOE's nuclear safety enforcement system, the operator of every nuclear weapons facility must develop its own rigorous plan for addressing safety questions, and since government safety experts have to approve these plans, they were generally adequate. When I sent inspectors out following a report of an accident or an inadvertent release of radiation, the first thing the inspector did was to determine whether the managers were meeting the facility's own plan. If not, they were in violation. End of discussion.

We need the equivalent system in which *every* employer and *every* polluter develops its own hazard abatement plan that is signed off by the corporation's CEO (call it "Sarbanes-Oxley for Safety and Health"). Each firm would be required to survey its facilities for the presence of hazards, both real and potential. Based on the results of this survey, the managers would develop a plan that addresses all hazards—from digging trenches safely to limiting chemical spills and from having well-marked unlocked exits to educating all workers about the unique risks of their job. (The government could set exposure limits for the worst and the most widely used chemicals.) Does this sound utopian? In fact, it is no more than companies should be doing right now under OSHA and EPA regulations, and responsible employers—thousands of them—are in full compliance. What's missing is systematic compliance, including regular self-inspections and effective enforcement. Today recalcitrant businesses do not bother to comply until OSHA catches them. Who knows when that will be, and, besides, the penalty for noncompliance will surely be trivial.

Under the new system, each business's plan would be public, available to workers and community residents to examine and critique. It would be certified by the government, state or federal, depending on the details, or perhaps certification could fall to private sector organizations (like insurance carriers) that would bear some of the risk if a plan were found to be inadequate.

As always, the devil would be in the details, and I am under no illusions about the political difficulty of putting such a sensible, reasonable plan into place. However, just think how a plan would clarify matters for all concerned. Public health protection would boil down to the enforcement of two questions:

- Does the corporation have a plan that is adequate to protect workers, its neighbors, and the environment?
- Is the corporation meeting the requirements of its own plan?

Such clarity would benefit regulators and responsible employers and would give irresponsible companies a clear direction for improvement.

10. Embrace ALARA ("As Low as Reasonably Achievable")

By law, some exposure standards have built-in safety margins. On the question of pesticide contamination in our food, the Food Quality Protection Act requires the EPA to determine a level that ensures "reasonable certainty that no harm will result" if the general public encounters amounts below that level. The agency then builds in an additional tenfold margin of safety to protect infants and children.[37] This helps protect us from one particular set of hazard, but many standards meant to protect us from other types of exposures—pollutants in the air we breathe, chemicals in the work environment—provide smaller or no safety margins. Instead, the agency scientists try to pick an exposure level that has been associated with few or, better yet, no cases of disease and declare this the safe level.

This approach does not work for many exposures because we do not know (and probably cannot know) whether a safe level actually exists. And for many other chemicals, the best science to date tells us there is no safe exposure.[38]

As we have seen, beryllium causes disease at unthinkably low exposure levels. We know this only because chronic beryllium disease is easily identified and cannot be mistaken for any other disease. If this toxic metal caused emphysema or another common lung ailment, we would never know. Studies of children who have been exposed to lead have consistently found an inverse relationship between blood lead level and intelligence measure. There is no evidence that there is a "threshold" or safe level of pediatric lead exposure, below which lead has no effect on children's intelligence.[39] Likewise, as air pollution epidemiology becomes more sophisticated, it appears that there is no clear safe level of exposure to fine and ultrafine airborne particles.[40] Finally, scientists charged with protecting workers and the public from radiation recognized many years ago that it would be both wrong and counterproductive to designate a single number to represent a safe level for exposure to radiation. With the exception of a small group of wacky scientists who believe that small doses are good for us, most scientists who are familiar with the studies on the ability of ionizing radiation to cause cancer subscribe to the "linear, no threshold" theory. This theory holds that there is no safe level or threshold for radiation, and that cancer risk increases with exposure in a linear fashion, so twice as much exposure doubles the risk.[41]

There are standards for radiation exposure. Under the current standard, DOE workers in the nuclear weapons industry are permitted to receive up to 5 rem (a measure of radiation exposure) a year, but this number is widely acknowledged as outdated and mostly ignored. Instead, everyone attempts to reduce exposure to as low as reasonably achievable (ALARA). This number is invariably lower than 5 rem. During 2000, the last full year I served at DOE, only three out of more than one hundred thousand monitored workers received more than 2 rem, and these three had been exposed during accidental releases.[42]

Radiation experts have embraced the ALARA goal because they understand that a safe level for radiation exposure is unknowable, and may not exist. The same fact holds for other substances. At least on a theoretical basis, it is true of all carcinogens and for many other chemicals as well. It is possible that exposure to tiny amounts can cause disease; we just cannot study this proposition because, at very low levels, few extra cases would occur in large populations. The goal should always be ALARA.

II. Take Down the Stovepipes: Integrate the Control of Environmental and Workplace Toxic Exposures

The EPA staff members who are concerned with benzene in water have little to do with those who are working on airborne benzene, and neither of these units coordinates with yet other personnel assigned to benzene in toxic waste dumps. This is not surprising. The legislation that authorizes the EPA to improve the air we breathe and the water we drink makes little attempt to harmonize standards or coordinate approaches. And this is just the beginning of the problem. The uncoordinated environmental protection systems in EPA are parallel to, but utterly unconnected with, the system of regulating workplace health and safety anchored in OSHA and MSHA. These three public health agencies all have different rules, regulations, and enforcement cultures—while addressing similar problems.

Few employers operate this way (staffing separate operations for environmental and occupational hazards). Why should they? It is generally the same machines or processes that put the same toxic chemicals into the air of both the workplace (OSHA's responsibility) and the surrounding community (EPA's responsibility). The solvents and metals that contaminate so many drinking water aquifers are the same chemicals from the same factories that cause disease among the exposed workers. The pesticide that sterilized the California factory workers went on to lower the sperm counts of farmworkers who were applying the chemical.[43] The same lead that poisons men and women working in lead smelters also slows the neurological development of children growing up nearby.[44]

Nor does this symbiosis pertain only to facilities susceptible to chemical exposures. One of the nation's top petroleum industry polluters is BP's Texas City, Texas, plant (so much for the company's "beyond petroleum" advertising campaign). In 2004 that plant alone released more than ten million pounds of polluting chemicals.[45] In March 2005 an explosion at the facility took the lives of fifteen workers and resulted in a record OSHA fine: $21 million. Or consider McWane, Inc., one of the nation's leading manufacturers of industrial, water, and sewer pipes. The firm's horrendous worker safety record—thousands of injuries and several easily preventable deaths—earned it a long exposé in the *New York Times*.[46–48] Meanwhile, McWane's environmental policies were so egregious that it was not merely fined by EPA; a jury in Alabama convicted the company and several of its executives of conspiracy to violate the Clean Water Act. The company also pleaded guilty to felony violations of the Clean Air Act. In all, the company has been fined more than $14 million for violating environmental and safety laws, and four executives have been convicted on felony charges.[49]

How can we best deal with such outrages and such companies? Integrate the regulation and enforcement of workplace and environmental exposures. The proposal appears to be radical, but there is evidence it can reduce hazardous exposures. When the EPA issued regulations that forced factories to control emissions into the environment of volatile organic compounds, factory managers found ways to use less toxic and smaller quantities of solvents on the production line, thereby protecting the workers, as well as the neighbors. Still, such an apparently major change in the structure of the regulatory system is unlikely because too many stakeholders are quite adept at manipulating the existing system to their benefit. They want less rigorous enforcement, not more. But the goal is worth fighting for because closer coordination of the systems holds the promise of significant gains in effectiveness and efficiency. Environmental and workplace coordination might be a good pilot project for a state to develop under my next proposal.

12. Make the States Public Health Protection "Laboratories."

Long before the federal health and safety agencies were created beginning in the 1960s, some state governments, particularly in industrial states, were pioneers in developing public health protection programs. Before the creation of the National Highway Traffic Safety Administration, New York State led the fight for seat belts and safer tires in the 1960s. The power to declare public health emergencies and quarantines has always been a state, not a federal, prerogative. State and, through them, county health departments have significant power to shut down facilities that endanger public health. All in all, public health authority in the United States has traditionally resided with the individual state governments, but these powers are rarely used today and seem almost to have been forgotten.

Some federal laws even give states powers they have chosen not to use. The legislation that established OSHA, for example, allows states to set and enforce occupational safety and health standards as long as they are at least as strong as OSHA's, but most of the twenty-one states that have elected to set their own standards have simply adopted the federal benchmarks. We know how inadequate these can be. While state governments work closely with the EPA in enforcing national environmental standards, they rarely issue their own regulations if the federal ones are weak or nonexistent.

The exception is California. Since the 1960s the state has had the authority (subject to limited EPA review) to set vehicle emission standards. It has also attempted to compel automobile manufacturers to produce more fuel-efficient cars. Similarly, California is slowly developing its own chemical protection policy. Proposition 65, voted into law by a statewide initiative in 1986, requires the labeling of chemicals known to cause cancer, birth defects, or other reproductive harm.[50]

The Bush administration supports the principle of devolving power to the states but acts on this rhetoric very selectively. It has opposed state initiatives that strengthen public health protections and has focused in particular on California's activities. Standards issued in 2006 by the U.S. Department of Transportation assert exclusive federal authority to set fuel economy standards, thus preempting California's vehicle emissions rules.[51] Through the misleadingly named "National Uniformity for Food Act," the administration attempted to overturn Proposition 65 by prohibiting states from requiring warning labels on food packages.[52]

Still, California is poised to move forward. Recognizing that federal policies are not sufficient to protect Californians and the environment from toxic chemicals, two state legislature committees commissioned a study by the California Policy Research Center (part of the office of the president of the University of California) for expert assistance. The center's report concluded that "a modern comprehensive chemicals policy is essential to placing California on the path to a sustainable future" and recommended that the state develop a comprehensive approach "that corrects long-standing federal chemicals policy weaknesses and builds the foundation for new productive capacity in green chemistry—the design, manufacture, and use of chemicals that are safer for biological and ecological systems."[53]

Other states need to join California in becoming living public health laboratories, too, even if it means battling federal authorities. In some states this will not happen, I know, but it could in others, including some red states; I don't think the red/blue political division is replicated in public attitudes about public health and the environment.

* * *

Through federal regulation we have made great progress in reducing toxic exposures and protecting the public's health, but that progress must not stop. We have the laws to further prevent disease and death. We have the regulatory agencies. We have the scientists (for the most part, though some are leaving). However, political will and creative leadership are missing. As a direct result, our most important federal public health protection programs are being destroyed in an amazingly short period of time by antiregulatory zealots, most of them working at the behest of the corporations who require this regulation most of all.

Industry has skillfully turned what should be a debate over policy into a debate over science. The retreat from regulation is fueled by the product defense experts who specialize in manufacturing uncertainty and creating not sound science, as they disingenuously claim, but something that sounds like science in order to allow toxic exposures to go unregulated and victims of these chemicals to go uncompensated. Decades down the line, we will surely view their campaign on its many fronts with the same dismay and outrage with which we now look back on the deceits Big Tobacco perpetrated. But will decades down the line be too late? On the matter of global warming, certainly, it might be.

It is vital that those charged with protecting the public's health understand that the alleged desire for absolute scientific certainty is both counterproductive and futile. To wait for certainty is to wait forever. The fundamental paradigm of public health is and must be to protect people on the basis of the best evidence currently available. The manufacture and magnification of scientific uncertainty endangers both the public's health and programs to protect that health and compensate victims. It is time to return to first principles: Use the best science available; do not demand certainty where it does not and cannot exist.

Acknowledgments

This book is an outgrowth of my work over the last decade, first as Assistant Secretary for Environment, Safety, and Health at the U.S. Department of Energy, then as director of the Project on Scientific Knowledge and Public Policy (SKAPP), based at the George Washington University School of Public Health and Health Services. Celeste Monforton has been an irreplaceable collaborator at SKAPP and George Washington University for more than four years. Her insight and assistance have been an all-important contribution to this book. I have also benefited immeasurably from my work with our other SKAPP colleagues who have made SKAPP a tremendously exciting initiative: Eula Bingham, Les Boden, Liz Borkowski, Rebecca Jensen Bruhl, Dick Clapp, Sarah Donahue, Polly Hoppin, Molly Jacobs, Shelly Krimsky, Dave Ozonoff, Tony Robbins, and Susan Wood. I am also grateful for the support SKAPP has received from the Common Benefit Trust, a fund established pursuant to a court order in the Silicone Gel Breast Implant Products Liability litigation. SKAPP accepts only unrestricted funding; we do not provide our funders the opportunity to review or approve any of our work products.

At George Washington University, Dean Ruth Katz has been unswerving in her support of SKAPP and my work. Christina Morgan tirelessly fact-checked and prepared the book's references. Most importantly, Mike Bryan worked with me on the manuscript itself, and his stylistic contributions have improved the book considerably.

I am fortunate to have many friends and colleagues whose work contributed to the book and who were also willing to critique early drafts of my writings: Jordan Barab, Eula Bingham, Les Boden, Liz Borkowski, Joe Cecil, Dick Clapp, Gina Davis, Gail Dratch, Peter Lurie, Ned Miltenberg, Celeste Monforton, Jackie Nowell, Naomi Oreskes, Mark Parascandola, Bob Rinsky, Tony Robbins, David Rosner, Josh Silverman, Dava Sobel, David Vladeck, Steve Wodka, Susan Wood, and Mary Jo Zacchero.

Special thanks to my mother, Ruth Gruber, for her editorial help. Few authors are fortunate to have mothers who can also edit their work. She is a truly remarkable woman: At the age of 96, she has just published her latest book, *Witness: One of the Great Correspondents of the Twentieth Century Tells Her Story.*

There are many others whose work and ideas have also helped shape my thinking about science and public policy. I want to thank Margaret Berger, Lisa Bero, Barry Castleman, Vincent Cogliano, Ernie Drucker, Nancy Dubler, David Egilman, Jim Ellenberger, Tony Fletcher, Jack Geiger, Lynn Goldman, Merrill Goozner, Susan Haack, Bob Harrison, Lisa Heinzerling, Sheila Jasanoff, David Kriebel, Jerry Markowitz, Steven Markowitz, Anne-Marie Mazza, the late Tony Mazzocchi, Tom McGarity, Frank Mirer, Richard Miller, Chris Mooney, Drummond Rennie, Kathy Rest, Linda Rosenstock, Barbara Seaman, Peg Seminario, Stuart Shapiro, Michael Silverstein, Emily Spieler, Rena Steinzor, Neil Vidmar, Greg Wagner, Wendy Wagner, Laura Welch, and Steve Zoloth.

I am grateful to Joe Spieler, my agent, and to Wendy Wolf, both of whom answered all the questions of this novice in the trade. At Oxford University Press, editor Carrie Pedersen cared enough about my subject to acquire this book, and her successor, William Lamsback, has supported it enthusiastically the rest of the way.

Despite the best efforts of all of these wonderful, dedicated people, there will certainly be mistakes in the book. They are mine.

This book is very much shaped by my personal experiences. I have conducted epidemiologic studies on the effects of exposure to asbestos, lead, solvents, inks, and engine exhaust and have been involved in court cases (mostly on the plaintiff's side) involving diseases caused by aromatic amines, asbestos, benzene, beryllium, and vinyl chloride. Several chapters include materials I acquired through this work, as well as through my service as the union representative on the Lead Health Committee at the DuPont Chambers Works. Other chapters contain material related to my activities with the Department of Energy and subsequently as a consultant to the Department of Labor.

The origin of this book is my article "Doubt is Their Product," published in *Scientific American* in 2005. Parts of the book are adapted from my papers and studies that have appeared in *Science*, *The American Journal of Public Health*, *Law and Contemporary Problems*, *Environmental Health Perspectives*, *Public Health Reports*, and other academic journals.

The publication of this book gives me an opportunity to thank some of my colleagues in federal agencies who worked so hard to advance the Energy Employees Occupational Illness Compensation Program Act (EEOICPA), the historic program (see chapter sixteen) that provides compensation payments to civilian nuclear weapons workers who have developed work-related illnesses. These colleagues are the following: at the Energy Department—Bob Alvarez, Lori Azim, David Berick, Gina Griego Cano, Jeff Eagan, Gary Falle, Matt Greenwald, Geoff Judge, Kate Kimpan, Andy Lawrence, Ted Pulliam, Paul Seligman, Josh Silverman, Loretta Young, and Mary Jo Zacchero; at the Labor Department—Carol DeDeo, Shelby Hallmark, Michael Kerr, Jeff Nesvet, Tom Markey, and Pete Turcic; at the Department of Health and Human Services—Kathy Rest, Gail Robarge, Bill Raub, Kathy Rest, Linda Rosenstock, Rosie Sokas, and Greg Wagner; at the Department of Justice—David Fishback and Richard Jerome; and at the White House—Bill Dauster, Ron Mintz, John Pfeiffer, and Bill Samuel.

EEOICPA would not have gone from dream to reality without the commitment and hard work of Senators Jeff Bingaman, Jim Bunning, Mike DeWine, Ted Kennedy, Mitch McConnell, Harry Reid, Fred Thompson, and George Voinovich, as well as Representatives Shelly Berkley, Lindsey Graham, Paul Kanjorski, Ted Strickland, Mark Udall, Tom Udall, Zach Wamp, and Ed Whitfield. Union staff Jim Ellenberger, Sylvia Kieding, the late Jay Power, Peg Seminario, and especially Richard Miller worked long hours generating support for the program and advising us on ways to improve it. Journalists Pete Eisler, Sam Roe, and Joby Warrick wrote insightful articles that greatly influenced the development of the program. And special thanks go to former Secretary of Energy (now New Mexico governor) Bill Richardson, who pushed so hard to make peace with the past.

Most importantly, I could not have written this book without the loving encouragement and patient support of my wife, Gail Dratch. I write with the dream of a safer world for my own extraordinary children, Joel and Lila Michaels, and for children everywhere.

Abbreviations and Acronyms

ACS	American Cancer Society
AEC	Atomic Energy Commission
AIA	Asbestos Information Association
ALARA	as low as reasonably achievable
AMA	American Medical Association
API	American Petroleum Institute
ASB	Army Science Board
ASH	Action on Smoking and Health
B&W	Brown and Williamson Tobacco Corporation
BISAC	Beryllium Industry Scientific Advisory Committee
BMJ	*British Medical Journal*
BNA	beta-naphthylamine
CAPM	Chinese Academy of Preventive Medicine
CBD	chronic beryllium disease
CBI	confidential business information
CDC	Centers for Disease Control and Prevention
CDER	Center for Drug Evaluation and Research
CIAR	Center for Indoor Air Research
CPSC	Consumer Product Safety Commission
CTR	Council for Tobacco Research
DBCP	1,2-dibromo-3-chloropropane
DCB	dichlorobenzidine

DOE	Department of Energy
DOJ	Department of Justice
DQA	Data Quality Act
EEOICPA	Energy Employees Occupational Illness Compensation Program Act
EPA	Environmental Protection Agency
ETS	Environmental Tobacco Smoke
FACA	Federal Advisory Committee Act
FDA	Food and Drug Administration
FEMA	Flavor and Extract Manufacturers Association
GRAS	generally recognized as safe
H&K	Hill and Knowlton
HIV	human immunodeficiency virus
HPV	high-production volume
IARC	International Agency for Research on Cancer
ICBA	International Carbon Black Association
ILO	International Labour Organization
IOM	Institute of Medicine
IPCC	Intergovernmental Panel on Climate Change
ISEE	International Society for Environmental Epidemiology
ISRTP	International Society of Regulatory Toxicology and Pharmacology
JAMA	*Journal of the American Medical Association*
JOEM	*Journal of Occupational and Environmental Medicine*
MCA	Manufacturing Chemists Association
MOCA	4,4 methylenemethlyene-bis (2-chloroaniline)
mppcf	million parts per cubic foot
MSHA	Mine Safety and Health Administration
MTBE	methyl tertiary-butyl ether
NAS	National Academy of Sciences
NASA	National Aeronautics and Space Administration
NCI	National Cancer Institute
NEJM	*New England Journal of Medicine*
NIH	National Institutes of Health
NIOSH	National Institute for Occupational Safety and Health
NOAA	National Oceanic and Atmospheric Administration
NRC	National Research Council
NSAID	nonsteroidal anti-inflammatory drug
NHTSA	National Highway Traffic Safety Administration
OIRA	Office of Information and Regulatory Affairs
OMB	Office of Management and Budget
OSHA	Occupational Safety and Health Administration
OT	ortho-toluidine

PCB	polychlorinated biphenyls
PDUFA	Prescription Drug User Fee Act
PEL	permissible exposure limit
PFOA	perfluorooctanoic acid
PhRMA	Pharmaceutical Research and Manufacturers of America
PPA	phenylpropanolamine
ppm	parts per million
PVC	polyvinyl chloride
REACH	Registration, Evaluation, and Authorization of Chemicals (European Union legislation)
RECA	Radiation Exposure Compensation Act
RJR	RJ Reynolds Tobacco Company
RSI	repetitive strain injury
SBREFA	Small Business Regulatory Enforcement Fairness Act
SEC	Securities and Exchange Commission
SSRI	selective serotonin reuptake inhibitor
STD	sexually transmitted disease
TASSC	The Advancement of Sound Science Coalition
TIRC	Tobacco Industry Research Committee
TSCA	Toxic Substances Control Act
TRI	Toxics Release Inventory
WHO	World Health Organization

References

INTRODUCTION

1. Belay ED, Bresee JS, Holman RC et al. Reye's syndrome in the United States from 1981 through 1997. *NEJM.* 1999;340(18):1377–82.
2. U.S. Food and Drug Administration. Advanced notice of proposed rule-making: Labeling for salicylate-containing products. *Fed. Reg.* 1982;47: 57886.
3. Lurie P, Wolfe S. Aspirin and Reye's syndrome. In *Paradigms for change: A public health textbook for medical, dental, pharmacy, and nursing students.* Washington, DC: Public Citizen Health Research Group, unpublished.
4. Hilts P. *Protecting America's Health: The FDA, Business, and One Hundred Years of Regulation.* New York: Knopf, 2003.
5. Brown and Williamson. *Smoking and health proposal.* Brown and Williamson document no. 680561778–1786, 1969. Available at: http://legacy.library.ucsf .edu/tid/nvs40foo. Accessed in June 2007.
6. Whitman CT. Effective policy making: The role of good science. Remarks at the National Academy of Science's Symposium on Nutrient Over-enrichment of Coastal Waters. October 13, 2000. Available at: http://www.usembassy.it/ file2001_01/alia/a0010407.htm. Accessed in June 2007.
7. Michaels D, Bingham E, Boden L. et al. Advice without dissent. *Science.* 2002;298(5594):703.

8. Luntz F. Memo: The environment: A cleaner, safer, healthier America; ca. 2003. Available at: http://www.ewg.org:16080/briefings/luntzmemo. Accessed in October 2006.

9. Herrick C, Jamieson D. Junk science and environmental policy: Obscuring public debate with misleading discourse. *Philos Public Policy Q.* 2001;21: 11–16.

CHAPTER ONE

1. *Smoking and Health.* Report of the Advisory Committee to the Surgeon General of the Public Health Service. U.S. Department of Health Education and Welfare: Public Health Service, 1964. Public Health Service publication no. 1103.

2. Parascandola M. Science, industry, and tobacco harm reduction: A case study of tobacco industry scientists' involvement in the National Cancer Institute's Smoking and Health Program, 1964–1980. *Public Health Rep.* 2005;120:338–49.

3. Brown and Williamson. Project Truth: The smoking/health controversy: A view from the other side. Prepared for the *Courier-Journal* and *Louisville Times.* February 8, 1971. Brown and Williamson document no. 2110.06. Available at: http://legacy.library.ucsf.edu/tid/xpb72doo. Accessed in June 2007.

4. Sandefur T. Testimony: Hearing on the regulation of tobacco products. U.S. House Committee on Energy and Commerce, Subcommittee on Health and the Environment; April 14, 1994. Available at: http://www.jeffreywigand.com/insider/7ceos.html. Accessed in June 2007.

5. Brenner M. The man who knew too much. *Vanity Fair.* May 1996: 170–192.

6. Kessler D. *A Question of Intent: A Great American Battle with a Deadly Industry.* New York: Public Affairs, 2001.

7. Brandt AM. *The Cigarette Industry: The Rise, Fall, and Deadly Persistence of the Product That Defined America.* New York: Basic Books, 2007.

8. Glantz S, Slade J, Bero L et al. *The Cigarette Papers.* Berkeley: University of California Press, 1996.

9. Kluger R. *Ashes to Ashes: America's Hundred-Year Cigarette War, the Public Health, and the Unabashed Triumph of Philip Morris.* New York: Random House, 1996.

10. *Reducing the Health Consequences of Smoking: 25 Years of Progress.* Report of the Surgeon General. U.S. Department of Health and Human Services, 1989. DHHS publication no. (CDC) 89–8411.

11. *The Health Consequences of Smoking.* Report of the Surgeon General. U.S. Department of Health and Human Services, 2004.

12. Pearl R. Tobacco smoking and longevity. *Science.* 1938;87:216–17.

13. George Seldes on tobacco: Fifty years ahead of his time (A collection of more than fifty articles from Seldes's newsletter, *In Fact* (1940–1950)). Available at: http://www.brasscheck.com/seldes/tobac.html. Accessed in June 2007.

14. Doll R, Hill A. Smoking and carcinoma of the lung: Preliminary report. *BMJ.* 1950:739–48.

15. Levin ML, Goldstein H, Gerhardt PR. Cancer and tobacco smoking: A preliminary report. *JAMA.* 1950;143:336–38.

16. Mills CA, Porter MM. Tobacco smoking habits and cancer of the mouth and respiratory system. *Cancer Research.* 1950;10:539–42.

17. Schrek R, Baker LA, Ballard GP et al. Tobacco smoking as an etiologic factor in disease. Part 1: Cancer. *Cancer Research.* 1950;10:49–58.

18. Wynder EL, Graham EA. Tobacco smoking as a possible etiologic factor in bronchiogenic carcinoma. *JAMA.* 1950;143:329–36.

19. Parascandola M. Skepticism, statistical methods, and the cigarette: A historical analysis of a methodological debate. *Perspect Biol Med.* 2004;47(42): 244–61.

20. Hill and Knowlton, Inc. Background material on the cigarette industry client. December 15, 1953. Tobacco documents, R. J. Reynolds document no. 519124023/4027. Available at: http://legacy.library.ucsf.edu/tid/ssq31doo. Available in June 2007.

21. Miller KS. *Voice of Power: Hill and Knowlton and Postwar Public Relations.* Chapel Hill, NC: University of North Carolina Press, 1999.

22. Wilson BS. Legislative history of the Pesticide Residues Amendments of 1954 and the Delaney Clause of the Food Additives Amendment of 1958. In: *Regulating Pesticides in Food: The Delaney Paradox.* Washington, DC: National Academy Press, 1987:161–73.

23. U.S. News and World Report. Coverage at AMA convention (June 21, 1954). *U.S. News and World Report.* July 2, 1954:64–67.

24. Hammond E, Horn D. The relationship between human smoking habits and death rates. *JAMA.* 1954;155(15):1316–28.

25. Hill and Knowlton, Inc. Press release: Re: Dr. Clarence Cook Little appointed director of Tobacco Industry Research Committee. Issued June 15, 1954. Available at: http://legacy.library.ucsf.edu/tid/arx49coo. Accessed in June 2007.

26. Thompson C (Hill and Knowlton, Inc.). Memorandum to Kloepfer W Jr. (Tobacco Institute). Subject: *Tobacco and Health Research* procedural memo. October 18, 1968. Tobacco Institute document no. TIMN0071488/1491. Available at: http://legacy.library.ucsf.edu/tid/upv92foo. Accessed in June 2007.

27. Tobacco Industry Research Committee (TIRC). *Reports on Tobacco and Health Research.* July–August 1963. Available at: http://legacy.library.ucsf .edu/tid/avz60aoo. Accessed in June 2007.

28. TIRC. *Research Reports on Tobacco and Health*. October 1960. Available at: http://legacy.library.ucsf.edu/tid/xof19doo. Accessed in June 2007.

29. TIRC. *Research Reports on Tobacco and Health*. April–May 1961. Available at: http://legacy.library.ucsf.edu/tid/ayx19doo. Accessed in June 2007.

30. TIRC. *Research Reports on Tobacco and Health*. September–October 1962. Available at: http://legacy.library.ucsf.edu/tid/jlf99doo. Accessed in June 2007.

31. TIRC. *Research Reports on Tobacco and Health*. December 1962. Available at: http://legacy.library.ucsf.edu/tid/fwf19doo. Accessed in June 2007.

32. TIRC. *Reports on Tobacco and Health Research*. November–December 1963. Available at: http://legacy.library.ucsf.edu/tid/dpl94foo. Accessed in June 2007.

33. TIRC. *Reports on Tobacco and Health Research*. March–April 1964. Available at: http://legacy.library.ucsf.edu/tid/bvz60aoo. Accessed in June 2007.

34. TIRC. *Reports on Tobacco and Health Research*. Winter 1964–1965. Available at: http://legacy.library.ucsf.edu/tid/jvz60aoo. Accessed in June 2007.

35. TIRC. *Reports on Tobacco and Health Research*. September–October 1964. Available at: http://legacy.library.ucsf.edu/tid/civ75foo. Accessed in June 2007.

36. Sterling TM. The Effects of Interview Bias on the Attempts to Measure the Relationship between Smoking and Health. Report no. 2: Evaluation of the Analysis and Procedures of the NHS Interview Data and Methods. [Report done under Special Project of the Council for Tobacco Research.] Council for Tobacco Research document no. CTRSP/FILES003743/3765. Available at: http://legacy.library.ucsf.edu/tid/xpd8aaoo. Accessed in July 2007.

37. Proposal to study interviewer bias. Philip Morris document no. 2075715519/5520. Available at: http://legacy.library.ucsf.edu/tid/coj37doo. Accessed in July 2007.

38. A proposal to explore the role of memory in epidemiologic studies, develop practical standards of significance, and improve scientific communication. Philip Morris document no. 2064229233/9247. Available at: http://legacy.library.ucsf.edu/tid/ayv93coo. Accessed in July 2007.

39. Koop CE. Foreword. In Glantz SA, Slade J, Bero L et al. *The Cigarette Papers*. Berkeley: University of California Press, 1996. Accessed in June 2007.

40. Haselbach C, Libert O. A tentative hypothesis on nicotine addiction. Report produced for the British-American Tobacco Co., May 30, 1963.

41. Federal Cigarette Labeling and Advertising Act of 1965: Public law 89–92; 1965.

42. Drew EB. The quiet victory of the cigarette lobby: How it found the best filter yet: Congress. *Atlantic Monthly*. 1965;216(3):76–80.

43. Brown and Williamson. *Smoking and health proposal*. Brown and Williamson document no. 680561778–1786, 1969. Available at: http://legacy.library.ucsf.edu/tid/nvs40foo. Accessed in June 2007.

44. Panzer F. Letter to Kornegay HR. Subject: The Roper proposal. American Tobacco document no. 963012260–2263. May 1, 1972. Available at: http://legacy.library.ucsf.edu/tid/crn15foo. Accessed in June 2007.

CHAPTER TWO

1. International Labour Organization, World Health Organization. Press release: Number of work-related accidents and illnesses continues to increase: ILO and WHO join in call for prevention strategies. Issued April 28, 2005. Available at: http://www.ilo.org/global/About_the_ILO/Media_and_public_information/Press_releases/lang–en/WCMS_005161. Accessed in June 2007.
2. Brodeur P. *Asbestos and Enzymes.* New York: Ballantine, 1972.
3. Brodeur P. *Expendable Americans.* New York: Viking, 1973.
4. Brodeur P. *Outrageous Misconduct: The Asbestos Industry on Trial.* New York: Pantheon, 1985.
5. Castleman B. *Asbestos: Medical and Legal Aspects,* 5th ed. New York: Aspen, 2005.
6. Ozonoff D. Failed warnings: Asbestos-related disease and industrial medicine In: Bayer R, ed. *Case Studies in the Politics of Professional Responsibility.* New York: Oxford University Press, 1988:139–218.
7. Schneider A, McCumber D. *An Air That Kills: How the Asbestos Poisoning of Libby, Montana, Uncovered a National Scandal.* New York: Putnam, 2004.
8. Egilman D, Fehnel C, Bohme SR. Exposing the "myth" of ABC, "anything but chrysotile": A critique of the Canadian asbestos mining industry and McGill University chrysotile studies. *Am J Ind Med.* 2003;44(5):540–57.
9. Tweedale G. *Magic Mineral to Killer Dust.* New York: Oxford University Press, 2000.
10. McCulloch J. *Asbestos: Its Human Cost.* New York: University of Queensland Press, 1986.
11. Frist W. Asbestos litigation crisis (Senate proceedings, November 22, 2003). *Congressional Record.* 2003:S15514–S15515.
12. *Annual report of Her Majesty's Lady Inspectors. In Annual Report of the Chief Inspector of Factories and Workshops for the Year 1898.* Part II: Reports. London: Her Majesty's Stationery Office, 1898:172.
13. Hoffman FL. Mortality from respiratory diseases from dusty trades (inorganic dusts) [bulletin]. U.S. Department of Labor, Bureau of Labor Statistics. Whole no. 231, Industrial Accidents and Hygiene Series no. 17. June 1918.
14. Cherniak M. *The Hawk's Nest Incident: America's Worst Industrial Disaster.* New Haven, CT: Yale University Press, 1986.

15. Trudeau Institute History. Available at: http://www.trudeauinstitute.org/info/history/history.htm. Accessed in June 2007.

16. Dreessen WC, Dallavalle JM, Edwards TI et al. A study of asbestosis in the asbestos textile industry. U.S. Treasury Department, Public Health Service. Public Health bulletin no. 241. August 1938.

17. Industrial Hygiene Foundation of America. Report of preliminary dust investigation for Asbestos Textile Institute. June 18, 1947. Pittsburgh, PA.

18. Brown V. The management viewpoint: Discussion. In: Vorwald AJ, ed. *Pneumoconiosis: Beryllium, Bauxite Fumes, Compensation.* New York: Hoeber, 1950;567–72.

19. Hueper W. *Occupational Tumors and Allied Diseases.* Baltimore, MD: Thomas, 1942.

20. Asbestosis and cancer of the lung. [Editorial]. *JAMA.* 1949;140(9):1219–20.

21. Conklin G. Cancer and the environment. *Sci Am.* 1949;180(1):11–15.

22. Proctor RN. *The Nazi War on Cancer.* Princeton, NJ: Princeton University Press, 1999.

23. Vorwald AJ, Durkan TM, Pratt PC. Experimental studies of asbestosis. *AMA Arch Ind Hyg Occup Med.* 1951;3(1):1–43.

24. Asbestos Textile Institute Air Hygiene and Manufacturing Committee. Meeting minutes. March 7, 1957.

25. Pritchard J (Pathologist, Wayne State University College of Medicine, Department of Industrial Medicine and Hygiene). Pathology report: William Cooling (Autopsy conducted at Montreal General Hospital, January 1949).

26. *Smoking and Health.* Report of the Advisory Committee to the Surgeon General of the Public Health Service. U.S. Department of Health Education and Welfare: Public Health Service, 1964. Public Health Service publication no. 1103.

27. Selikoff IJ, Churg J, eds. Biological effects of asbestos. *Ann NY Acad Sci.* 1965;132(1):1–766.

28. Brodeur P. The magic mineral. *New Yorker.* October 12, 1968.

29. Cadwalader, Wickersham, and Taft (lawyers for Asbestos Textile Institute). Letter to Selikoff I. October 26, 1964.

30. About the speaker: Matthew M. Swetonic. Addendum to meeting minutes for Asbestos Textile Institute general meeting. Key Bridge Marriott, Arlington, VA, June 7, 1973.

31. Hill and Knowlton, Inc. Division of Scientific, Technical, and Environmental Affairs; ca. 1989. Available at: http://www.defendingscience.org/upload/HK_1989.pdf. Accessed in December 2007.

32. Hill and Knowlton, Inc. Division of Scientific, Technical, and Environmental Affairs. Case study: Asbestos and human health; ca. 1989. Available at: http://www.defendingscience.org/upload/HK_1989.pdf. Accessed in December 2007.

33. Filteau PA (General Manager, Quebec Asbestos Mining Association [QAMA]). Special winter meeting, Grand Bahama Hotel and Country Club. January 31, 1968: 8.
34. Selikoff IJ, Hammond E, Churg J. Asbestos exposure, smoking, and neoplasia. *JAMA.* 1968;204(2):106–12.
35. Evans EE (director, Medical Division, Chambers Works) on behalf of Brothers WC (manager, Chambers Works). Letter to Mangelsdorff A (Calco Chemical Co.). June 18, 1947. Available at: http://www.defending science.org/upload/Evans_1947.pdf. Accessed in December 2007.
36. Scott TS. *Carcinogenic and Chronic Toxic Hazards of Aromatic Amines.* New York: Elsevier, 1962.
37. Norton TH. *Dyestuffs for American Textile and Other Industries.* U.S. Department of Commerce, Bureau of Foreign and Domestic Commerce Special Agents Series, no. 96, 1915.
38. National Academy of Engineering. *Technology and Environment.* Washington, DC: National Academy Press, 1989.
39. Dietrich H, Dietrich B. Ludwig Rehn (1849–1930). Pioneering findings on the aetioliogy of bladder cancers. *World J Urol.* 2000;19:151–53.
40. Hueper W. *Occupational and Environmental Cancers of the Urinary System.* New Haven, CT: Yale University Press, 1969.
41. International Labour Organization. *Cancer of the Bladder among Workers in Aniline Factories.* Studies and Reports Series F, no. 1. February 1921.
42. U.S. Tariff Commission. *Dyes.* (Prepared in response to requests from the Committee on Finance of the U.S. Senate and the Committee on Ways and Means of the House of Representatives). War Changes in Industry Series, report no. 19, 1946.
43. *DuPont, the Autobiography of an American Enterprise.* New York: Scribner, 1952.
44. Hounshell D, Smith JK Jr. *Science and Corporate Strategy: Du Pont R&D, 1902–1980.* New York: Cambridge University Press, 1988.
45. Smith DT (supervisor, Protection Division). Letter to Queener JS (manager, Safety and Fire Protection Division). Subject: History of beta-naphthylamine manufacture: Chamber Works. September 22, 1958. Available at: http://www.defendingscience.org/upload/Smith_1958.pdf. Accessed in December 2007.
46. Michaels D. Waiting for the body count: Corporate decision making and bladder cancer in the U.S. dye industry. *Med Anthro Q.* 1988;2:215–232.
47. Michaels D. When science isn't enough: Wilhelm Hueper, Robert A.M. Case and the limits of scientific evidence in preventing occupational bladder cancer. *Int J Occup Environ Health.* 1995;1:278–288.
48. Washburn V. Abstract of discussion. *JAMA.* 1936;107:1438–39.
49. Wignall TH. Incidence of disease of the bladder in workers in certain chemicals. *BMJ.* 1929;2:291–93.
50. Agran L. *The Cancer Connection.* Boston, MA: Houghton Mifflin, 1977.

51. Hueper WC. Wilhelm Hueper's autobiography. Unpublished manuscript.

52. Hueper WC, Wiley FH, Wolfe HD. Experimental production of bladder tumors in dogs by administration of beta-naphthylamine. *J Ind Hyg Toxicol.* 1938;20:46–84.

53. Evans E. Causative agents and protective measures in the anilin tumor of the bladder. *J Urol.* 1936;38:212–15.

54. Agran L. Interview with Dr. Wilhelm C. Hueper, MD; December 1975. In: Breslow L, ed. *A History of Cancer Control in the United States, 1946–1971.* DHEW publication no. (NIH) 79–1519, 1979.

55. Bent S. Tetraethyl lead fatal to makers. *New York Times.* June 22, 1925:3.

56. Markowitz G, Rosner D. *Deceit and Denial: The Deadly Politics of Industrial Pollution.* Berkeley, CA: University of California Press, 2002.

57. Schwartz BS, Bolla KI, Stewart W et al. Decrements in neurobehavioral performance associated with mixed exposure to organic and inorganic lead. *Am J Epidemiol.* 1993;137(9):1006–21.

58. Schwartz BS, Stewart WF, Bolla KI et al. Past adult lead exposure is associated with longitudinal decline in cognitive function. *Neurology.* 2000; 55:1144–50.

59. Otto GB. Operation of new plant/chronological history: Manufacture of beta napthylamine. Unpublished report. April 13, 1953. Available at: http://www.defendingscience.org/upload/Otto_1953.pdf. Accessed in December 2007.

60. Weiss RJ. Email to Fayerweather WE and Karns E. October 25, 1991.

61. Epstein S. Presentation of the first award of the Society for Occupational and Environmental Health to Dr. Wilhelm C. Hueper. *Ann NY Acad Sci.* 1975;271:457–59.

62. Case R. The misbegotten camel. Unpublished manuscript. 1983.

63. Case R. Tumors of the urinary tract as an occupational disease in several industries. *Ann Royal College Surgery.* 1966;39:213–35.

64. Case RAM. Incidence of death from tumours of the urinary bladder. *Br J Prev Soc Med.* 1953;7(1):14–19.

65. Case R, Hosker M, McDonald D et al. Tumors of the urinary bladder in workmen engaged in the manufacture and use of certain dyestuff intermediates in the British chemical industry: Part 1: The role of aniline, benzidine, alpha-naphthylamine, and beta-naphthylamine. *British J Ind Med.* 1954;11:75–96.

66. Case RAM, Hosker ME. Tumour of the urinary bladder as an occupational disease in the rubber industry in England and Wales. *British J Prev Soc Med.* 1954;48:39–50.

67. Ward E, Carpenter A, Markowitz S et al. Excess number of bladder cancers in workers exposed to ortho-toluidine and aniline. *J Natl Cancer Inst.* 1991; 83(7):501–06.

68. Gehrmann GH, Foulger JH, Fleming AJ. Occupational tumours of the bladder. Paper presented at Ninth International Congress on Industrial Medicine, 1948. London, 1949.

69. Case RAM (Chester Beatty Research Institute, London). Letter to the Editor *(Washington Post)*. July 30, 1979. Printed in Corporate Criminal Liability Hearing Report for Sessions 1 and 2. U.S. House of Representatives (96th Cong.), Committee on the Judiciary, Subcommittee on Crime. 71: 101–03. Washington, DC: U.S. Government Printing Office, 1981.

70. Castleman B. DuPont's record in business ethics: Another view. *Washington Post.* July 15, 1979:E4.

71. Spitz S, Maguigan WH, Dobriner K. The carcinogenic action of benzidine. *Cancer.* 1950;3(5):789–804.

72. Ferber KH, Hill WJ, Cobb DA. An assessment of the effect of improved working conditions on bladder tumor incidence in a benzidine manufacturing facility. *Am Ind Hyg Assoc J.* 1976;37(1):61–68.

73. Johnson W, Parnes W. Beta-naphthylamine and benzidine: Identification of groups at high risk of bladder cancer. *Ann NY Acad Sci.* 1979;329:277–84.

74. Scott TS. The incidence of bladder tumours in a dyestuffs factory. *Br J Ind Med.* 1952;9(2):127–32.

75. Bingham E. Personal communication, April 26, 1988.

76. Zavon M, Hoegg U, Bingham E. Benzidine exposure as a cause of bladder tumors. *Arch Environ Health.* 1973;27(1):1–7.

77. Mancuso T, El-Attar A. Cohort study of workers exposed to beta-naphthylamine and benzidine. *J Occup Med.* 1967;9:277–85.

78. Fleming A, D'Alonzo C, Zapp J. *Modern Occupational Medicine.* Philadelphia: Lea and Febiger, 1954.

79. Mason T, Prorock P, Neeld W et al. Screening for bladder cancer at the DuPont Chamber Works: Initial findings. *J Occup Med.* 1986;28:1011–16.

80. Temkin IS. *Industrial Bladder Carcinogenesis.* New York: Pergamon, 1963.

81. Stern FB, Murthy LI, Beaumont JJ et al. Notification and risk assessment for bladder cancer of a cohort exposed to aromatic amines. III. Mortality among workers exposed to aromatic amines in the last beta-naphthylamine manufacturing facility in the United States. *J Occup Med.* 1985;27(7):495–500.

CHAPTER THREE

1. Carson R. *Silent Spring.* Boston, MA: Houghton Mifflin, 1962.

2. Presidential Science Advisory Committee. Use of pesticides [report]. Issued May 15, 1963.

3. *Smoking and Health.* Report of the Advisory Committee to the Surgeon General of the Public Health Service. U.S. Department of Health Education and Welfare: Public Health Service, 1964. Public Health Service publication no. 1103.

4. Selikoff IJ, Churg J, eds. Biological effects of asbestos. *Ann NY Acad Sci.* 1965;132(1):1–766.

5. The cities: The price of optimism. *Time.* August 1, 1969:41–44.

6. U.S. Environmental Protection Agency. Press release: DDT ban takes effect. Issued December 31, 1972. Available at: http://www.epa.gov/history/topics/ddt/01.htm. Accessed in June 2007.

7. EPA. Press release: Government ban on fluorocarbon gases in aerosol products begins October 15. Issued October 15, 1978. Available at: http://www.epa.gov/history/topics/ozone/01.htm. Accessed in June 2007.

8. Press release: EPA bans PCB manufacture; phases out uses. Issued April 19, 1979. Available at: http://www.epa.gov/history/topics/pcbs/01.htm. Accessed in June 2007.

9. Press release: U.S. sues Hooker Chemical at Niagara Falls, New York. Issued December 20, 1979. Available at: http://www.epa.gov/history/topics/lovecanal/02.htm. Accessed in June 2007.

10. Gibbs LM. *Love Canal: The Story Continues.* Gabriola Island, BC, Canada and Stony Creek, CT: New Society Publishers, 1998.

11. U.S. Environmental Protection Agency, Office of Air Quality and Standards, Air Quality Strategies and Standards Division. National Air Quality and Emissions Trends Report, Special Studies Edition. 2003. EPA publication no. 454/R-03-005.

12. Davis D, Hanig J. *Song of the Canary* [film]. 1978.

13. Torkelson TR, Sadek SE, Rowe VK et al. Toxicologic investigations of 1,2-dibromo-3-chloropropane. *Toxicol Appl Pharmacol.* September 1961;3: 545–59.

14. U.S. Occupational Safety and Health Administration. Occupational exposure to 1,2-dibromo-3-chloropropane (DBCP): Emergency temporary standard; Hearing. *Fed. Reg.* 1977;42:45535.

15. AFL-CIO. *Death on the Job: The Toll of Neglect. A National and State-by-State Profile of Worker Safety and Health in the United States.* April 2007. 16th ed. Available at: http://www.aflcio.org/issues/safety/memorial/upload/doj_2007.pdf. Accessed in July 2007.

16. OSHA. Hazard communication. Final rule. *Fed. Reg.* 1983;48:53280.

17. OSHA. Identification, classification, and regulation of toxic substances posing a potential occupational carcinogenic risk. Proposed rule and notice of hearing. *Fed. Reg.* 1977;42:54148.

18. *Industrial Union Department vs. American Petroleum Institute,* 44 U.S. 607 (July 2, 1980). Available at: http://www.publichealthlaw.net/Reader/docs/IndustUnion.pdf. Accessed in June 2007.

19. *AFL-CIO vs. OSHA,* 965 F.2d 962 (July 7, 1992).

20. U.S. House of Representatives (91st Cong., 1st sess.). Report on H.R. 13950, Federal Coal Mine Health and Safety Act. Committee on Education and Labor; 1969. House Report no. 91–563. Available at: http://

www.msha.gov/SOLICITOR/COALACT/69hous.htm. Accessed in June 2007.

21. Federal Coal Mine Health and Safety Act. Public law no. 91–173, 1969.

22. NIOSH Safety and Health Topic: Occupational Respiratory Disease Surveillance. Available at: http://www.cdc.gov/niosh/topics/surveillance/ORDS/CoalMineHealthSafetyAct35Years.html. Accessed in July 2007.

23. Mine Safety and Health Administration (MSHA). History of mine safety and health legislation. Available at: http://www.msha.gov/MSHAINFO/MSHAINF2.HTM. Accessed in June 2007.

24. PVC rolls out of jeopardy, into jubilation. *Chemical Week.* September 15, 1976:34.

25. Torkelson TR, Oyen F, Rowe VK. The toxicity of vinyl chloride as determined by repeated exposure of laboratory animals. *Am Ind Hyg Assoc J.* 1961;22:354–61.

26. Cook WA, Giever P, Dinman BD et al. Occupational acroosteolysis: Part 2. An industrial hygiene study. *Arch Environ Health.* 1971;22(1):74–82.

27. Markowitz G, Rosner D. *Deceit and Denial: The Deadly Politics of Industrial Pollution.* Berkeley, CA: University of California Press, 2002.

28. Viola PL. Cancerogenic effect of vinyl chloride. Paper presented at the Tenth International Cancer Congress, Houston, TX, May 22–29, 1970.

29. Viola P, Bigotti A, Caputo A. Oncogenic response of rat skin, lungs, and bones to vinyl chloride. *Cancer Res.* 1971;31:516–22.

30. Meeting minutes: Manufacturing Chemists Association, vinyl chloride research coordinators. January 30, 1973.

31. Elliott DM (general manager, Production, Solvents and Monomers Group, Imperial Chemical Industries Limited, Mond Division). Letter to Best GE (Manufacturing Chemists Association). October 30, 1972.

32. Siegel AC (Tenneco Chemicals, Inc.). Memorandum to Rozland GI (Tenneco Chemicals, Inc.). Subject: Vinyl chloride technical task group meeting; November 16, 1972.

33. Meeting minutes: Manufacturing Chemists Association, vinyl chloride research coordinators. May 21, 1973. Available at: http://www.defendingscience.org/upload/MCA_1973.pdf. Accessed in December 2007.

34. Kusnetz HL (manager of Industrial Hygiene, Head Office, Shell Oil Co.). Notes on the meeting of the VCM committee. July 17, 1973. Available at: http://www.defendingscience.org/upload/Kusnetz_1973.pdf. Accessed in December 2007.

35. Wheeler RN Jr. (Union Carbide). Memorandum to Carvajal JL, Dernehl CU, Hanks GJ, Lane KS, Steele AB, Zutty NL. Subject: Vinyl chloride research: MCA report to NIOSH; July 19, 1973. Available at: http://www.defendingscience.org/upload/Wheeler_1973.pdf. Accessed in December 2007.

36. Angiosarcoma of the liver among polyvinyl chloride workers. *Morbidity and Mortality Weekly Report.* 1974;23(6):49–50.

37. Maltoni C, Lefemine G. Carcinogenicity bioassays of vinyl chloride: Current results. *Ann NY Acad Sci.* 1975;246:195–218.

38. OSHA. Press release: News: OSHA investigating Goodrich cancer fatalities. Issued January 24, 1974.

39. OSHA. Transcript: Informal fact-finding hearings on possible hazards of polyvinyl chloride manufacture and use. February 15, 1974. Available at: http://www.chemicalindustryarchives.org/search/pdfs/vinyl/19740215_ 001_00000495.PDF (124–40). Accessed in June 2007.

40. OSHA. Vinyl chloride: proposed standard. *Fed. Reg.* 1974;39(92):16896.

41. Key MM. Deposition in the United States District Court for the Western District of New York, in the matter of *Holly M. Smith v. the Dow Chemical Company; PPG Industries, Inc., and Shell Oil Company v. the Goodyear Tire and Rubber Company.* CA no. 94-CV-0393 (September 19, 1995).

42. Hill and Knowlton, Inc. Recommendations for public affairs program for SPI's vinyl chloride committee, Phase 1: Preparation for OSHA hearings; June 1974. Available at: www.defendingscience.org/upload/HK_1974.pdf. Accessed in December 2007.

43. Weaver PH. On the horns of the vinyl chloride dilemma. *Fortune.* October 1974:150.

44. OSHA. Standard for exposure to vinyl chloride. *Fed. Reg.* 1974;39(194): 35890.

45. *The Society of the Plastics Industry, Inc. v. OSHA,* 509 F.2d 1301 (January 31, 1975).

46. OSHA. Standard for exposure to vinyl chloride; effective date. *Fed. Reg.* 1975;40(58):13211.

47. U.S. Congress, Office of Technology Assessment. Gauging control technology and regulatory impacts in occupational safety and health: An appraisal of OSHA's analytic approach OTA-ENV-635. Washington, DC: U.S. Government Printing Office, 1995.

CHAPTER FOUR

1. Markowitz G, Rosner D. *Deceit and Denial: The Deadly Politics of Industrial Pollution.* Berkeley, CA: University of California Press, 2002.

2. Lanphear BP, Hornung R, Khoury J et al. Low-level environmental lead exposure and children's intellectual function: An international pooled analysis. *Environ Health Perspect.* 2005;113(7):894–99.

3. Schwartz J. Low-level lead exposure and children's IQ: A meta-analysis and search for a threshold. *Environ Res.* 1994;65(1):42–55.

4. Lead-based Paint Poisoning Prevention Act. Public law no. 91–695. January 13, 1971.
5. U.S. Consumer Product Safety Commission, Office of Information and Public Affairs. Press release: CPSC announces decision on lead-in-paint issue raised by Congress. Issued December 17, 1976. Available at: http://www.cpsc.gov/CPSCPUB/PREREL/prhtml76/76087.html. Accessed in June 2007.
6. Mishra R. Rhode Island wins lead paint suit. *Boston Globe*. February 23, 2006.
7. Warren C. *Brush with Death: A Social History of Lead Poisoning*. Baltimore, MD: Johns Hopkins University Press, 2000.
8. Bent S. Tetraethyl lead fatal to makers. *New York Times*. June 22, 1925:3.
9. Odd gas kills one, makes four insane. *New York Times*. October 27, 1924.
10. Sullivan W. Warning is issued on lead poisoning. *New York Times*. September 12, 1965:71.
11. National Research Council. *Toxicological Effects of Methylmercury*. Washington, DC: National Academy Press, 2000.
12. U.S. Food and Drug Administration, U.S. Environmental Protection Agency. Consumer advisory: What you need to know about mercury in fish and shellfish. March 2004. Report no. EPA-823-F-04–009.
13. Hamburger T, Miller AC. Mercury emissions rule geared to benefit industry, staffers say. *Los Angeles Times*. March 16, 2004.
14. Pianin E. Proposed mercury rules bear industry mark: EPA language similar to that in memos from law firm representing utilities. *Washington Post*. January 31, 2004:A4.
15. Trasande L, Schechter C, Haynes KA et al. Applying cost analyses to drive policy that protects children: Mercury as a case study. *Ann NY Acad Sci*. 2006;1076:911–23.
16. Patterson C. Contaminated and natural lead environments of man. *Arch Environ Health*. 1965;11:350.
17. Kimberly JL (executive vice president, Lead Industries Association, Inc.) Letter to board of directors and industry development committee. Subject: Survey on Public Knowledge and Attitudes on Lead. March 7, 1967.
18. U.S. Environmental Protection Agency. Regulation of fuels and fuel additives: Notice of proposed rulemaking. *Fed. Reg.* 1972;37:3882.
19. *Ethyl Corp. v. EPA,* 541 F.2d 1 (March 19, 1976).
20. Houk VN (director, Center for Environmental Health, Centers for Disease Control, Public Health Service), Testimony before the Committee on Environment and Public Works, U.S. Senate (98th Cong., 2d sess.) on S.2609: Airborne Lead Reduction Act of 1984. Senate hearing no. 98–978, June 22, 1984.
21. S.2609. Airborne Lead Reduction Act of 1984. Introduced April 30, 1984, by Sen. Durenberger D (R-MN).

22. Sen. Durenberger D (R-MN). Testimony before the Committee on Environment and Public Works, U.S. Senate (98th Cong., 2d sess.) on S.2609: Airborne Lead Reduction Act of 1984. Senate hearing no. 98–978, June 22, 1984.

23. Needleman HL (director, Behavioral Sciences Division, Children's Hospital of Pittsburgh). Testimony before the Committee on Environment and Public Works, U.S. Senate (98th Cong., 2d sess.) on S.2609: Airborne Lead Reduction Act of 1984. Senate hearing: 98–978, June 22, 1984.

24. Needleman HL, Gunnoe C, Leviton A et al. Deficits in psychologic and classroom performance of children with elevated dentine lead levels. *NEJM.* 1979;300(13):689–95.

25. Cole JF (president, International Lead Zinc Research Organization, Inc.) Testimony before the Committee on Environment and Public Works, U.S. Senate (98th Cong., 2d sess.) on S.2609: Airborne Lead Reduction Act of 1984. Senate hearing: 98–978, June 22, 1984.

26. Needleman HL. The removal of lead from gasoline: Historical and personal reflections. *Environ Res.* 2000;84(1):20–35.

27. Clean Air Act Amendments of 1990. Public law no. 101–549, November 15, 1990.

28. Grosse SD, Matte TD, Schwartz J et al. Economic gains resulting from the reduction in children's exposure to lead in the United States. *Environ Health Perspect.* 2002;110(6):563–69.

CHAPTER FIVE

1. Hill and Knowlton, Inc. Division of Scientific, Technical, and Environmental Affairs; ca. 1989. Available at: http://www.defendingscience.org/upload/HK_1989.pdf. Accessed in December 2007.

2. Hill and Knowlton, Inc. Division of Scientific, Technical, and Environmental Affairs. Case study: Vinyl chloride and cancer; ca. 1989. Available at: http://www.defendingscience.org/upload/HK_1989.pdf. Accessed in December 2007.

3. Molina MJ, Rowland FS. Stratospheric sink for chlorofluoromethanes: Chlorine atomc-atalyzed [*sic*] destruction of ozone. *Nature.* 1974;249:810–12.

4. Hill and Knowlton, Inc. Division of Scientific, Technical, and Environmental Affairs. Case study: Fluorocarbons and ozone depletion; ca. 1989. Available at: http://www.defendingscience.org/upload/HK_1989.pdf. Accessed in December 2007.

5. Egilman DS, Bohme SR. Author reply to Paustenbach DJ. Scientific method questioned. *Int J Occup Environ Health.* 2006;12(3):290–92.

6. Exponent, Inc. Form 10-K filed with the U.S. Securities and Exchange Commission for fiscal year ended December 29, 2006. Available at: http://

www.sec.gov/Archives/edgar/data/851520/000119312507049476/d10k.htm. Accessed in June 2007.

7. Robertson LM. *The Expert Witness Scam*. Lulu.com, 2006.

8. Exponent, Inc. Announcement of merging of three companies (Failure Analysis Associates, PTI Environmental Services, and Environmental Health Strategies) to Exponent. 1998. Available at: http://legacy.library .ucsf.edu/tid/wtt93c00. Accessed in June 2007.

9. Office of Environmental Health Hazard Assessment (OEHHA). California public health goal for methyl tertiary butyl ether (MTBE) in drinking water. March 1999. Available at: http://www.oehha.ca.gov/water/phg/pdf/ mtbe_f.pdf. Accessed in June 2007.

10. Jones, Day, Reavis & Pogue (Methanex Corporation Counsel). Claimant Methanex Corporation's second amended statement of claim in the matter of *Methanex Corp. v U.S.* Submitted November 5, 2002. Exhibit E: *Evaluation of UST/LUST Status in California and MTBE in Drinking Water.* Prepared by Exponent, Inc., 2002. Available at: http://www.state.gov/ documents/organization/15035.pdf. Accessed in June 2007.

11. Martinson M, Davidson J. Analysis of MTBE groundwater cleanup costs: A report to the American Petroleum Institute. June 2005.

12. Braksiek RJ, Roberts DJ. Amusement park injuries and deaths. *Ann Emerg Med.* 2002;39(1):65–72.

13. Exponent, Inc. Investigation of amusement park and rollercoaster injury likelihood and severity. [Report] August 9, 2002.

14. Six Flags. Press release: Roller coasters, theme parks extraordinarily safe, according to two comprehensive, scientific studies. 2002.

15. Ginevan ME. Soft drinks and obesity. *J Pediatrics.* 2004;144(4):555–56.

16. Forshee RA, Storey ML, Ginevan ME. A risk analysis model of the relationship between beverage consumption from school vending machines and risk of adolescent overweight. *Risk Analysis.* 2005;25(5):1121.

17. Burros M, Warner M. Bottlers agree to a school ban on sweet drinks. *New York Times.* May 4, 2006.

18. National Research Council. Health implications of perchlorate ingestion. Washington, DC: National Academies Press, 2005.

19. Kelsh MA, Buffler PA, Daaboul JJ et al. Primary congential hypothyroidism, newborn thyroid function, and environmental perchlorate exposure among residents of a southern California community. *J Occup Environ Med.* 2003;45(10):1116–27.

20. Buffler PA, Kelsh MA, Lau EC et al. Thyroid function and perchlorate in drinking water: An evaluation among California newborns, 1998. *Environ Health Perspect.* 2006;114(5):798–804.

21. MacLennan PA, Delzell E, Sathiakumar N et al. Cancer incidence among triazine herbicide manufacturing workers. *J Occup Environ Med.* 2002;44 (11):1048–58.

22. Hessel PA, Kalmes R, Smith TJ, Lau E, Mink PJ, Mandel J. A nested case-control study of prostate cancer and atrazine exposure. *J Occup Environ Med.* 2004;46(4):379–85.

23. Li AA, Mink PJ, McIntosh LJ, Teta MJ, Finley B. Evaluation of epidemiologic and animal data associating pesticides with Parkinson's disease. *J Occup Environ Med.* 2005;47(10):1059–87.

24. Yarborough CM. Chrysotile as a cause of mesothelioma: An assessment based on epidemiology. *Crit Rev Toxicol.* 2006;36(2):165–87.

25. Hessel PA, Teta MJ, Goodman M, Lau E. Mesothelioma among brake mechanics: An expanded analysis of a case control study. *Risk Analysis.* 2004;24(3):547–52.

26. Goodman M, Morgan RW, Ray R, Malloy CD, Zhao K. Cancer in asbestos-exposed occupational cohorts: A meta-analysis. *Cancer Causes Control.* 1999;10(5):453–65.

27. Huggard J. (Weinberg Group, LLC). Asbestos, tobacco, pharmaceuticals—We're all next! (PowerPoint presentation). June 18, 2003. Available at: http://www.defendingscience.org/upload/Huggard_slides.pdf. Accessed in December 2007.

28. Weinberg Group. The Weinberg Group: Case studies: Analyzed existing studies to find any design flaws to support legal defense. 2001. Available at: http://www.defendingscience.org/upload/Weinbergcs.pdf. Accessed in December 2007.

29. Gaffney PT (vice president, Product Defense, the Weinberg Group). Letter to Brooks J (vice president, Special Initiatives, DuPont de Nemours). Re: Perfluorooctanoic acid (PFOA). April 29, 2003. Available at: http://www.defendingscience.org/upload/Gaffney_PFOA.pdf. Accessed in December 2007.

30. U.S. Environmental Protection Agency. Science Advisory Board (SAB) review of EPA's draft risk assessment of potential human health effects associated with perfluorooctanoic acid (PFOA) and its salts. May 30, 2006. Report no. EPA-SAB-06–006.

31. Thacker PD. The Weinberg proposal. *Environ Sci Technol.* February 22, 2006.

32. Hurley D. As ephedra ban nears, a race to sell last supplies. *New York Times.* April 11, 2004.

33. Levy P, Roth HD, Hwang PMT, Powers TE. Beryllium and lung cancer: A reanalysis of a NIOSH cohort mortality study. *Inhalation Toxicology.* 2002;14(10):1003–15.

34. Levy PS. Workplace exposures to ETS and lung cancer: Presentation of meta-analysis findings to the NTP Board of Scientific Counselors, Report on Carcinogens Subcommittee, December 1, 1998. Available at: http://ntp.niehs.nih.gov/files/levy-12–01–98.pdf. Accessed in June 2007.

35. Philip Morris. H. Daniel Roth, Ph.D. 1985. Philip Morris document no. 2023082974. Available at: http://legacy.library.ucsf.edu/tid/hyl52doo. Accessed in June 2007.

36. Brissenden McFarland Wagoner & Fuccella, Inc. Confidential executive summary on H. Daniel Roth, candidate for the position of executive director for the Center of Indoor Air Research (CIAR). Prepared for the Board of Directors of CIAR. September 1987. Tobacco Institute document no. TI0065–0534. Available at: http://tobaccodocuments.org/nysa_ti_s1/TI00650534.html. Accessed in June 2007.

37. Roth HD (Roth Associates, Inc.). Letter to Hall T (Division of Consumer Affairs, OSHA). Subject: Occupational Safety and Health Association's [*sic*] notice of proposed rulemaking and notice of public hearing on indoor air quality, April 5, 1994, 59 *Fed. Reg.* 15966, and the extension of comment period and rescheduling of public hearing. 59 *Fed. Reg.* 30560. August 12, 1994. R. J. Reynolds document no. 515918609/8611. Available at: http://legacy.library.ucsf.edu/tid/qwc92d00. Accessed in June 2007.

38. Roth HD. A survey of health effects: Mercury emissions from North Dakota lignite-fired power plants [report prepared for North Dakota Industrial Commission]. August 28, 1996. Available at: http://www.defending science.org/upload/Roth_1996.pdf. Accessed in December 2007.

39. Roth HD, Viren JR, Colucci AV. Evaluation of *CHESS:* New York Asthma Data 1970–1971. Vol. 1: Findings and supporting tables. EPRI EA-450 (Research project 681–1). Report prepared for the Electric Power Research Institute. 1977. R.J. Reynolds document no. 501558651/8808. Available at: http://legacy.library.ucsf.edu/tid/lsp39d00. Accessed in December 2007.

40. U.S. Department of Justice. United States' final proposed findings of fact. Filed July 1, 2004, for *U.S. v. Philip Morris* (civil action no. 99-CV-02496 [GK]). Available at: http://www.library.ucsf.edu/tobacco/litigation/usvpm/uspm.pdf. Accessed in June 2007.

41. Roth HD, Levy PS, Shi L, Post E. Alcoholic beverages and breast cancer: Some observations on published case-control studies. *J Clin Epidemiol.* 1994;47(2):207–16.

42. Roth HD, Levy PS. Response to MP Longnecker, *J Clin Epidemiol.* 1995; 48(4):497–500.

43. Clapp RW. Industry influence in the dioxin reassessment (PowerPoint presentation), July 12, 2004. Available at: http://www.cspinet.org/integrity/cf/visualclapp.pdf. Accessed in June 2007.

44. Paustenbach DJ, Finley BL, Lu ET et al. Environmental and occupational health hazards associated with the presence of asbestos in brake linings and pads (1900 to present): A "state-of-the-art" review. *J Toxicol Environ Health Part B.* 2004;7(1):25–80.

45. Paustenbach DJ, Richter RO, Finley BL et al. An evaluation of the historical exposures of mechanics to asbestos in brake dust. *Appl Occup Environ Hyg.* 2003;18(10):786–804.

46. Paustenbach DJ (vice president, McLaren/Hart; national director, Chem-Risk division). Letter to Project Officer- Environmental Tobacco Smoke,

Technical Information Staff, Office of Health and Environmental Assessment, U.S. Environmental Protection Agency. Subject: Health effects of passive smoking—assessment of lung cancer in adults and respiratory disorders in children. (External review draft). September 27, 1990. Available at: http://ltdlimages.library.ucsf.edu/imagesr/r/s/m/rsm92d00/Srsm92d00 .pdf. Accessed in July 2007.

47. Waldman P. Study tied pollutant to cancer; then consultants got hold of it. *Wall Street Journal.* December 23, 2005:A1.

48. Lane A. Weakened rules a boon to 3 polluters: Work of scientist paid by the firms viewed skeptically by other experts. *Newark (NJ) Star Ledger.* March 7, 2004.

49. Zhang J, Li X. Chromium pollution of soil and water in Jinzhou. *J Chinese Prevent Med.* 1987;2(5):262–64.

50. Zhang J, Li S. Cancer mortality in a Chinese population exposed to hexavalent chromium in water. *J Occup Environ Med.* 1997;39(4):315–19.

51. Environmental Working Group. Chrome-plated fraud: How PG&E's scientists-for-hire reversed findings of cancer study. 2005. Available at: http://www.ewg.org/reports/chromium/index.php. Accessed in June 2007.

52. Brandt-Rauf P. Editorial retraction. *J Occup Environ Med.* 2006;48(7): 749.

53. Beaumont J, Sedman R, Reynolds S et al. Analysis of cancer mortality data from five villages in China with hexavalent chromium-contaminated drinking water. *Am J Epidemiol.* 2006;163(Suppl):S115.

54. Phillips ML. Journal retracts chromium study. *Scientist.* June 7, 2006.

55. *Wall Street Journal* accused of wrongdoing on Erin Brockovich story credited as key in $295 million settlement, says Dr. Shukun Li. *Businesswire .com.* December 6, 2006.

56. Henz KL, Karch KJ, Ginevan ME. Statistical analysis of binned data without access to raw data [abstract for the Society for Risk Analysis annual meeting], 2003. Available at: http://www.birenheide.com/sra/2003AM/ program/singlesession.php3?sessid=T9. Accessed in June 2007.

57. International Agency for Research on Cancer. IARC Monographs on the Evaluation of Carcinogenic Risks to Humans: Preamble. January 2006. Available at: http://monographs.iarc.fr/ENG/Preamble/CurrentPreamble .pdf. Accessed in June 2007.

58. Garne D, Watson M, Chapman S, Byrne F. Environmental tobacco smoke research published in the journal *Indoor and Built Environment* and associations with the tobacco industry. *Lancet.* 2005;365(9461):804–09.

59. Axelson O, Balbus JB, Cohen G et al. Correspondence regarding publication ethics and *Regulatory Toxicology and Pharmacology. Int J Occup Environ Health.* 2003;9(4):386–89.

60. Weinberg Group. Terry Quill, Esq. 2005. Available at: http://www .defendingscience.org/upload/Quill_bio.pdf. Accessed in December 2007.

61. Quill TF (Beveridge Diamond). Memorandum prepared by outside legal counsel to the tobacco companies concerning a report on the EPA's ETS risk assessment providing confidential information to industry counsel to aid in the rendering of legal advice in connection with ongoing regulatory proceedings. RJ Reynolds document no. 517572542 -2542. Available at: http://legacy.library.ucsf.edu/tid/hz083a00.

62. Packett KT (Tobacco Institute). Memorandum to Gleason M, Stunz S (Tobacco Institute). Analysis of scientific affairs budget for the 1991 calendar year, Appendix A (analysis of expenses incurred for scientific projects). June 24, 1991. Available at: http://tobaccodocuments.org/nysa_ti_m2/TI10011124.html or http://tdo.roswellpark.org/ti/TIDN0018313–8319.pdf. Accessed in June 2007.

63. Cole P, Rodu B. Epidemiologic studies of chrome and cancer mortality: A series of meta-analyses. *Regul Toxicol Pharmacol.* 2005;43(3):225–31.

64. Wellmann J, Weiland S, Neiteler G et al. Cancer mortality in German carbon black workers, 1976–1998. *Occup Environ Med.* 2006;63:513–21.

65. Büchte S, Morfeld P, Wellmann J et al. Lung cancer mortality and carbon black exposure: A nested case-control study at a German carbon black production plant. *J Occup Environ Med.* 2006;48(12):1242–52.

66. Morfeld P, Büchte SF, Wellmann J et al. Lung cancer mortality and carbon black exposure: Cox regression analysis of a cohort from a German carbon black production plant. *J Occup Environ Med.* 2006;48(12):1230–41.

67. Morfeld P, Büchte SF, Wellmann J et al. Lung cancer mortality and carbon black exposure: Uncertainties of SMR analyses in a cohort study at a German carbon black production plant. *J Occup Environ Med.* 2006;48(12):1253–64.

68. Conference program: Particles and cancer. Massachusetts Institute of Technology, Biological Engineering Division. January 10–11, 2006. Available at: http://web.mit.edu/be/pc-conference/program.html. Accessed in June 2007.

69. Baan R, Straif K, Grosse V et al. Carcinogenicity of carbon black, titanium dioxide, and talc. *Lancet Oncol.* 2006;7(4):295–96.

70. Moynihan DP. Defining deviancy down: How we've become accustomed to alarming levels of crime and destructive behavior. *American Scholar.* 1993; 62:17–30.

71. Council on Water Quality. 2007. Available at: http://www.councilon waterquality.org/. Accessed in June 2007.

72. Environment California. The politics of rocket fuel pollution: Executive summary. December 1, 2006. Available at: http://www.environmentcalifornia.org/reports/clean-water/clean-water-program-reports/the-politics-of-rocket-fuel-pollution. Accessed in June 2007.

73. SourceWatch. Category: Front groups. 2005. Available at: http://www.sourcewatch.org/index.php?title=Category:Front_groups. Accessed in June 2007.

74. Stauber J, Rampton S. *Toxic Sludge Is Good for You: Lies, Damn Lies, and the Public Relations Industry.* Monroe, ME: Common Courage Press, 1995.

75. Rampton S, Stauber J. *Trust Us, We're Experts! How Industry Manipulates Science and Gambles with Your Future.* New York: Center for Media and Democracy, 2001.

76. SourceWatch. Center for Consumer Freedom. 2006. Available at: http://www.sourcewatch.org/index.php?title=Center_for_Consumer_Freedom. Accessed in June 2007.

77. Center for Consumer Freedom. FishScam.com. Available at: http://www.fishscam.com. Accessed in June 2007.

78. SourceWatch. Foundation for Clear Air Progress. 2006. Available at: http://www.sourcewatch.org/index.php?title=Foundation_for_Clean_Air_Progress. Accessed in June 2007.

79. Fialka JJ. Panel judging EPA's proposed air regulations receives most of its funding from the regulated. *Wall Street Journal.* January 16, 1997:A20.

80. ExxonSecrets.org. Factsheet: The Annapolis Center for Science-based Public Policy. 2005. Available at: http://www.exxonsecrets.org/html/orgfactsheet.php?id=13. Accessed in June 2007.

81. Mooney C. Some like it hot. *Mother Jones.* May/June 2005.

82. Southern Co. Services. Annual report U-13–60, filed with Securities and Exchange Commission for 12/31/03. April 30, 2004. SEC file 49–00059; accession no. 92122–4-17. Available at: http://www.secinfo.com/d2Puw.151.htm. Accessed in June 2007.

83. Southern Co. Services. Annual report U-13–60, filed with Securities and Exchange Commission for 12/31/04. April 29, 2005. SEC file 49–00059; accession no. 217216–5-2. Available at: http://www.secinfo.com/d6k4f.zd.htm. Accessed in June 2007.

84. Lipfert FW. *The "Particle Wars" and a Path to Peace.* Annapolis Center for Science-Based Public Policy, 2003.

85. Edison Electric Institute. Comments submitted to Docket EPA-HQ-OAR-2001–0017 (National Ambient Air Quality Standards for Particulate Matter, proposed rule, 71 *Fed. Reg.* 2620–708, January 17, 2006). April 17, 2006. Document no. EPA-HQ-OAR-2001–0017-2193.1.

86. Utility Air Regulatory Group (UARG). Comments submitted to Docket EPA-HQ-OAR-2001–0017 (National Ambient Air Quality Standards for Particulate Matter, Proposed Rule, 71 *Fed. Reg.* 2620, January 17, 2006), and EPA-HQ-OAR-2004–0018 (Revisions to Ambient Air Monitoring Requirements, 71 *Fed. Reg.* 2710, Jan. 17, 2006). April 17, 2006. Document no. EPA-HQ-OAR-2001–0017-1629.1.

87. Pope III CA. Particulate pollution and health: A review of the Utah valley experience. *J Expo Anal Environ Epidemiol.* 1996;6(1):23–34.

88. Samet J. Air pollution and epidemiology: "Déjà vu all over again?" *Epidemiology.* 2002;13(2):118–19.

89. Rom WN, Samet JM. Small particles with big effects. *Am J Respir Crit Care Med.* 2006;173(4):365–66.

90. Samet JM, Zeger SL, Dominici F, et al. The National Morbidity, Mortality, and Air Pollution Study. Part 2: Morbidity and mortality from air pollution in the United States. Cambridge, MA: Health Effects Institute: June 2000, no. 94. Available at: http://pubs.healtheffects.org/view.php?id=118. Accessed in June 2007.

91. Samet JM, Dominici F, Curriero FC et al. Fine particulate air pollution and mortality in 20 U.S. cities, 1987–1994. *NEJM.* 2000;343(24):1742–49.

92. Huber P. W. *Galileo's Revenge: Junk Science in the Courtroom.* New York: Basic Books, 1993:2–3.

93. Junkscience.com. Junk science at large: Junk scientists, 1997. Available at: http://www.junkscience.com/roster. Accessed in November 2007.

94. The Advancement of Sound Science Coalition fact sheet. Philip Morris document no. 2046989061, 1993. Available at: http://legacy.library.ucsf.edu/tid/zyh09e00. Accessed in June 2007.

95. The Advancement of Sound Science Coalition (TASSC). Press release: National watchdog organization launched to fight unsound science used for public policy comes to Texas. Issued December 13, 1993. Philip Morris document no. 2046988980/8982. Available at: http://legacy.library.ucsf.edu/tid/eko42e00. Accessed in June 2007.

96. Merlo E (Philip Morris). Memorandum to Campbell WI (Philip Morris). Philip Morris document no. 2070039928/9930; February 17, 1993. Available at: http://legacy.library.ucsf.edu/tid/fup16c00. Accessed in June 2007.

97. Ong EK, Glantz SA. Constructing "sound science" and "good epidemiology": Tobacco, lawyers, and public relations firms. *Am J Public Health.* 2001;91(11):1749–57.

98. Office of Management and Budget (OMB). Draft 2006 report to Congress on the costs and benefits of federal regulations. 2006. Available at: http://www.whitehouse.gov/OMB/inforeg/reports/2006_draft_cost_benefit_report.pdf. Accessed in June 2007.

99. U.S. Environmental Protection Agency. Press release: New report shows benefits of 1990 Clean Air Amendments outweigh costs by four-to-one margin. Issued November 16, 1999. Available at: http://www.epa.gov/air/sect812/r-140.html. Accessed in June 2007.

100. The quote was a line written by Jane Wagner and delivered by Lily Tomlin in the play, *The Search for Signs of Intelligent Life in the Universe.* See Keyes R. *The Quote Verifier: Who Said What, When, and Where.* New York: St. Martin's Press, 2006:39.

CHAPTER SIX

1. International Agency for Research on Cancer. IARC Monographs on the Evaluation of Carcinogenic Risks to Humans, Vol. 88: Formaldehyde, 2-Butoxyethanol, and 1-tert-Butoxypropan-2-ol. December 2006.

2. Schull WJ. *Effects of Atomic Radiation: A Half-Century of Studies from Hiroshima and Nagasaki.* New York: Wiley-Liss, 1995.

3. Hernberg S. "Negative" results in cohort studies: How to recognize fallacies. *Scand J Work Environ Health.* 1981;7(suppl.4):121–26.

4. Axelson O. Negative and non-positive epidemiological studies. *Int J Occup Med Environ Health.* 2004;17(1):115–21.

5. Ward E, Carpenter A, Markowitz S et al. Excess number of bladder cancers in workers exposed to ortho-toluidine and aniline. *J Natl Cancer Inst.* 1991; 83(7):501–6.

6. Angiosarcoma of the liver among polyvinyl chloride workers. *Morbidity and Mortality Weekly Report.* 1974;23(6):49–50.

7. Peto R, Gray R, Brantom P et al. Nitrosamine carcinogenesis in 5,120 rodents: Chronic administration of sixteen different concentrations of NDEA, NDMA, NPYR, and NPIP in the water of 4,440 inbred rats, with parallel studies on NDEA alone of the effect of age of starting (3, 6, or 20 weeks) and of species (rats, mice, or hamsters). *IARC Sci Publ.* 1984;57:627–65.

8. Littlefield NA, Farmer JH, Gaylor DW et al. Effects of dose and time in a long-term, low-dose carcinogenic study. *J Environ Pathol Toxicol.* 1980; 3(3 Spec No.):17–34.

9. Peto R, Gray R, Brantom P et al. Effects on 4,080 rats of chronic ingestion of N-nitrosodiethylamine or N-nitrosodimethylamine: A detailed dose-response study. *Cancer Res.* 1991;51(23 Pt 2):6415–51.

10. Peto R, Gray R, Brantom P et al. Dose and time relationships for tumor induction in the liver and esophagus of 4,080 inbred rats by chronic ingestion of N-nitrosodiethylamine or N-nitrosodimethylamine. *Cancer Res.* 1991;51(23 Pt 2):6452–69.

11. Contini S, Amendola A, Ziomas I. Benchmark exercise on major hazard analysis. Vol. 1: Description of the project; Discussion of the results and conclusions. Final Report. Luxembourg: Commission of European Communities; 1991. EUR 13386 EN.

12. Ruckelshaus WD. Risk in a free society. *Environ Law Reporter.* 1984;14: 10190.

13. U.S. Environmental Protection Agency. National Priorities List (NPL). Available at: http://www.epa.gov/superfund/sites/npl/index.htm. Accessed in June 2007.

14. Hamilton A. Benzene (benzol) poisoning. *Arch Pathol.* 1931:434–54 and 601–37.

15. Hunter FT. Chronic exposure to benzene (benzol). Part 2: The clinical effects. *J Ind Hyg Toxicol.* 1939;21(8):331–54.

16. Mallory TB, Gall EA, Brickley WJ. Chronic exposure to benzene (benzol). Part 3: The pathologic results. *J Ind Hyg Toxicol.* 1939;21(8):355–93.

17. Erf LA, Rhoads CP. The hematological effects of benzene (benzol) poisoning. *J Ind Hyg Toxicol.* 1939;21(8):421–35.

18. Conklin G. Cancer and the environment. *Sci Am.* 1949;180(1):11–15.

19. Hueper WC. Cancer in its relation to occupation and environment. *Bull Am Soc Control Cancer.* June 1943;25:63–69.

20. Hueper WC. Environmental cancer [report]. Environmental Cancer Section, Cancer Control Branch, National Cancer Institute; November 1948.

21. Hueper WC. Industrial management and occupational cancer. *JAMA.* 1946;131:738–41.

22. Hueper WC. Clinical aspects of occupational cancer. *Public Health Rep.* 1948:157–65.

23. Hueper WC. Occupational cancer hazards found in industry. *Ind Hygiene Newsletter.* 1949;9(12):7–9.

24. American Petroleum Institute. API Toxicological Review: Benzene. New York, 1948.

25. Eckardt RE. Recent developments in industrial carcinogens. *J Occup Med.* November 1973;15(11):904–07.

26. Infante PF, Rinsky RA, Wagoner JK, et al. Leukaemia in benzene workers. *Lancet.* 1977;2(8028):76–78.

27. OSHA. Occupational exposure to benzene: Emergency temporary standard. *Fed. Reg.* 1977;42(85):22516–29.

28. *Industrial Union Department v. American Petroleum Institute,* 44 U.S. 607 (July 2, 1980). Available at: http://www.publichealthlaw.net/Reader/docs/IndustUnion.pdf. Accessed in June 2007.

29. Rinsky RA, Smith AB, Hornung R et al. Benzene and leukemia: An epidemiologic risk assessment. *NEJM.* 1987;316(17):1044–50.

30. OSHA. Occupational exposure to benzene: Final rule. *Fed. Reg.* 1987;52:34460–578.

31. Lamm SH. Heterogeneity of the Akron and St. Mary's plants. September 1, 1977. Post-hearing comments submitted to OSHA Docket H059, Exhibit no. 217-21-E.

32. McCraw DS, Joyner RE, Cole P. Excess leukemia in a refinery population. *J Occup Med.* 1985;27(3):220–22.

33. Austin H, Cole P, McCraw DS. A case-control study of leukemia at an oil refinery. *J Occup Med.* 1986;28(11):1169–73.

34. Honda Y, Delzell E, Cole P. An updated study of mortality among workers at a petroleum manufacturing plant. *J Occup Environ Med.* 1995;37(2):194–200.

35. Wong O, Morgan RW, Bailey WJ et al. An epidemiological study of petroleum refinery employees. *Br J Ind Med.* 1986;43(1):6–17.

36. Wong O, Harris F, Rosamilia K et al. An updated mortality study of workers at a petroleum refinery in Beaumont, Texas, 1945 to 1996. *J Occup Environ Med.* 2001;43(4):384–401.

37. Wong O, Harris F, Rosamilia K et al. Updated mortality study of workers at a petroleum refinery in Torrance, California, 1959 to 1997. *J Occup Environ Med.* 2001;43(12):1089–102.

38. Huebner WW, Wojcik NC, Rosamilia K et al. Mortality updates (1970–1997) of two refinery/petrochemical plant cohorts at Baton Rouge, Louisiana, and Baytown, Texas. *J Occup Environ Med.* 2004;46(12):1229–45.

39. Raabe GK, Wong O. Leukemia mortality by cell type in petroleum workers with potential exposure to benzene. *Environ Health Perspect.* 1996;104 (suppl 6):1381–92.

40. Lamm SH, Walters AS, Wilson R, Byrd DM, Grunwald H. Consistencies and inconsistencies underlying the quantitative assessment of leukemia risk from benzene exposure. *Environ Health Perspect.* 1989;82:289–97.

41. Paxton MB, Chinchilli VM, Brett SM et al. Leukemia risk associated with benzene exposure in the Pliofilm cohort. Part 1: Mortality update and exposure distribution. *Risk Analysis.* 1994;14(2):147–54.

42. Paxton MB, Chinchilli VM, Brett SM et al. Leukemia risk associated with benzene exposure in the Pliofilm cohort. Part 2: Risk estimates. *Risk Analysis.* 1994;14(2):155–61.

43. Paxton MB. Leukemia risk associated with benzene exposure in the Pliofilm cohort. *Environ Health Perspect.* 1996;104(suppl 6):1431–36.

44. Schnatter AR, Nicolich MJ, Bird MG. Determination of leukemogenic benzene exposure concentrations: Refined analyses of the Pliofilm cohort. *Risk Analysis.* 1996;16(6):833–40.

45. van Raalte HGS, Grasso P. Hematological, myelotoxic, clastogenic, carcinogenic, and leukemogenic effects of benzene. *Regul Toxicol Pharmacol.* 1982;2:153–76.

46. Paustenbach DJ, Price PS, Ollison W et al. Reevaluation of benzene exposure for the Pliofilm (rubberworker) cohort (1936–1976). *J Toxicol Environ Health.* 1992;36:177–231.

47. Utterback DF, Rinsky RA. Benzene exposure assessment in rubber hydrochloride workers: A critical evaluation of previous estimates. *Am J Ind Med.* 1995;27(5):661–76.

48. Williams PRD, Paustenbach DJ. Reconstruction of benzene exposure for the Pliofilm cohort (1936–1976) using Monte Carlo techniques. *J Toxicol Environ Health,* Part A. 2003;66(8):677–781.

49. Nilsson RI, Nordlinder R, Hörte L-G et al. Leukaemia, lymphoma, and multiple myeloma in seamen on tankers. *Occup Environ Med.* 1998;55:517–21.

50. ChemRisk. Contemporary projects of the month: Case involving benzene and the development of AML. July 2005. Available at: http://www .chemrisk.com/archives/july2005.htm. Acessed in October 2007.

51. Williams PRD, Robinson K, Paustenbach DJ. Benzene exposures associated with tasks performed on marine vessels (ca. 1975–2000). *J Occup Environ Hygiene.* 2005;2:586–99.

52. Hayes RB, Yin SN, Dosemeci M et al. Benzene and the dose-related incidence of hematologic neoplasms in China. Chinese Academy of Preventive Medicine, National Cancer Institute Benzene Study Group. *J Natl Cancer Inst.* 1997;89(14):1065–71.

53. Lan Q, Zhang L, Li G et al. Hematotoxicity in workers exposed to low levels of benzene. *Science.* December 3, 2004;306:1774–76.

54. Hurtley S, Szuromi P, eds. This week in *Science*: A little is still too much. *Science.* December 3, 2004;306:1647.

55. Hricko A. Rings of controversy around benzene. *Environ Health Perspect.* 1994;102(3):276.

56. Wong O. A critique of the exposure assessment in the epidemiologic study of benzene-exposed workers in China conducted by the Chinese Academy of Preventive Medicine and the U.S. National Cancer Institute. *Regul Toxicol Pharmacol.* 1999;30(3):259–367.

57. Budinsky RA, DeMott RP, Wernke MJ et al. An evaluation of modeled benzene exposure and dose estimates published in the Chinese-National Cancer Institute Collaborative Epidemiology Studies. *Regul Toxicol Pharmacol.* 1999;30:244–58.

58. Wong O. Investigations of benzene exposure, benzene poisoning, and malignancies in China. *Regul Toxicol Pharmacol.* 2002;35(1):126–35.

59. Wong O, Fu H. Exposure to benzene and non-Hodgkin lymphoma: An epidemiologic overview and an ongoing case-control study in Shanghai. *Chem Biol Interact.* 2005;153–54:33–41.

60. Wang L, Zhou Y, Liang Y et al. Benzene exposure in the shoemaking industry in China: A literature survey, 1978–2004. *Regul Toxicol Pharmacol.* 2006;46(2):149–56.

61. Twerdok L, Beatty P. Proposed studies on the risk of benzene-induced diseases in China: Costs and funding. Available at http://www.defending science.org/upload/Benzene_proposal.pdf. Accessed in December 2007.

62. Benzene Health Research Consortium. The Shanghai Health Study (Power-Point presentation). February 1, 2003. Available at http://www.defending science.org/upload/Benzene_Shanghai.pdf. Accessed in December 2007.

63. Parker CM (Marathon Oil). Memorandum to manager of Toxicology and Product Safety (Marathon Oil). Subject: International leveraged research proposal, 2000. Available at http://www.defendingscience.org/upload/ Parker_proposal.pdf. Accessed in December 2007.

CHAPTER SEVEN

1. Kornegay HR. New directions: A presentation of the Tobacco Institute staff by Horace R. Kornegay, chairman to the Executive Committee; June 25, 1981 Tobacco Institute document no. TIMN0074974/4990. Available at: http://legacy.library.ucsf.edu/tid/gyv92foo. Accessed in June 2007.

2. Hill and Knowlton, Inc. Background material on the cigarette industry client; December 15, 1953. R.J. Reynolds document no. 519124023/4027. Available at: http://legacy.library.ucsf.edu/tid/ssq31doo. Accessed in June 2007.

3. Hill and Knowlton, Inc. Press release: Re: Dr. Clarence Cook Little appointed director of Tobacco Industry Research Committee. Issued June 15, 1954. Available at: http://legacy.library.ucsf.edu/tid/arx49coo. Accessed in June 2007.

4. Diethelm P, McKee M. Lifting the smokescreen: Tobacco industry strategy to defeat smoke free policies and legislation. Brussels: Report prepared for the European Respiratory Society and Institut National du Cancer (INCa, France). February 2006. Available at: http://www.ersnet.org/ers/show/default.aspx?id_attach=13552. Accessed in June 2007.

5. Roper Organization, Inc. A study of public attitudes toward cigarette smoking and the tobacco industry in 1978, vol. 1. Brown and Williamson document no. 501000285/0340; May 1978. Available at: http://legacy.library.ucsf.edu/tid/cns10foo. Accessed in June 2007.

6. Hirayama T. Non-smoking wives of heavy smokers have a higher risk of lung cancer: A study from Japan. *BMJ* (clinical research ed.). 1981;282 (6259):183–85.

7. Tobacco Merchants Association. Tobacco: Its Economic Performance. Part VIII: Government Impact on Consumption: Executive summary. October 28, 1983. Lorillard document no. 93137245/7256. Available at: http://legacy.library.ucsf.edu/tid/cbc60eoo. Accessed in June 2007.

8. Workplace smoking restrictions: Communications and lobbying support program. February 1984. Brown and Williamson document no. 521046145/6174. Available at: http://legacy.library.ucsf.edu/tid/soc43foo. Accessed in June 2007.

9. Proposal for the organization of the Whitecoat Project. 1988. Philip Morris document no. 2501254705/4708. Available at: http://legacy.library.ucsf.edu/tid/atj32eoo. Accessed in June 2007.

10. Boyse S. Note on a special meeting of the UK industry on environmental tobacco smoke, London, February 17, 1988. Philip Morris document no. 2063791176/1180. Available at: http://legacy.library.ucsf.edu/tid/dof53aoo. Accessed in June 2007.

11. Diethelm PA, Rielle J-C, McKee M. The whole truth and nothing but the truth? The research that Philip Morris did not want you to see. *Lancet*. 2005;366(9479):86–92.

12. Drope J, Chapman S. Tobacco industry efforts at discrediting scientific knowledge of environmental tobacco smoke: A review of internal industry documents. *J Epidemiol Community Health.* 2001;55:588–94.

13. Tobacco Institute. Public smoking issue: Consulting scientists on ETS and IAQ. Undated. Tobacco Institute document no. TIDN0003162-TIDN 0003164. Available at: http://legacy.library.ucsf.edu/tid/dym91f00. Accessed in June 2007.

14. Bero LA, Glantz SA, Rennie D. Publication bias and public health policy on environmental tobacco smoke. *JAMA.* 1994;272(2):133–36.

15. Schroeder TD (Womble, Carlyle, Sandridge, & Rice). Letter to Gold SM (Magistrate Judge, U.S. District Court for the Eastern District of New York). Re: *Falise et al. v. American Tobacco Co. et al.* (CV99–73492) (JBW). February 29, 2000. Available at: http://legacy.library.ucsf.edu/tid/eyl62d00. Accessed in June 2007.

16. Wiggins E, McKenna J. Researchers' reactions to compelled disclosure of scientific information. *Law and Contemporary Problems.* 1996;59(3):67–93.

17. R.J. Reynolds Outside Legal Counsel. Smoking and health litigation: Integrated exposure and hazard assessment initiative. Descriptive project proposal and working notes. Draft: January 20, 1987. R.J. Reynolds Document no. 507916450/6480. Available at: http://legacy.library.ucsf.edu/tid/0gm95a00. Accessed in June 2007.

18. Colucci AV (R.J. Reynolds). Memorandum to Newton G (R.J. Reynolds). Subject: Planning of strategic analyses. January 2, 1986. R.J. Reynolds Document no. 515838456/8457. Available at: http://legacy.library.ucsf.edu/tid/ouj95a00. Accessed in June 2007.

19. Colucci AV (R.J. Reynolds). Memorandum to Newton G (R.J. Reynolds). Subject: Consultants and witnesses status, February 25, 1985.

20. Life Systems, Inc. Alternate causation: ICAIR. October 21, 1985. R.J. Reynolds Document no. 515872625/2864. Available at: http://legacy .library.ucsf.edu/tid/znj95a00. Accessed in June 2007.

21. *Action on Smoking and Health v. U.S. Occupational Safety and Health Administration (OSHA),* 1991 U.S. App. LEXIS 10487; 15 OSHC (BNA) 1030. Unpublished disposition filed May 10, 1991.

22. OSHA. Occupational exposure to indoor air pollutants: Request for information. *Fed. Reg.* 1991;56(183):47892–97.

23. OSHA. Indoor air quality: Notice of proposed rulemaking; notice of informal public hearing. *Fed. Reg.* 1994;59(65):15968–16039.

24. Bryan-Jones K, Bero LA. Tobacco industry efforts to defeat the Occupational Safety and Health Administration indoor air quality rule. *Am J Public Health.* 2003;93(4):585–92.

25. Philip Morris. Draft, 7/8/94, CAC presentation #4. Philip Morris document no. 2041183751/3790; 1994. Available at: http://legacy.library.ucsf.edu/tid/vnf77e00. Accessed in June 2007.

26. Smith C, Vizcaino T (R.J. Reynolds). Memorandum to Simmons S (R.J. Reynolds). Subject: October 28, 1988, meeting with Dr. Neil [H. Daniel] Roth. November 3, 1988. R. J. Reynolds document no. 508234343/4344. Available at: http://legacy.library.ucsf.edu/tid/lvc04doo. Accessed in June 2007.

27. Stern FB, Halperin WE, Hornung RW et al. Heart disease mortality among bridge and tunnel officers exposed to carbon monoxide. *Am J Epidemiol.* 1988;128(6):1276–88.

28. Roth HD (Roth Associates, Inc.). Letter to Hall T (Division of Consumer Affairs, OSHA). Subject: Occupational Safety and Health Association's [*sic*] notice of proposed rulemaking and notice of public hearing on indoor air quality, April 5, 1994, 59 *Fed. Reg.* 15966, and the extension of comment period and rescheduling of public hearing, June 14, 1994, 59 *Fed. Reg.* 30560. August 12, 1994. R.J. Reynolds document no. 515918609/8611. Available at: http://legacy.library.ucsf.edu/tid/qwc92doo. Accessed in June 2007.

29. Roth HD. Comments submitted to OSHA re: analysis of the ETS lung cancer and heart disease data. August 12, 1994. Available at: http://legacy.library.ucsf.edu/tid/swc92doo. Accessed in June 2007.

30. International Agency for Research on Cancer (IARC). IARC Monographs on the evaluation of carcinogenic risks to humans, Volume 83: Tobacco smoke and involuntary smoking. 2002. Available at: http://monographs.iarc.fr/ENG/Monographs/vol83/volume83.pdf. Accessed in July 2007.

31. *The Health Consequences of Involuntary Exposure to Tobacco Smoke.* Report of the Surgeon General. U.S. Department of Health and Human Services, 2006.

32. Dreyer LP. Wash Tech Conference Call. (Handwritten notes of Philip Morris in-house memorializing meeting between Philip Morris in-house counsel and Philip Morris regulatory consultants regarding proposed OSHA rulemaking.) Philip Morris document no. 2023896207. April 12, 1994. Available at: http://legacy.library.ucsf.edu/tid/cfn12aoo. Accessed in June 2007.

33. U.S. Environmental Protection Agency. Respiratory health effects of passive smoking: Lung cancer and other disorders. December 1992. Available at: http://cfpub2.epa.gov/ncea/cfm/recordisplay.cfm?deid=2835. Accessed in June 2007.

34. Philip Morris. Task force review of [Young & Rubicam] ETS materials. January 20, 1994. Available at: http://legacy.library.ucsf.edu/tid/cyl24eoo. Accessed in June 2007.

35. Philip Morris. ETS media strategy. Philip Morris document no. 2023920090/0101. 1993. Available at: http://legacy.library.ucsf.edu/tid/sav88eoo. Accessed in June 2007.

36. Rampton S, Stauber J. *Trust Us, We're Experts! How Industry Manipulates Science and Gambles with Your Future.* New York: Center for Media and Democracy, 2001.

37. Roth HD, Viren JR, Colucci AV. Evaluation of *CHESS:* New York asthma data 1970–1971. Vol. 1: Findings and supporting tables. EPRI EA-450 (Research Project 681–1). Report prepared for Electric Power Research Institute. 1977. R.J. Reynolds document no. 501558651/8808. Available at: http://legacy.library.ucsf.edu/tid/lsp39d00. Accessed in December 2007.

38. Center for Indoor Air Research (CIAR). CIAR presentation; ca. 1995. Philip Morris document no. 2057790853/0866. Available at: http://legacy .library.ucsf.edu/tid/wjm42d00. Accessed in June 2007.

39. Ong EK, Glantz SA. Tobacco industry efforts subverting International Agency for Research on Cancer's second-hand smoke study. *Lancet.* 2000; 355(9211):1253–59.

40. Rupp JP (counsel to the Center for Indoor Air Research). Letter to Sadler P (Imperial Tobacco Limited). Lorillard document no. 87602316/2319. 1993. Available at: http://legacy.library.ucsf.edu/tid/nml11e00. Accessed in June 2007.

41. Barnes DE, Bero LA. Industry-funded research and conflict of interest: An analysis of research sponsored by the tobacco industry through the Center for Indoor Air Research. *J Health Polit Policy Law.* 1996;21(3):515–42.

42. Barnes DE, Bero LA. Why review articles on health effects of passive smoking reach different conclusions. *JAMA.* 1998;279(19):1566–70.

43. Lee PN. "Marriage to a smoker" may not be a valid marker of exposure in studies relating environmental tobacco smoke to risk of lung cancer in Japanese non-smoking women. *Int Arch Occup Environ Health.* 1995;67(5): 287–94.

44. Hong M-K, Bero LA. How the tobacco industry responded to an influential study of the health effects of secondhand smoke. *BMJ.* 2002;325 (7377):1413–16.

45. Oldaker III GB (Center for Indoor Air Research). Letter to Rodricks JV (ENVIRON Corp.). Re: agreement between CIAR and ENVIRON re: Hirayama study to be performed by Michael E. Ginevan. July 14, 1988. Available at: http://legacy.library.ucsf.edu/tid/cme04d00. Accessed in June 2007.

46. Ward ME (R.J. Reynolds Tobacco Co.). Letter to Rupp J (Covington and Burling). Re: CIAR-sponsored investigation of John Viren's Hirayama analysis by Michael E. Ginevan, ENVIRON Corp. March 22, 1988. Lorillard document no. 87676622/6623. Available at: http://legacy.library.ucsf .edu/tid/moq21e00. Accessed in June 2007.

47. Viren JR (R.J. Reynolds). Letter to Goold JA (R.J. Reynolds). Status report: June to the present. July 18, 1988. R. J. Reynolds document no. 515788650–8652. Available at: http://legacy.library.ucsf.edu/tid/ezj95a00. Accessed in June 2007.

48. Layard MW (Failure Analysis Associates). Letter to Oldecker G (acting director, Indoor Air Quality Institute). December 10, 1987. Tobacco In-

stitute document no. TI01230757. Available at: http://legacy.library.ucsf.edu/tid/zle04doo. Accessed in June 2007.

49. Viren JR (R.J. Reynolds). Status report: July 17–29, 1988. R.J. Reynolds document no. 515788653/8655. Available at: http://legacy.library.ucsf.edu/tid/dzj95a00. Accessed in June 2007.

50. Viren JR (R.J. Reynolds). Letter to Goold JA. Re: Status report. R.J. Reynolds document no. 51578 8665. February 22, 1989. Available at: http://legacy.library.ucsf.edu/tid/bzj95a00. Accessed in June 2007.

51. Ong E, Glantz SA. Hirayama's work has stood the test of time. *Bull World Health Organ.* 2000;78(7):938–39.

52. Eriksen MP, LeMaistre CA, Newell GR. Health hazards of passive smoking. *Annu Rev Public Health.* 1988;9:47–70.

53. Fontham ET, Correa P, WuWilliams A et al. Lung cancer in nonsmoking women: A multicenter case-control study. *Cancer Epidemiol Biomarkers Prev.* 1991;1(1):35–43.

54. Fontham ETH, Correa P, Chen VW. Passive smoking and lung cancer. *J La State Med Soc.* 1993;145(4):132–36.

55. Fontham ET, Correa P, Reynolds P et al. Environmental tobacco smoke and lung cancer in nonsmoking women: A multicenter study. *JAMA.* 1994; 271(22):1752–59.

56. Baba A, Cook DM, McGarity TO et al. Legislating "sound science": The role of the tobacco industry. *Am J Public Health.* 2005;95(suppl 1):S20–S27.

57. Meeting minutes: The National Toxicology Program (NTP) Board of Scientific Counselors' Report on Carcinogens (BSC RoC) subcommittee meeting. December 2–3, 1998.

58. Meeting transcript: National Toxicology Program Board of Scientific Counselors' Report on Carcinogens subcommittee meeting. December 2–3, 1998. Available at: http://legacy.library.ucsf.edu/tid/epw60doo. Accessed in June 2007.

59. Chemical Manufacturers Association Epidemiology Task Force. Guidelines for good epidemiology practices for occupational and environmental epidemiologic research. 1991. Available at: http://legacy.library.ucsf.edu/tid/ifi73e00. Accessed in June 2007.

60. Federal Focus, Inc. Principles for evaluating epidemiologic data in regulatory risk assessment: Developed by an expert panel at a conference in London, England. Philip Morris document no. 2065386542/6612. October 1996. Available at: http://legacy.library.ucsf.edu/tid/vwv77doo. Accessed in June 2007.

61. Weiss R. "Data quality" law is nemesis of regulation. *Washington Post.* August 16, 2004:A1.

62. IARC tools. Philip Morris document no. 2029059645/9652. 1994. Available at: http://legacy.library.ucsf.edu/tid/wwd83e00. Accessed in June 2007.

63. *Flue-cured Tobacco Cooperative Stabilization Corp. v. EPA*, 4 F Supp. 2d 435 (July 17, 1998).

64. McGarity T. On the prospect of *"Daubert*izing" judicial review of risk assessment. *Law and Contemporary Problems.* 2003;66(155).

65. Blot WJ, McLaughlin JK. Passive smoking and lung cancer risk: What is the story now? *J Natl Cancer Inst.* 1998;90(19):1416–17.

66. Barnoya J, Glantz SA. Cardiovascular effects of secondhand smoke: Nearly as large as smoking. *Circulation.* 2005;111(20):2684–98.

67. Glantz S, Slade J, Bero L et al. *The Cigarette Papers.* Berkeley: University of California Press, 1996.

68. U.S. House of Representatives (103rd Cong., 2^d sess.) Committee on Energy and Commerce, Subcommittee on Health and the Environment. *Hearing: Regulation of Tobacco Products,* Part 3. June 21 and 23, 1994. Serial no. 103–71. Available at: http://legacy.library.ucsf.edu/tid/dojo5coo. Accessed in June 2007.

69. *Brown and Williamson Tobacco Corp. v. Regents of the University of California,* Super. Ct. for County of San Francisco, no. 967298 (May 25, 1995).

70. Koop CE. Foreward. In Glantz SA, Slade J, Bero L et al. *The Cigarette Papers.* Berkeley: University of California Press, 1996.

71. Glantz SA, Barnes DE, Bero L et al. Looking through a keyhole at the tobacco industry: The Brown and Williamson documents. *JAMA.* 1995;274(3):219–24.

72. Slade J, Bero LA, Hanauer P et al. Nicotine and addiction: The Brown and Williamson documents. *JAMA.* 1995;274(3):225–33.

73. Hanauer P, Slade J, Barnes DE et al. Lawyer control of internal scientific research to protect against products liability lawsuits: The Brown and Williamson documents. *JAMA.* 1995;274(3):234–40.

74. Bero L, Barnes DE, Hanauer P et al. Lawyer control of the tobacco industry's external research program: The Brown and Williamson documents. *JAMA.* 1995;274(3):241–47.

75. Barnes DE, Hanauer P, Slade J et al. Environmental tobacco smoke: The Brown and Williamson documents. *JAMA.* 1995;274(3):248–53.

76. Graham T. The Brown and Williamson documents: The company's response. *JAMA.* 1995;274(3):254–55.

77. Todd JS, Rennie D, McAfee RE et al. The Brown and Williamson Documents: Where do we go from here? *JAMA.* 1995;274(3):256–58.

78. Kessler D. *A Question of Intent: A Great American Battle with a Deadly Industry.* New York: Public Affairs, 2001.

79. *U.S. Food and Drug Administration v. Brown and Williamson Tobacco Corporation,* 529 U.S. 120 (March 21, 2000).

80. Tobacco use among adults: United States, 2005. *Morbidity and Mortality Weekly Report* 2006;55(42):1145–48.

81. *The Health Consequences of Smoking.* Report of the Surgeon General. U.S. Department of Health and Human Services, 2004.

82. World Health Organization, Western Pacific Region. Country profiles for tobacco or health, 2000.

83. Hanai K. A sham anti-smoking program. *Japan Times.* May 28, 2001.

CHAPTER EIGHT

1. Public Citizen Health Research Group of the Oil, Chemical, and Atomic Workers International Union. Petition to request a zero tolerance for ten carcinogens through an emergency temporary standard issued under the authority of the Occupational Safety and Health Act. December 29, 1972.

2. U.S. Occupational Safety and Health Administration (OSHA). Emergency temporary standard on certain carcinogens. *Fed. Reg.* 1973;38(85):10929–30.

3. Synthetic Organic Chemical Manufacturers. Association (SOCMA) Benzidine Task Force. Comments on the production and use of benzidine. March 9, 1973.

4. OSHA. Carcinogens. *Fed. Reg.* 1974;39(20):3756–97.

5. Walker B, Gerber A. Occupational exposure to aromatic amines: Benzidine and benzidine-based dyes. *Natl Cancer Inst Monogr.* 1981;58:11–13.

6. U.S. National Institute for Occupational Safety and Health (NIOSH). Special occupational hazard review for benzidine-based dyes. 1980. DHHS (NIOSH) publication no. 80–109. Available at: http://www.cdc.gov/niosh/80-109.html. Accessed in June 2007.

7. Ward E, Carpenter A, Markowitz S et al. Excess number of bladder cancers in workers exposed to ortho-toluidine and aniline. *J Natl Cancer Inst.* 1991; 83(7):501–06.

8. Morigami S, Nisimura I. Experimental studies on aniline bladder tumors. *GANN.* 1940;34:146–47.

9. Strombeck J. Azotoluene bladder tumors in rats. *J Path Bact.* 1946;58:275–78.

10. Ekman B, Strombeck J. Demonstration of tumorigenic decomposition products of 2,3 azotoluene. *Acta Physiol Scand.* 1947;14:43–50.

11. Hartwell JL, ed. Survey of Compounds Which Have Been Tested for Carcinogenic Activity. 2nd ed. Washington, DC: U.S. Public Health Service publication no. 149, 1951: 88.

12. Foulger JH (director, Medical Research). Letter to Rice RM (executive director, Medical Research, Lilly Research Laboratories, Eli Lilly and Co.). September 15, 1958.

13. Zapp Jr. JA. Deposition in U.S. District Court for the Northern District of Texas, Dallas Division, in the matter of *Dorothy Schiro et al. v. E. I. Du Pont de Nemours.* Civil action no. 3–85–0339-T. Scottsdale, AZ: March 2, 1987: 69–71.

14. Cousett J (Association of British Chemical Manufacturer). Letter to Mates E (National Aniline Division, Allied Chemical and Dye Corporation). Re: A.B.C.M. papilloma research scheme. October 11, 1954. Available at http://www.defendingscience.org/upload/ABCM_1954.pdf. Accessed in December 2007.

15. Ferber KH (superintendent, Tests and Inspection Department, Buffalo Plant, Allied Chemical Corporation). Letter to Rahall VH (safety coordinator, New York Office, Allied Chemical Corporation). Subject: MCA safety data sheet: Toluidine. November 25, 1958. Available at http://www.defendingscience.org/upload/Allied_1958.pdf. Accessed in December 2007.

16. Manufacturing Chemists Association (MCA). Officers, board of directors, committees, members. September 1961. Available at http://www.defendingscience.org/upload/MCA_Officers.pdf. Accessed in December 2007.

17. Stephenson FG (secretary, General Safety Committee, Manufacturing Chemists Association, Inc.). Letter to Fleming GG, Kelly RE, Ferber KH, Gois HH (Celanese Corporation of America, Monsanto Chemical Company, National Aniline Division–Allied Chemical Corporation, and American Cyanamid Corporation, respectively). Enclosure: Galley proof for proposed chemical safety data sheet on toluidine. February 24, 1961. Available at http://www.defendingscience.org/upload/MCA_1961.pdf. Accessed in December 2007.

18. Case RA, Pearson JT. Tumours of the urinary bladder in workmen engaged in the manufacture and use of certain dyestuff intermediates in the British chemical industry. Part 2: Further consideration of the role of aniline and of the manufacture of auramine and magenta (fuchsine) as possible causative agents. *Br J Ind Med.* 1954;11(3):213–16.

19. Scott TS. *Carcinogenic and Chronic Toxic Hazards of Aromatic Amines.* New York: Elsevier, 1962.

20. Borneff J. Carcinoma of the bladder found in workers employed in tar distilleries. *Zentralblatt fur Arbeitsmedizin und Arbeitsschutz.* 1965;15:288–92.

21. Khlebnikova M, Gladkova Y, Kurenko L et al. Problems of labor hygiene and the state of health of workers in the production of o-toluidine. Published and translated to English by the Institute of Idustrial Hygiene and Occupational Diseases, 1971.

22. Rubino GF, Scansetti G, Piolatto G et al. The carcinogenic effect of aromatic amines: An epidemiological study on the role of o-toluidine and 4,4′-methylene bis (2-methylaniline) in inducing bladder cancer in man. *Environ Res.* 1982;27(2):241–54.

23. Genin VA, Pliss GB, Pylev LN et al. Prevention of occupational bladder tumors in toluidine manufacture. *Gig Tr Prof Zabol.* 1978;7:10–14.

24. Ferber KH (superintendent, Tests and Inspection Department, Buffalo Plant, Allied Chemical Corporation). Memorandum to Daly JF (plant manager, Buffalo plant, Allied Chemical Corporation.) Subject: Biochemical research: Product toxicity ortho toluidine. August 2, 1962.

25. Neeld Jr. WE (director, Medical Division, E. I. Du Pont de Nemours and Co.). Chemical cyanosis cases from Ortho-toluidine August 18, 1975.

26. Homburger F, Friedell G, Weisburger E et al. Carcinogenicity of simple aromatic amine derivatives in mice and rats [abstract]. *Toxicol Appl Pharmacol.* 1972;22:280–81.

27. Russfield A, Homburger F, Weisburger J et al. Further studies on carcinogenicity of environmental chemicals including simple aromatic amines [abstract]. *Toxicol Appl Pharmacol.* 1973;25:446–47.

28. U.S. National Cancer Institute (NCI). Bioassay of *o*-toluidine hydrochloride for possible carcinogenicity. National Institutes of Health. 1979. DHEW publication no. (NIH) 79–1709.

29. International Agency for Research on Cancer. IARC Monographs on the Evaluation of the Carcinogenic Risks to Humans, Vol. 27: Some Aromatic Amines, Anthraquinones and Nitroso Compounds, and Inorganic Fluorides used in Drinking-water and Dental Preparations. April 1982.

30. Hunt NJ (Haskell Laboratory for Toxicology and Industrial Medicine, Central Research Department, E. I. Du Pont de Nemours and Co.). Letter to Schultz EF (product manager, Intermediate Sales, Organic Chemicals Department, E. I. Du Pont de Nemours and Co.). Subject: Ortho-toluidine carcinogenicity. June 12, 1974.

31. Schultz EF (technical manager, Intermediates Division, Organic Chemicals Department, Dyes and Chemicals Division, E. I. Du Pont de Nemours and Co.). Letter to LeCain R (manager, Purchases, Goodyear Tire and Rubber Co.). January 12, 1977.

32. McKusick BC (assistant director, Haskell Laboratory for Toxicology and Industrial Medicine, Central Research and Development Department, E. I. Du Pont de Nemours and Co.). Letter to Finklea JF (director, NIOSH). January 12, 1977.

33. Freudenthal RI, Stephens E, Anderson DP. Determining the potential of aromatic amines to induce cancer of the urinary bladder. *Int J Toxicol.* 1999;15:353–59.

34. Freudenthal RI, Anderson DP. Re: Monitoring of aromatic amine exposures in workers at a chemical plant with known bladder cancer excess. *J Natl Cancer Inst.* 1997;89(10):734; author reply 735–36.

35. Freudenthal RI, Anderson DP. A reexamination of recent publications suggesting *o*-toluidine may be a human bladder carcinogen. *Regul Toxicol Pharmacol.* 1995;21:199–202.

36. Tannenbaum SR. Bladder cancer in workers exposed to aniline. *J Natl Cancer Inst.* 1991;83(20):1507; author reply 1507–8.

37. Stephens ER. Re: Monitoring of aromatic amine exposures in workers at a chemical plant with a known bladder cancer excess. *J Natl Cancer Inst.* 1997;89(10):734–35; author reply 735–36.

38. Ferber KH. Examination before trial in the matter of *Sullivan v. E. I. Du Pont de Nemours and Co., Inc.,* in the U.S. District Court for the Eastern District of Texas, Beaumont Division. Transcript prepared by Jack W. Hunt and Associates, Inc., p. 30. October 27, 1989.

39. NIOSH Alert: Request for assistance in preventing bladder cancer from exposure to o-toluidine and aniline. December 1990. Publication no. DHHS (NIOSH) 90–116.

40. DuPont. Material safety data sheet no. DU000271: O-toluidine. Revision date: October 4, 1990.

41. Vogler W. Confidential Du Pont memorandum to be filed, re: AA-9737 [thirty-four-year-old employee with bladder tumor]. July 10, 1990.

42. Weiss RJ. Email to Fayerweather WE and Karns E. October 25, 1991.

43. Murray W. Affidavit concerning 3,3'-dichlorobenzidine (May 15, 1973). Submitted to OSHA's Standards Advisory Committee on Carcinogens, by Morgan DL (Cleary, Gottlieb, Steen, and Hamilton), June 26, 1973.

44. Ouellet-Hellstrom R, Rench JD. Bladder cancer incidence in arylamine workers. *J Occup Environ Med.* 1996;38(12):1239–47.

45. Schwieger KE. Testimony of the National Association of Manufacturers on the Emergency Temporary Standard for Certain Carcinogens 29-CFR 1910.93C as revised on July 27, 1973, before a Department of Labor Hearing Officer. September 12, 1973. OSHA Docket H-003, Exhibit no. 24.

46. Korbitz B. Affidavit on OSHA's proposed standard on 4,4'-methylenebis (2-chloroaniline. March 10, 1975. Submitted to OSHA Docket OSH-70 on behalf of the Polyurethane Manufacturers Association by Wahl EJ (Michael, Best, and Friedrich).

47. Ward E, Halperin W, Thun M et al. Bladder tumors in two young males occupationally exposed to MBOCA. *Am J Ind Med.* 1988;14(3):267–72.

48. Ward E, Halperin W, Thun M et al. Screening workers exposed to 4,4'-methylenebis (2-chloroaniline) for bladder cancer by cystoscopy. *J Occup Med.* 1990;32(9):865–68.

49. Dietrich H, Dietrich B. Ludwig Rehn (1849–1930): Pioneering findings on the aetioliogy of bladder cancers. *World J Urol.* 2000;19:151–53.

50. International Labour Organization. Cancer of the bladder among workers in aniline factories. February 1921. Studies and Reports Series F, no. 1.

51. Xue-Yun Y, Ji-Gang C, Yong-Ning H. Studies on the relation between bladder cancer and benzidine or its derived dyes in Shanghai. *Br J Ind Med.* 1990;47(8):544–52.

52. Bi W, Hayes RB, Feng P et al. Mortality and incidence of bladder cancer in benzidine-exposed workers in China. *Am J Ind Med.* 1992;21(4):481–89.

53. Samuels SW. *The International Context of Carcinogen Regulation: Benzidine. Banbury Report,* vol. 9, 497–512. Cold Spring Harbor Laboratory, Cold Spring Harbor, New York, 1981.

CHAPTER NINE

1. Public Citizen Health Research Group of the Oil, Chemical, and Atomic Workers International Union. Petition requesting a reduced tolerance for chromium (VI) (hexavalent chromium) through an emergency temporary standard issued under the authority of the Occupational Safety and Health Act. July 19, 1993. Available at: http://dockets.osha.gov/vg001/V026A/01/01/54.PDF. Accessed in June 2007.

2. U.S. Occupational Safety and Health Administration (OSHA). Occupational exposure to hexavalent chromium: Final rule. *Fed. Reg.* 2006;71(39): 10099–10385.

3. U.S. National Institute for Occupational Safety and Health (NIOSH). Criteria for a recommended standard: Occupational exposure to chromium (VI). 1975. DHHS (NIOSH) publication no. 76–129.

4. Nelson S, Vladeck DC for the Public Citizen Litigation Group. Brief of petitioners: *Public Citizen Health Research Group, and Paper, Allied-Industrial, Chemical and Energy Workers International Union v. Elaine Chao, Secretary of Labor, and Occupational Safety and Health Administration.* February 2002. Available at: http://www.citizen.org/documents/HexchromBrief.pdf. Accessed in June 2007.

5. Mancuso TF, Hueper WC. Occupational cancer and other health hazards in a chromate plant: A medical appraisal. Part 1: Lung cancers in chromate workers. *Ind Med Surg.* 1951;20(8):358–63.

6. Mancuso TF. *Consideration of Chromium as an Industrial Carcinogen.* Proceedings of the International Conference on Heavy Metals in the Environment, Toronto, Ontario, Canada, October 27–31, 1975.

7. Mancuso TF. Chromium as an industrial carcinogen: Part 1. *Am J Ind Med.* 1997;31(2):129–39.

8. OSHA History, Part 3: Dunlop/Corn Administration, 1975–1977: Reform and professionalization. Available at: http://www.dol.gov/oasam/programs/history/osha13corn.htm. Accessed in June 2007.

9. OSHA. Occupational exposure to hexavalent chromium: Proposed standards. *Fed. Reg.* 1976;41(90):18869–71.

10. *Industrial Union Department v. American Petroleum Institute,* 44 U.S. 607 (July 2, 1980). Available at: http://www.publichealthlaw.net/Reader/docs/IndustUnion.pdf. Accessed in June 2007.

11. *Public Citizen Health Research Group v. Chao*, 314 F.3d 143 (December 24, 2002). Available at: http://www.citizen.org/documents/hexavalentchromium opinion.pdf. Accessed in June 2007.

12. Occupational Safety and Health Act. Public law no. 91–596, December 29, 1970.

13. Dear JA (assistant secretary of Labor for Occupational Safety and Health). Letter to Wolfe SM (director, Public Citizen's Health Research Group). March 8, 1994.

14. OSHA. DOL semiannual agenda of regulations (Part 12). *Fed. Reg.* 1994; 59(79):20602–55.

15. OSHA. DOL semiannual agenda of regulations (Part 12). *Fed. Reg.* 1994; 59(79):57800.

16. OSHA. DOL semiannual agenda of regulations. *Fed. Reg.* 1995;60(88): 23536.

17. Dear JA (assistant secretary of Occupational Safety and Health). Letter to Wolfe SM (director, Public Citizen Health Research Group). Re: May 22 letter on behalf of Public Citizen Health Reearch Group and the Oil Chemical and Atomic Workers Union. June 30, 1995.

18. OSHA. DOL semiannual agenda of regulations (Part 12). *Fed. Reg.* 1995;60(228):60246–85.

19. K. S. Crump Division (under contract no. 7–9-F-1–0066 with the Occupational Safety and Health Administration). Evaluation of epidemiological data and risk assessment for hexavalent chromium. May 1995.

20. Hayes RB, Lilienfeld AM, Snell LM. Mortality in chromium chemical production workers: A prospective study. *Int J Epidemiol.* 1979;8(4):365–74.

21. Gibb HJ, Lees PSJ, Pinsky PF et al. Lung cancer among workers in chromium chemical production. *Am J Ind Med.* 2000;38:115–26.

22. Meeting minutes: Chrome Coalition meeting. November 14, 1995. Available at http://www.defendingscience.org/upload/CC_1995.pdf. Accessed in December 2007.

23. Meeting minutes: Chrome Coalition and ad hoc PEL committee, special meeting with ChemRisk. February 13, 1996. Available at http://www.ehjournal.net/content/supplementary/1476-069x-5-5-s2.pdf. Accessed in December 2007.

24. Buczynski MA (OxyChem). Memorandum to Stephenson DB (OxyChem). Subject: Recent activities of the Chrome Coalition OSHA/PEL ad hoc committee, April 4, 1996. Available at http://www.defendingscience.org/upload/OxyChem_1996.pdf. Accessed in December 2007.

25. Chrome Coalition. Contract between Collier, Shannon, Rill, & Scott, PLLC, on behalf of the Chrome Coalition, and ChemRisk, a division of the McLaren/Hart Environmental Engineering Corporation. September 10, 1996. Available at http://www.ehjournal.net/content/supplementary/1476-069x-5-5-s3.pdf. Accessed in December 2007.

26. Wittenborn J (Collier Shannon Scott PLC). Email to Barnhart J (Chrome Coalition). Subject: OSHA info request. August 29, 2002. Available at http://www.defendingscience.org/upload/Wittenborn_2002.pdf. Accessed in December 2007.

27. Chrome Coalition. Meeting summary. September 12, 2002. Available at http://www.ehjournal.net/content/supplementary/1476-069x-5-5-s4.pdf. Accessed in December 2007.

28. Finley BL, Kerger BD, Dodge DG et al. Assessment of airborne hexavalent chromium in the home following use of contaminated tapwater. *J Expo Anal Environ Epidemiol.* 1996;6(2):229–45.

29. Kerger BD, Paustenbach DJ, Corbett GE et al. Absorption and elimination of trivalent and hexavalent chromium in humans following ingestion of a bolus dose in drinking water. *Toxicol Appl Pharmacol.* 1996;141(1):145–58.

30. Kerger BD, Richter RO, Chute SM et al. Refined exposure assessment for ingestion of tapwater contaminated with hexavalent chromium: Consideration of exogenous and endogenous reducing agents. *J Expo Anal Environ Epidemiol.* 1996;6(2):163–79.

31. Kuykendall JR, Kerger BD, Jarvi EJ et al. Measurement of DNA-protein cross-links in human leukocytes following acute ingestion of chromium in drinking water. *Carcinogenesis.* 1996;17(9):1971–77.

32. Mirsalis JC, Hamilton CM, O'Loughlin KG et al. Chromium (VI) at plausible drinking water concentrations is not genotoxic in the in vivo bone marrow micronucleus or liver unscheduled DNA synthesis assays. *Environ Mol Mutagen.* 1996;28(1):60–63.

33. Paustenbach DJ, Hays SM, Brien BA et al. Observation of steady state in blood and urine following human ingestion of hexavalent chromium in drinking water. *J Toxicol Environ Health.* 1996;49(5):453–61.

34. Corbett GE, Finley BL, Paustenbach DJ et al. Systemic uptake of chromium in human volunteers following dermal contact with hexavalent chromium (22 mg/l). *J Expo Anal Environ Epidemiol.* 1997;7(2):179–89.

35. Finley BL, Kerger BD, Katona MW et al. Human ingestion of chromium (VI) in drinking water: Pharmacokinetics following repeated exposure. *Toxicol Appl Pharmacol.* 1997;142(1):151–59.

36. Kerger BD, Finley BL, Corbett GE et al. Ingestion of chromium(VI) in drinking water by human volunteers: Absorption, distribution, and excretion of single and repeated doses. *J Toxicol Environ Health.* 1997;50(1):67–95.

37. Proctor DM, Fredrick MM, Scott PK et al. The prevalence of chromium allergy in the United States and its implications for setting soil cleanup: A cost-effectiveness case study. *Regul Toxicol Pharmacol.* 1998;28(1):27–37.

38. Fowler JF Jr., Kauffman CL, Marks Jr. JG et al. An environmental hazard assessment of low-level dermal exposure to hexavalent chromium in solution among chromium-sensitized volunteers. *J Occup Environ Med.* 1999; 41(3):150–60.

39. Proctor DM, Panko JM, Finley BL et al. Need for improved science in standard setting for hexavalent chromium. *Regul Toxicol Pharmacol.* 1999; 29(2 Pt 1):99–101.

40. Proctor DM, Otani JM, Finley BL et al. Is hexavalent chromium carcinogenic via ingestion? A weight-of-evidence review. *J Toxicol Environ Health,* Part A. 2002;65:701–46.

41. Crump C, Crump K, Hack E et al. Dose-response and risk assessment of airborne hexavalent chromium and lung cancer mortality. *Risk Analysis.* 2003;23(6):1147–63.

42. Luippold RS, Mundt KA, Austin RP et al. Lung cancer mortality among chromate production workers. *Occup Environ Med.* 2003;60(6):451–57.

43. Paustenbach DJ, Finley BL, Mowat FS et al. Human health risk and exposure assessment of chromium (VI) in tap water. *J Toxicol Environ Health,* Part A. 2003;66(14):1295–1339.

44. Proctor DM, Panko JP, Liebig EW et al. Workplace airborne hexavalent chromium concentrations for the Painesville, Ohio, chromate production plant (1943–1971). *Appl Occup Environ Hyg.* 2003;18(6):430–49.

45. Proctor DM, Panko JP, Liebig EW et al. Estimating historical occupational exposure to airborne hexavalent chromium in a chromate production plant: 1940–1972. *J Occup Environ Hyg.* 2004;1:752–67.

46. Tritchler JP, Mundt KA (Applied Epidemiology, Inc.). Epidemiological study of six modern chromate production facilities: A unified strategy for updating mortality experience through 1998: A draft proposal prepared for the Industrial Hygiene Foundation's Chromium Chemicals Health and Environmental Committee members. March 17, 1997.

47. Applied Epidemiology, Inc. Draft protocol: Collaborative cohort mortality study of five chromate production facilities, 1958–1998. Prepared for the Industrial Health Foundation, Inc. April 23, 1999.

48. Pastides H, Austin R, Lemeshow S et al. A retrospective-cohort study of occupational exposure to hexavalent chromium. *Am J Ind Med.* 1994;25: 663–75.

49. Matzzie CG, Wolfe SM (staff attorney for Public Citizen Litigation Group and director of Public Citizen Health Research Group, respectively). Letter to Watchman G (acting assistant secretary of Labor for OSHA). March 3, 1997.

50. OSHA. DOL semiannual agenda of regulations (Part 12). *Fed. Reg.* 1997; 62(80):21934–80.

51. *Oil, Chemical, and Atomic Workers Union v. OSHA,* 145 F.3d 120 (filed March 16, 1998).

52. OSHA. DOL semiannual agenda of regulations (Part 12). *Fed. Reg.* 1997;62(209):57714–56.

53. OSHA. DOL semiannual agenda of regulations (Part 12). *Fed. Reg.* 1997;64(224):64622–71 (see 64628 and 64664–65).

54. OSHA. DOL semiannual agenda of regulations (Part 12). *Fed. Reg.* 65(321):74072–124 (see 74110).

55. OSHA. DOL semiannual agenda of regulations (Part 12). *Fed. Reg.* 2001; 66(232):61839–86 (see 61846 and 61879–80).

56. Exponent, Inc. Critique of two studies by Gibb et al.: Lung cancer among workers in chromium chemical production, clinical findings of irritation smong chromium chemical production workers. Prepared for Chrome Coalition, c/o Collier Shannon and Scott, LLP by Exponent, Inc. June 2002. OSHA Docket H054A, Exhibit no. 31–18–14.

57. OSHA. Occupational exposure to hexavalent chromium: Request for information. *Fed. Reg.* 2002;67:54389–94.

58. Exponent, Inc. Reanalysis of lung cancer mortality study for workers in the Baltimore chromium production facility. Study sponsored by Elementis Chromium, Engelhard Corporation, Honeywell, Lockheed Martin, and Tierra Solutions, Inc.; November 20, 2002. OSHA docket H054A, Exhibit no. 31–18–15–1.

59. Exponent, Inc. Technical Memorandum: Comments on the OSHA Hexavalent Chromium Rulemaking for the Aerospace Industries Association. Prepared for the Aerospace Industries Association. December 27, 2004. OSHA docket H054A, Exhibit no. 38-215-2.

60. OSHA. Occupational exposure to hexavalent chromium; proposed rule, request for comments and scheduling of informal public hearings. *Fed. Reg.* 2004;69(191):59306–404.

61. Luippold R, Mundt KA, Dell LD et al. Low-level hexavalent chromium exposure and rate of mortality among U.S. chromate production employees. *J Occup Environ Med.* 2005;47(4):381–85.

62. Spraycar M (managing editor, *JOEM*). Email to Michaels D (George Washington University). Subject: *JOEM* dates of Luippold study. May 16, 2005.

63. Tampio C (director of Employment Policy, Human Resources Policy at the National Association of Manufacturers). Letter to OSHA Docket Office. Re: Comments to proposed rule on occupational exposure to hexavalent chromium. *Fed. Reg.* October 4, 2004; 69:59305. January 3, 2005. OSHA Docket H054A, Exhibit no. 39–53.

64. Dweck A, Lurie P, Michaels D. Hexavalent chromium study's conclusions unjustified. *J Occup Environ Med.* 2005;47(10):980–81.

65. Howe SR (senior technical director, Worker Health and Safety, Society of the Plastics Industry). Letter to OSHA Docket Office. Re: Post-hearing brief, proposed rule on occupational exposure to hexavalent chromium. 60 *Fed. Reg.* 59305 (October 4, 2004). April 20, 2005. OSHA docket H054A, Exhibit no. 47–24–1.

66. McMahon-Lohrer K, Nelson K (Collier Shannon Scott, PLLC; counsel for the Speciality Steel Industry of North America). Post-hearing brief. April 20, 2005. OSHA docket H054A, Exhibit 47–27–1.

67. Richter CM, Hannapel JS (The Policy Group). Post-hearing comments of the Surface Finishing Industry Council. April 20, 2005. OSHA docket H054A, Exhibit no. 47–35–1.

68. Barnhart J. Affidavit. December 17, 2004. In re: Industrial Health Foundation, Inc., U.S. Bankruptcy Court for the Western District of Pennsylvania, 2004.

69. Applied Epidemiology, Inc. Collaborative cohort mortality study of four chromate production facilities, 1958–1998: Final report. Prepared for the Industrial Health Foundation, Inc. September 27, 2002.

70. Mundt KA, Luippold R, Dell L. Reply to Dweck, Lurie, and Michaels: Hexavalent chromium study's conclusions unjustified. *J Occup Environ Med.* 2005;47(10):980–81. *J Occup Environ Hygiene.* 2005;47(10):981.

71. Mundt K (principal, Environ Health Sciences). Email to Edens M (OSHA). Subject: Occupational hexavalent chromium exposure (with attached manuscript on German cohort mortality study). October 17, 2005. OSHA docket H054A, Exhibit no 48-4-1.

72. Birk T, Mundt KA, Dell LD et al. Lung cancer mortality in the German chromate industry, 1958 to 1998. *J Occup Environ Med.* 2006;48(4):426–33.

CHAPTER 10

1. U.S. National Institute for Occupational Safety and Health (NIOSH). NIOSH Investigation of Gilster Mary Lee. August 22, 2001. HETA no. 2000–0401; interim report.

2. Roberts DW (director, Section for Environmental Public Health, Missouri Department of Health). Letter to Gaines M (OSHA). May 19, 2000.

3. U.S. Occupational Safety and Health Administration (OSHA). Inspection report: Jasper Popcorn Company. Health narrative: CSHO workplace findings. May 23, 2000. Report ID no. 0728500, inspection no. 303206387.

4. Freshwater M (senior environmental health engineer, Wausau [Insurance Companies]). Letter to Cook J (Popcorn Plant, Jasper Foods, Inc.). Loss control services report: Environmental Health Engineering Service. May 10, 1996.

5. Fixed obstructive lung disease in workers at a microwave popcorn factory— Missouri, 2000–2002. *Morbidity and Mortality Weekly Report.* 2002;51(16): 345–47.

6. Kreiss K, Gomaa A, Kullman G et al. Clinical bronchiolitis obliterans in workers at a microwave-popcorn plant. *NEJM* 2002;345(5):330–38.

7. Shipley S. Study showed chemical was toxic. *St. Louis Post–Dispatch.* February 28, 2004.

8. Hubbs AF, Battelli LA, Goldsmith WT et al. Necrosis of nasal and airway epithelium in rats inhaling vapors of artificial butter flavoring. *Toxicol Appl Pharmacol.* 2002;185:128–35.

9. BASF. Report: Study on the acute inhalation toxicity LC50 of diacetyl FCC as a vapor in rats: 4-hour exposure. Project no. 1310247/927010 (June 8, 1993). Unpublished manuscript. Available at: http//www.defending science.org/case_studies/upload/BASF-study.pdf. Accessed in December 2007.

10. NIOSH. Important worker health notice about the popcorn plant in Jasper, Missouri (September 9, 2001).

11. Powell AR (Humphrey, Farrington, McClain, and Edgar, P.C.). Letter to Rick Roberts (OSHA Kansas City Area Office). Re: Gilster–Mary Lee Corp. OSHA complaint and request for records. December 19, 2001.

12. OSHA. Complaint/inspection case file activity diary, Kansas City Area Office. Company name: Glister [sic]-Mary Lee Corporation. December 20, 2001. Complaint no. 203783865, inspection no. 304306483.

13. OSHA. Inspection report: Glister [sic]-Mary Lee Corporation. December 20, 2001. Report ID no. 0728500, inspection no. 304306483.

14. Olmedo M (area director, OSHA Kansas City Area Office). Letter to Powell AR (Humphrey, Farrington, McClain, and Edgar, P.C.). February 28, 2002.

15. Occupational Safety and Health Act. Public law no. 91–596, December 29, 1970.

16. Page JA, O'Brien M-W. *Bitter Wages: Ralph Nader's Study Group Report on Disease and Injury on the Job.* New York: Grossman, 1973.

17. Moure-Eraso R. Primary prevention and precaution in hazard identification in the NIEHS/NTP: Body in the morgue approach. *Public Health Rep.* November–December 2002;117:564–73.

18. *Industrial Union Department v. American Petroleum Institute,* 44 U.S. 607 (July 2, 1980). Available at: http://www.publichealthlaw.net/Reader/docs/IndustUnion.pdf. Accessed in June 2007.

19. OSHA. Coke oven emissions: Final standard. *Fed. Reg.* 1976;41:46742.

20. Michaels D, Ashford NA, Baker D et al. Letter to Chao EL (secretary, U.S. Department of Labor). July 26, 2006. Available at: http://defending science.org/upload/Scientists%20Letter%20to%20OSHA%20on%20Diacetyl 07262006.pdf. Accessed in June 2007.

21. Fixed obstructive lung disease among workers in the flavor-manufacturing industry—California, 2004–2007. *Morbidity and Mortality Weekly Report* 2007;56(16):389–393.

22. NIOSH alert: Preventing lung disease in workers who use or make flavorings. December 2003. DHHS (NIOSH) publication no. 2004–110.

23. Schneider A. Disease is swift, response is slow. *Baltimore Sun.* April 23, 2006.

24. Asssociated Press. Testimony ends in second trial on claim that popcorn flavoring caused injury. April 30, 2004.

25. OSHA. Chemical sampling information: Diacetyl. 2007. Available at: http://www.osha.gov/dts/chemicalsampling/data/CH_231710.html. Accessed in June 2007.

26. Bowman C. Investigative report: Flavoring agent destroys lungs. *Sacramento Bee.* July 30, 2006.

27. United Food and Commercial Workers International Union, International Brotherhood of Teamsters. Letter to Chao E (OSHA). Subject: Petition for an OSHA emergency temporary standard for diacetyl. July 26, 2006. Available at: http://defendingscience.org/case_studies/upload/Union_Petition_to_CHAO_on_Diacetyl.pdf. Accessed in June 2007.

28. Flavor and Extract Manufacturers Association of the United States. Respiratory Health and Safety in the Flavor Manufacturing Workplace. August 2004. Available at: http://www.ifraorg.org/Enclosures/News/RespiratoryRpt.pdf. Accessed in June 2007.

29. OSHA. Agreement establishing an alliance between the Occupational Safety and Health Administration, U.S. Department of Labor Region VII, and the Popcorn Board. September 22, 2002. Available at: http://www.osha.gov/dcsp/alliances/regional/reg7/popcorn.html. Accessed in June 2007.

30. OSHA. Fact sheet: OSHA Alliance Program. August 2005. Available at: http://www.osha.gov/dcsp/alliances/. Accessed in June 2007.

31. OSHA. The Alliance Program. Power Point Presentation. Available at: http://www.osha.gov/dcsp/alliances/presentations/alliance_final/index.html. Accessed in July 2007.

32. OSHA. Press release: OSHA signs alliance with the International Society of Canine Cosmetologists. Issued 2005. Available at: http://www.osha.gov/pls/oshaweb/owadisp.show_document?p_table=NEWS_RELEASES&p_id=11616. Accessed in July 2007.

33. Adkins CE (regional administrator, OSHA). Letter to Michaels D (George Washington University). Re: FOIA request. June 4, 2004.

34. U.S. House of Representatives, Committee on Education and Labor, Subcommittee on Workforce Protections. Hearing: Have OSHA standards kept up with workplace hazards? April 24, 2007. Available at: http://edlabor.house.gov/hearings/wp042407.shtml. Accessed in June 2007.

35. U.S. Senate, Committee on Health, Education, Labor and Pensions, Subcommittee on Employment and Workplace Safety. Hearing: Is OSHA working for working people? April 26, 2007. Available at: http://help.senate.gov/Hearings/2007_04_26/2007_04_26.html. Accessed in June 2007.

36. Foulke Jr. EG (assistant secretary, OSHA). Testimony before the House Subcommittee on Workforce Protections. April 24, 2007. Available at: http://edlabor.house.gov/testimony/042407EdwinFoulketestimony.pdf. Accessed in July 2007.

37. Van Rooy GBGJ, Rooyackers JM, Prokop M et al. Bronchiolitis obliterans syndrome in chemical workers producing diacetyl for food flavorings. *Am J Respir Crit Care.* 2007;176:498–504.

38. Ettlinger S. *Twinkie, Deconstructed.* New York: Hudson Street Press, 2007.

39. H.R. 2693. Popcorn Workers Lung Disease Prevention Act. Introduced June 13, 2007, by Rep. Woolsey L (D-CA-6). Available at: http://www .defendingscience.org/case_studies/upload/2693_Markup.pdf. Accessed in June 2007.

40. Foulke Jr. EG (assistant secretary, OSHA). Letter to Rep. Miller G (Chairman, U.S. House Committee on Education and Labor). June 19, 2007. Available at: http://www.defendingscience.org/case_studies/upload/ 2693_Foulke_Letter.pdf. Accessed in June 2007.

41. Flavor and Extract Manufacturers Association of the United States. Press Release: The Flavor and Extract Manufacturers Association of the United States supports H.R. 2693, legislation to ensure workplace safety in flavor manufacturing. Issued June 13, 2007. Available at: http://www.femaflavor .org/downloads/PressReleases/FEMA_Statement_Diacetyl_061307.pdf. Accessed in June 2007.

42. Rep. McKeon HP (R-CA-25). Opening statement before the Committee on Education and Labor Markup of H.R. 2693, the Popcorn Workers Lung Disease Prevention Act. Available at: http://republicans.edlabor .house.gov/PRArticle.aspx?NewsID=185&IID=16. Accessed in June 2007.

43. U.S. House Committee on Education and Labor. Press Release: House Labor Committee passes legislation to protect food flavoring workers from severe lung disease. Issued June 20, 2007. Available at: http://www.house .gov/apps/list/speech/edlabor_dem/rel062007b.html. Accessed in June 2007.

44. Roberts JD, Galbraith DA, Finley BL (ChemRisk, Inc.). A comprehensive review of occupational exposure to diacetyl in microwave popcorn facilities. Poster presented at Society of Toxicology Meeting, 2007. Available at: http://defendingscience.org/case_studies/upload/ChemRisk_Poster_Diacetyl .pdf. Accessed in June 2007.

45. Kanwal R, Kullman G, Piacitelli C et al. Evaluation of flavorings-related lung disease risk at six microwave popcorn plants. *J Occup Environ Med.* 2006;48(2):149–57.

46. Montealegre J (Vice president for R & D, ConAgra Foods, Inc.) Email to Rosati J. September 9, 2003. Available at: http://www.defendingscience .org/upload/Meeting_request_from_ConAgra.pdf Accessed in June 2007.

47. Verduin P (Senior Vice President, Product Quality and Development, Con-Agra Foods, Inc.). Letter to Gilman G (Assistant Administrator for the Office of Research and Development, U.S. Environmental Protection Agency). November 29, 2004. Available at: http://www.defendingscience.org/upload/ Letter_from_ConAgra_regarding_progress.pdf. Accessed in June 2007.

48. Eaton S. Ohio popcorn plant workers say flavoring hurts lungs. *(Cleveland) Plain Dealer.* December 3, 2006: A1.

49. U.S. Food and Drug Administration. Overview of the Center for Food Safety and Applied Nutrition. February 2001. Available at: http://www .cfsan.fda.gov/~lrd/cfsan4.html. Accessed in June 2007.

50. Life Sciences Research Office of the Federation of American Societies for Experimental Biology (under contract no. FDA 223–75–2004 to the U.S. Food and Drug Administration). Evaluation of the health aspects of starter distillate and diacetyl as food ingredients. 1980.

51. U.S. Food and Drug Administration. Starter distillate and diacetyl; proposed GRAS status as direct human food ingredients: Proposed rule. *Fed. Reg.* 1982;47(152):34155–58.

52. Michaels D (director, Project on Scientific Knowledge and Public Policy [SKAPP], George Washington University). Letter to von Eschenbach AC (acting commissioner, U.S. Food and Drug Administration). Re: Petition to urge the FDA's prompt action to cancel the GRAS designation for diacetyl. September 8, 2006. FDA docket 2006P-0379. Available at: http://defendingscience.org/newsroom/upload/Petition_to_FDA_on_Diacetyl.pdf. Accessed in June 2007.

53. Rep. DeLauro RL (D-CT-3). Letter to von Eschenbach AC (commissioner, U.S. Food and Drug Administration). May 7, 2007. Available at: http://www.house.gov/delauro/press/2007/May/Diacetyl_FDA_05_07_07.html. Accessed in June 2007.

54. von Eschenbach AC (commissioner, U.S. Food and Drug Administration). Letter to DeLauro RL (D-CT-3). June 12, 2007. Available at: http://www.defendingscience.org/upload/FDA_DeLauro_response.pdf. Accessed in June 2007.

55. Michaels D. Popcorn lung coming to your kitchen? The FDA doesn't want you to know. The Pump Handle Blog. September 4, 2007. Available at: http://thepumphandle.wordpress.com/2007/09/04/popcorn-lung-coming-to-your-kitchen-the-fda-doesnt-want-to-know/. Accessed in September 2007.

56. Harris G. Doctor links a man's illness to a microwave popcorn habit. *New York Times.* September 5, 2007.

57. Rose C (acting head, Division of Environmental and Occupational Health Sciences National Jewish Medical and Research Center). Letter to Landa M, (deputy commissioner for Regulatory Affairs, Center for Food Safety and Applied Nutrition, U.S. Food and Drug Administration). July 18, 2007. Available at: http://www.defendingscience.org/case_studies/upload/National_Jewish_FDA_Letter.pdf. Accessed in September 2007.

58. Pop Weaver Popcorn Company. Press Release: Pop Weaver introduces first microwave popcorn with flavoring containing no diacetyl. Issued August 28, 2007. Available at: http://www.popweaver.com/NoDiacetylPressRelease.pdf. Accessed in September 2007.

59. Funk J. Popcorn makers work to remove chemical. *Associated Press.* September 5, 2007.

60. Swoboda F. U.S. acts to reduce repetitive motion injuries; Labor department's voluntary workplace standards to be basis for mandatory rules. *Washington Post.* August 31, 1990: A4.

61. U.S. Bureau of Labor Statistics. Highest incidence rates and number of disorders with repeated trauma, private industry, 2001. Table S10. Available at: http://www.bls.gov/iif/oshwc/osh/os/ostb1120.pdf. Accessed in June 2007.

62. OSHA. Advanced notice of proposed rulemaking on ergonomics safety and health management. *Fed. Reg.* 1992;57:34192.

63. National Research Council. Work-related musculoskeletal disorders: A review of the evidence. Washington, DC: National Academy Press, 1998.

64. OSHA. Ergonomics Program, Part 2: Proposed rule, request for comments; scheduling of informal public hearing. *Fed. Reg.* 1999;64(225): 65768.

65. Ivins M, Dubose L. *Bushwacked: Life in George W. Bush's America.* New York: Random House, 2003.

66. Cato Institute. Press release: Labor expert: OSHA's ergonomics regulations based on junk science. Issued May 15, 2000. Available at: http://www.cato.org/new/05-00/05-15-oor.html. Accessed in June 2007.

67. Scalia E. OSHA'S ergonomics litigation record: Three strikes and it's out. *Cato Policy Analysis.* May 15, 2000. Available at: http://www.cato.org/pubs/pas/pa-370es.html. Accessed in June 2007.

68. National Research Council, Institute of Medicine. *Musculoskeletal Disorders and the Workplace: Low Back and Upper Extremities.* Washington, DC: National Academy Press, 2001.

69. OSHA. Ergonomics Program: Final rule. *Fed. Reg.* 2000;65(220):68262.

70. Joint Resolution of Senate and House of Representatives to disapprove of OSHA's final rule on ergonomics. Public law no. 107-5, March 20, 2001.

71. OSHA. Press release: OSHA issues final rule on recordkeeping form. Issued June 30, 2003. Available at: http://www.osha.gov/pls/oshaweb/owadisp.show_document?p_table=NEWS_RELEASES&p_id=10281&p_text_version=FALSE. Accessed in June 2007.

72. Barab J. Egonomics injuries: Now you see 'em, now you don't. Confined Space Blog. July 1, 2003. Available at: http://spewingforth.blogspot.com/2003_06_29_spewingforth_archive.html#105710492409972876. Accessed in June 2007.

CHAPTER 11

1. Tepper LB, Hardy HL, and Chamberlain RI. *Toxicity of Beryllium Compounds.* New York: Elsevier, 1961.

2. Breslin AJ. Exposures and patterns of disease in the beryllium industry. In: Stokinger HE, ed. *Beryllium: Its Industrial Hygiene Aspects.* New York: Academic Press, 1966:19-43.

3. Eisenbud M, Wanta RC, Dustan C et al. Non-occupational berylliosis. *J Ind Hyg Toxicol.* 1949;31:282.

4. Tumbleson R (U.S. Atomic Energy Commission Public/Technical Information Service). Public relations problems in connection with occupational diseases in the beryllium industry. 1947.

5. Eisenbud M. *An Environmental Odyssey: People, Pollution, and Politics in the Life of a Practical Scientist.* Seattle, WA: University of Washington Press, 1990.

6. Sprince NL, Kazemi H. U.S. Beryllium Case Registry through 1977. *Environ Res.* 1980;21:44–47.

7. Roe S. Deadly alliance. *Toledo Blade.* Series of articles published March 28–April 2, 1999.

8. U.S. National Institute for Occupational Safety and Health (NIOSH). Criteria for a recommended standard to beryllium exposure. 1972. DHHS (NIOSH) publication no. 72–10268.

9. Stokinger HE. Recommended hygienic limits of exposure to beryllium. In: Stokinger HE, ed. *Beryllium: Its Industrial Hygiene Aspects.* New York: Academic Press, 1966:235–244.

10. Kohara T (director and general manager, Personnel Department, NGK Insulators, Ltd.). Letter to Piper HG (Vice President, Brush Wellman, Inc.). August 9, 1974.

11. Cullen MR, Kominsky JR, Rossman MD et al. Chronic beryllium disease in a precious metal refinery: Clinical epidemiologic and immunologic evidence for continuing risk from exposure to low-level beryllium fume. *Am Rev Respir Dis.* 1987;135(1):201–08.

12. Vorwald AJ. Animal methods. In: Vorwald AJ, ed. *Pneumoconiosis: Beryllium, Bauxite Fumes, Compensation.* New York: Hoeber, 1950:393–425.

13. Machle W. A further program. In: Vorwald AJ, ed. *Pneumoconiosis: Beryllium, Bauxite Fumes, Compensation.* New York: Hoeber, 1950:447–51.

14. Saranac Laboratory. Proposal on the co-carcinogenic potentialities of inhaled tobacco smoke in relation to beryllium-provoked lung cancer of the rat. Submitted to the Tobacco Industry Research Committee, October 1, 1954.

15. Mancuso TF, el-Attar AA. Epidemiological study of the beryllium industry: Cohort methodology and mortality studies. *J Occup Med.* 1969;11(8):422–34.

16. Mancuso TF. Relation of duration of employment and prior respiratory illness to respiratory cancer among beryllium workers. *Environ Res.* 1970; 3(3):251–75.

17. Mancuso TF, Coulter EJ. Methods of studying the relation of employment and long-term illness: Cohort analysis. *Am J Public Health.* 1959;49:1525–36.

18. Mancuso TF. Methodology in industrial health studies: Social Security disability data and the medical care system. *Am J Ind Med.* 1993;23(4):653–71.

19. Mancuso TF. Mortality study of beryllium industry workers' occupational lung cancer. *Environ Res.* 1980;21(1):48–55.

20. Wagoner JK, Infante PF, Bayliss DL. Beryllium: An etiologic agent in the induction of lung cancer, nonneoplastic respiratory disease, and heart disease among industrially exposed workers. *Environ Res.* 1980;21(1):15–34.

21. Finklea JF (director, NIOSH). Memorandum to assistant secretary for Occupational Safety and Health. Subject: Update of NIOSH criteria document on beryllium, December 10, 1975.

22. U.S. Occupational Safety and Health Administration (OSHA). Beryllium: Proposed occupational safety and health standard. *Fed. Reg.* 1975;40(202): 48814–27.

23. Baier EJ (NIOSH). Statement at OSHA's public hearing on the occupational standard for beryllium. August 19, 1977.

24. Brush Wellman. Briefing outline on OSHA. October 6, 1977. Bates no. BF009662–BF009677.

25. Newman JM Jr. (Jones, Day, Reavis, and Pogue on behalf of Brush Wellman, Inc.). Letter to OSHA Docket Office. Re: Public hearing on proposed beryllium standard. July 13, 1977.

26. Steenland K, Ward E. Lung cancer incidence among patients with beryllium disease: A cohort mortality study. *J Natl Cancer Inst.* 1991;83(19): 1380–85.

27. Ward E, Okun A, Ruder A et al. A mortality study of workers at seven beryllium processing plants. *Am J Ind Med.* 1992;22(6):885–904.

28. Sanderson WT, Ward EM, Steenland K et al. Lung cancer case-control study of beryllium workers. *Am J Ind Med.* 2001;39(2):133–44.

29. MacCarten P. Letter to Administrative Law Judge Lesser P, submitted by Jones, Day, Reavis, and Pogue (Counsel for Brush Wellman, Inc.), November 17, 1977. Document no. CDC 00027, 1977.

30. Roth HD. OSHA beryllium hearings: Analysis of epidemiological data; ca.1978. Document no. D087051.

31. MacMahon B, Roth N. An evaluation of Wagoner JK, Bayliss DL, Infante PF: Beryllium: An etiologic agent in the induction of lung cancer, nonneoplastic respiratory disease and heart disease among industrially exposed workers. Manuscript, May 23, 1978.

32. Powers MB. Statement of Brush Wellman, Inc., at the public hearings on OSHA's proposed beryllium standard, 1977.

33. Eisenbud M, Goldwater LJ, Higgins I et al. Letter to Califano JA, Marshall R (secretary of Health, Education, and Welfare and secretary of Labor, respectively). February 10, 1978. Bates no. ME007469 or TW103006.

34. Odorich J, Schwartz AE, Wright MJ (vice president; director, Safety and Health Department; and industrial hygienist, Safety and Health Department; respectively, of the United Steelworkers of America). Letter to Ca-

lifano JA, Marshall R (secretary of Health, Education, and Welfare and secretary of Labor, respectively). March 20, 1978.

35. Califano J Jr. (secretary of Health, Education, and Welfare). Letter to Sen. Eagleton TF (D-MO). August 21, 1978.

36. Shy CM (professor of Epidemiology and director, Institute for Environmental Studies, University of Northa Carolina–Chapel Hill). Letter to Foege WH (director, Center [*sic*] for Disease Control). October 12, 1978. Document no. 1011291).

37. Alsop R. Beryllium firm optimistic on fight to keep metal off carcinogen list. *Wall Street Journal*. March 7, 1978.

38. Schlesinger JR (secretary of Energy). Letter to Marshall RF (secretary of Labor). August 30, 1978.

39. International Agency for Research on Cancer. IARC Monograph on the Evaluation of Carcinogenic Risks to Humans, Volume 23: Some Metals and Metallic Compounds. July 1980.

40. National Toxicology Program. Second annual report on carcinogens. 1981.

41. Preuss OP. Long-term follow-up of workers exposed to beryllium. *Brit J Industr Med.* 1985;42:69.

42. Roth HD. Memorandum to Brush Wellman enclosing a critique of the EPA health assessment document for beryllium. February 22, 1985.

43. Roth HD. Evaluation of beryllium epidemiological data, prepared for beryllium industry. August 1987.

44. Roth N (Roth Associates, Inc.). Memorandum to Davis D, Markham T, Miller J, Newman J, Wolfe D (Brush Wellman, Inc.). Subject: NIOSH Meeting (March 31, 1988). April 13, 1988.

45. Powers MB, Preuss OP. Memorandum to Gulick JE. Subject: Proposed program of filling need for new and accurate beryllium health and safety literature. January 23, 1987. Available at http://www.defendingscience.org/upload/Powers_1987.pdf. Accessed in December 2007.

46. Rossman MD, Preuss OP, Powers MB, eds. *Beryllium: Biomedical and Environmental Aspects.* Baltimore, MD: Williams and Wilkins, 1991.

47. Hill and Knowlton, Inc. Letter to Gulick JE (vice president, Planning and Administration, Brush Wellman). February 21, 1989. Available at http://www.defendingscience.org/upload/HK_beryllium.pdf. Accessed in December 2007.

48. Swetonic M (Hill and Knowlton, Inc.) Memorandum to Allen P (RJR Nabisco). Subject: Hill and Knowlton ETS Assignment. July 23, 1987. Available at: http://legacy.library.ucsf.edu/tid/jid03doo. Accessed in July 2007.

49. Public Relations Plan: Liability Litigation. 1985. R.J. Reynolds document no. 505439316/9330. Available at: http://legacy.library.ucsf.edu/tid/mgw15doo. Accessed in July 2007.

50. Asebstos Textile Institute. General meeting minutes, June 7, 1973. Addendum: About the speaker: Matthew M. Swetonic.

51. Brush Wellman. Introduction; ca. 1993. Bates no. BF0010985-BF0010987. Available at http://www.defendingscience.org/upload/BW_intro.pdf. Accessed in December 2007.

52. Harnett GD (president, chief executive officer, Brush Wellman, Inc.). Letter to Millar JD (director, NIOSH). Re: A mortality study of workers at seven beryllium processing plants. Elizabeth Ward, PhD, and Andrea Okun, MS. July 18, 1991.

53. Saracci R. Beryllium and lung cancer: Adding another piece to the puzzle of epidemiologic evidence. *J Natl Cancer Inst.* 1991;83(19):1362–63.

54. Levy P, Roth HD, Hwang PMT et al. Beryllium and lung cancer: A reanalysis of a NIOSH cohort mortality study. *Inhal Toxicol.* 2002;14(10):1003–15.

55. Niwa Y (vice president, NGK Metals Corp.) Letter to Ratney R (chair, Committee on Dusts and Inorganic Substances, ACGIH). Re: Brush Wellman, Inc., and NGK Metal Corporation submission of information relevant to ACGIH guidelines for occupational beryllium exposure. July 9, 1993.

56. Hanes HD (vice president of Government Affairs, Brush Wellman, Inc.). Letter to Bruce RM (chemical manager, Office of Research and Development, U.S. Environmental Protection Agency). Re: IRIS pilot draft toxicological review of beryllium compounds. April 15, 1997.

57. Kolanz M, Roth HD. Supplemental comments of Brush Wellman, Inc., on the National Toxicology Board of Scientific Counselors January 20, 2000 review and recommendation regarding the appropriate classification of beryllium and beryllium compounds. June 5, 2000.

58. Trichopoulos D (Harvard School of Public Health). Letter to Jameson CW (National Toxicology Program). On the alleged human carcinogenicity of beryllium. June 1, 1999.

59. Kolanz M (director of Environment and Safety, Brush Wellman). Letter to Jameson CW (National Toxicology Program). June 1, 1999.

60. Jameson CW (NIEHS). Letter to Rep. Strickland T (D-OH-6). Re: NTP's review of beryllium for the report on carcinogens. August 2003.

61. Hanes H. Memorandum to Rozek B. Subject: Activity report, environmental and government affairs. July 23, 1992.

62. International Agency for Research on Cancer. IARC Monographs on the Evaluation of Carcinogenic Risks to Humans, Vol. 58: Beryllium, Cadmium, Mercury, and Exposures in the Glass Manufacturing Industry. 1993.

63. Egilman D, Bagley S, Connolly S. Anything but beryllium: The beryllium industry's corruption of safety information. *Am J Ind Med.* 2002;42(3):270–71.

64. Egilman DS, Bagley S, Biklen M et al. The beryllium "double standard" standard. *Int J Health Serv.* 2003;33(4):769–812.

65. Hanes HD (vice president of Government Affairs, Brush Wellman, Inc.). Memorandum to Eisenbud M, Kotin P, MacMahon B, Markham T,

Powers M, Trichopoulos D, Stonehouse J, and Valiquette J. Subject: What was unique about the processing of beryllium materials in the Brush-Lorain plant? January 31, 1994.

66. Stonehouse AJ (consultant). Leter to Hanes H (vice president of Governmental Affairs, Brush Wellman). Subject: Brief study of preparations at the Lorain plant of the Brush Beryllium Co. relative to unique health and safety issues. January 19, 1994.

67. Hanes HD (vice president of Governmental Affairs, Brush Wellman). Letter to Trichopoulos D (chairman and professor, Department of Epidemiology, Harvard School of Public Health). Re: Lorain plant paper. April 18, 1995.

68. Beryllium Industry Scientific Advisory Committee (BISAC). Draft minutes of meeting of the Beryllium Industry Scientific Advisory Committee, October 9–10, 1995.

69. BISAC. Is beryllium carcinogenic in humans? *J Occup Environ Med.* 1997; 39(3):205–08.

70. Cruzan G (ToxWorks). Facsimile to Hanes H (Brush Wellman). Subject: Recent articles of relevance to beryllium. June 13, 1997.

71. Sathiakumar N, Delzell E, Amoateng-Adjepong Y et al. Epidemiologic evidence on the rleationship between mists containing sulfuric acid and respiratory tract cancer. *Crit Rev Toxicol.* 1997;27(3):223–51.

72. Fehner TR, Gosling FG. Coming in from the cold: Regulating U.S. Department of Energy nuclear facilities, 1942–1996. *Environ Hist.* 1996;1(2):5–33.

73. Hanes HD (vice president of Environmental and Legislative Affairs, Brush Wellman). Letter to Weitzman DJ (director, Industrial Hygiene Programs Division, EH-412, Office of Health Physics and Industrial Hygiene, U.S. Department of Energy). January 10, 1992.

74. Hanes HD (vice president of Environmental and Legislative Affairs, Brush Wellman). Memorandum to Brophy J, Harnett G, Skoch D, Craig Harlan, Sandor A, Waite C. Subject: Beryllium supply to the government. March 12, 1992.

75. Kolanz M. Testimony at the Department of Energy's beryllium public forum in Albuquerque, NM. January 15, 1997.

76. Paustenbach DJ, Madl AK, Greene JF. Identifying an appropriate occupational exposure limit (OEL) for beryllium: Data gaps and current research initiatives. *Appl Occup Environ Hyg.* 2001;16(5):527–38.

77. Egilman D, Bohme SR. TLVs, threshold limit values: Should we trust them? *NECOEM Reporter.* 2003;2(7):1,4–5.

78. Kolanz M. Testimony at the Department of Energy Public hearing on the proposed Chronic Beryllium Disease Prevention Program. February 11, 1999.

79. Jeffress CN (assistant secretary, OSHA, to Peter Brush). Letter to Brush P (acting assistant secretary, Environment, Safety, and Health, U.S. Department of Energy). August 27, 1998.

80. OSHA. DOL semiannual agenda of regulations (Part 12). *Fed. Reg.* November 30, 2000;65(321):74072–124 (see 74110).

81. OSHA. DOL semiannual agenda of regulations (Part 12). *Fed. Reg.* December 3, 2001;66(232):61839–86 (see 61846 and 61879–80).

82. Cummings KJ, Deubner DC, Day GA et al. Enhanced preventive programme at a beryllium oxide ceramics facility reduces beryllium sensitisation among new workers. *Occup Environ Med.* 2007;64:134–40.

83. Day GA, Dufresne A, Stefaniak AB et al. Exposure pathway assessment at a copper-beryllium alloy facility. *Ann Occup Hyg.* 2007;51(1):67–80.

84. Stanton ML, Henneberger PK, Kent MS et al. Sensitization and chronic beryllium disease among workers in copper-beryllium distribution centers. *J Occup Environ Med.* 2006;48(2):204–11.

85. Schuler CR, Kent MS, Deubner DC et al. Process-related risk of beryllium sensitization and disease in a copper-beryllium alloy facility. *Am J Ind Med.* 2005;47(3):195–205.

86. Henneberger PK, Cumro D, Deubner DD et al. Beryllium sensitization and disease among long-term and short-term workers in a beryllium ceramics plant. *Int Arch Occup Environ Health.* 2001;74(3):167–76.

87. Rosenman K, Hertzberg V, Rice C et al. Chronic Beryllium Disease and sensitization at a beryllium processing facility. *Environ Health Perspect.* 2005;113(10):1366–72.

88. Madl AK, Unice K, Brown JL et al. Exposure-response analysis for beryllium sensitization and chronic beryllium disease among workers in a beryllium metal machining plant. *J Occup Environ Hyg.* 2007;4(6):448–66.

89. BISAC. Minutes of meeting, November 2–3, 1994.

90. BISAC. Minutes of meeting, April 23, 1996.

91. BISAC. Minutes of meeting, October 1, 1998.

92. BISAC. Minutes of meeting, November 11–12, 1999.

93. Kolanz M (Brush Wellman). Letter to Sanderson W (NIOSH). January 31, 2000.

94. Deubner DC, Lockey JL, Kotin P et al. Re: Lung cancer case-control study of beryllium workers. Sanderson WT, Ward EM, Steenland K, Petersen MR. *Am J Ind Med.* 2001;39:133–44. *Am J Ind Med.* 2001;40(3):284–85.

95. OSHA. Occupational exposure to beryllium: Request for information. *Fed. Reg.* 2002;67(228):70707.

96. National Toxicology Program. Tenth annual report on carcinogens. 2002.

97. Robin J-P. Beryllium health surveillance: The Quebec experience in the copper recycling industry (PowerPoint presentation on behalf of Noranda Inc./Falconbridge Ltd., at the International Beryllium Research Conference; March 8, 2005). Available at: http://irsst.qc.ca/files/documents/divers/Beryllium_ppt/SESSION2/2-Jean-Paul-Robin.pdf. Accessed in June 2007.

98. Brush Wellman, Inc. Supplementary documentation of Brush Wellman briefing outline on OSHA. October 11, 1977. Bates no. BF009665–77.

99. Brush Wellman, Inc., Health, Safety, and Environmental Strategic Plan. Presented by Rozek RH (vice president of Corporate Development, Brush Wellman, Inc.), at the board of directors' meeting, June 25, 1991.

100. Turcic P. Personal communication, October 30, 2006.

101. H.R. 1758: Reform of Energy Workers Compensation Act, Section 202: Coverage for lung cancer in covered beryllium employees. Introduced April 10, 2003, by Rep. Strickland T. (D-OH-6).

102. Schumacher RP (Brush Wellman). Letter to to Dallafior M (Office of Rep. Strickland T (D-OH-6). Re: Levy/Roth paper. June 2003.

103. Schoeters I (Eurometaux). Letter to Fassold E (European Chemicals Bureau). Re: Agenda point 8.1: Comments on new proposals from Norway (ECBI/09/95, Add. 20). April 7, 2000.

CHAPTER 12

1. Angell M. *The Truth about the Drug Companies: How They Deceive Us and What to Do about It.* New York: Random House, 2004.

2. Abramson J. *Overdosed America: The Broken Promise of American Medicine.* New York: HarperCollins, 2004.

3. Goozner M. *The $800 Million Pill: The Truth behind the Cost of New Drugs.* Los Angeles, CA: University of California Press, 2004.

4. Avorn J. *Powerful Medicines: The Benefits, Risks, and Costs of Prescription Drugs.* New York: Knopf, 2004.

5. Kassirer JP. *On the Take: How Medicine's Complicity with Big Business Can Endanger Your Health.* New York: Oxford University Press, 2005.

6. Krimsky S. *Science in the Private Interest: Has the Lure of Profits Corrupted Biomedical Research?* Lanham, MD: Rowman and Littlefield, 2003.

7. Krimsky S. The funding effect in science and its implications for the judiciary. *J Law Policy.* 2005;13(1):46–68.

8. Rochon PA, Gurwitz JH, Simms RW et al. A study of manufacturer-supported trials of nonsteroidal anti-inflammatory drugs in the treatment of arthritis. *Arch Intern Med.* 1994;154(2):157–63.

9. Stelfox HT, Chua G, O'Rourke K et al. Conflict of interest in the debate over calcium-channel antagonists. *NEJM.* 1998;338(2):101–06.

10. Vandenbroucke JP, Helmerhorst FM, Rosendaal FR. Competing interests and controversy about third generation oral contraceptives: *BMJ* readers should know whose words they read. *BMJ.* 2000;320(7231): 381–82.

11. Montgomery JH, Byerly M, Carmody T et al. An analysis of the effect of funding source in randomized clinical trials of second generation antipsychotics for the treatment of schizophrenia. *Control Clin Trials.* 2004;25(6):598–612.

12. Koepp R, Miles SH. Meta-analysis of tacrine for Alzheimer disease: The influence of industry sponsors. *JAMA*. 1999;281(24):2287–88.

13. Knox KS, Adams JR, Djulbegovic B et al. Reporting and dissemination of industry versus non-profit sponsored economic analyses of six novel drugs used in oncology. *Ann Oncol*. 2000;11(12):1591–95.

14. Bekelman JE, Li Y, Gross CP. Scope and impact of financial conflicts of interest in biomedical research: a systematic review. *JAMA*. 2003;289(4): 454–65.

15. Lexchin J, Bero LA, Djulbegovic B et al. Pharmaceutical industry sponsorship and research outcome and quality: Systematic review. *BMJ*. 2003; 326(7400):1167–70.

16. Mandelkern M. Manufacturer support and outcome. *J Clin Psychiatry*. 1999;60(2):122–23.

17. Yaphe J, Edman R, Knishkowy B et al. The association between funding by commercial interests and study outcome in randomized controlled drug trials. *Fam Pract*. 2001;18(6):565–68.

18. Smith R. Medical journals are an extension of the marketing arm of pharmaceutical companies. *PLoS Med*. 2005;2(5):0364–66.

19. Rochon PA, Berger PB, Gordon M. The evolution of clinical trials: Inclusion and representation. *CMAJ*. 1998;159(11):1373–74.

20. Wolfe SM, Sasich LD (Public Citizen's Health Research Group). Letter to Jefferys D (director, Licensing Division, Medicines Control Agency, United Kingdom). August 27, 1998. HRG publication no. 1454. Available at: http://www.citizen.org/publications/release.cfm?ID=6652. Accessed in June 2007.

21. Bombardier C, Laine L, Reicin A et al. Comparison of upper gastrointestinal toxicity of rofecoxib and naproxen in patients with rheumatoid arthritis. *NEJM*. 2000;343(21):1520–28.

22. Mukherjee D, Nissen SE, Topol EJ. Lack of cardioprotective effect of naproxen. *Arch Intern Med*. 2002;162(22):2637; author reply 2638–39.

23. Villalba ML. Statistical reviewing briefing document for the Advisory Committee. 2000. Available at: http://www.fda.gov/OHRMS/DOCKETS/ac/01/briefing/3677b2_04_stats.pdf. Accessed in June 2007.

24. Mukherjee D, Nissen SE, Topol EJ. Risk of cardiovascular events associated with selective COX-2 inhibitors. *JAMA*. 2001;286(8):954–59.

25. Waxman HA (Ranking member, U.S. House Committee on Governmental Reform, minority staff). Memorandum to Democratic members of Congress. Re: the marketing of Vioxx to physicians. May 5, 2005. Available at: http://www.democrats.reform.house.gov/Documents/20050505114932–41272 .pdf. Accessed in June 2007.

26. Singh G. Testimony before the Senate Finance Commitee. November 18, 2004. Available at: http://www.senate.gov/~finance/hearings/testimony/2004test/111804GStest.pdf. Accessed in June 2007.

27. Matthews AW, Martinez B. Warning signs: Emails suggest Merck knew Vioxx's dangers at early stage; as heart-risk evidence rose, officials played hardball; internal message: "DODGE!"; company says "out of context." *Wall Street Journal.* November 1, 2004:A1.

28. Bresalier RS, Sandler RS, Quan H et al. Cardiovascular events associated with rofecoxib in a colorectal adenoma chemoprevention trial. *NEJM.* 2005; 352(11):1092–1102.

29. Graham DJ, Campen D, Hui R et al. Risk of acute myocardial infarction and sudden cardiac death in patients treated with cyclo-oxygenase 2 selective and non-selective non-steroidal anti-inflammatory drugs: nested case-control study. *Lancet.* 2005;365(9458):475–81.

30. Graham DJ. Testimony before the Senate Finance Committee. November 18, 2004. Available at: http://www.senate.gov/~finance/hearings/testimony/2004test/111804dgtest.pdf. Accessed in June 2007.

31. Curfman GD, Morrissey S, Drazen JM. Expression of concern: Bombardier et al., "Comparison of upper gastrointestinal toxicity of rofecoxib and naproxen in patients with rheumatoid arthritis." *NEJM.* 2000;343:1520–28. *NEJM.* 2005;353(26):2813–14.

32. Curfman GD, Morrissey S, Drazen JM. Expression of concern reaffirmed. *NEJM.* 2006;354(11):1193.

33. Lagakos SW. Time-to-event analyses for long-term treatments: The APPROVe Trial. *NEJM.* 2006;355(2):113–17.

34. Tesoriero HW. New Vioxx study may cast doubt on Merck claims. *Wall Street Journal.* July 3, 2007:D2.

35. Lévesque LE, Brophy JM, Zhang B. Time variations in risk of myocardial infarction among elderly users of COX-2 inhibitors. *CMAJ.* 2006;174(11): 1563–69.

36. Psaty BM. Testimony before the Senate Finance Committee. November 18, 2004. Available at: http://www.senate.gov/~finance/hearings/testimony/2004test/111804bptest.pdf. Accessed in June 2007.

37. Bero LA, Rennie D. Influences on the quality of published drug studies. *Int J Technol Assess Health Care.* 1996;12(2):209–37.

38. Sackett DL, Oxman AD. HARLOT plc: An amalgamation of the world's two oldest professions. *BMJ.* 2003;327(7429):1442–45.

39. Bodenheimer T. Uneasy alliance: Clinical investigators and the pharmaceutical industry. *NEJM.* 2000;342(20):1539–44.

40. Safer DJ. Design and reporting modifications in industry-sponsored comparative psychopharmacology trials. *J Nerv Ment Dis.* 2002;190(9):583–92.

41. Johansen HK, Gotzsche PC. Problems in the design and reporting of trials of antifungal agents encountered during meta-analysis. *JAMA.* 1999;282 (18):1752–59.

42. Psaty BM, Weiss NS, Furberg CD. Recent trials in hypertension: Compelling science or commercial speech? *JAMA.* 2006;295(14):1704–06.

43. Tramèr MR, Reynolds DJ, Moore RA et al. Impact of covert duplicate publication on meta-analysis: A case study. *BMJ.* 1997;315(7109):635–40.

44. Silverstein FE, Faich G, Goldstein JL et al. Gastrointestinal toxicity with celecoxib vs. nonsteroidal anti-inflammatory drugs for osteoarthritis and rheumatoid arthritis: The CLASS Study: A randomized control trial. *JAMA.* 2000;284(10):1247–55.

45. Lichtenstein DR, Wolfe MM. COX-2-selective NSAIDs: New and improved? *JAMA.* 2000;284(10):1297–99.

46. Okie S. Missing data on Celebrex: Full study altered picture of drug. *Washington Post.* August 5, 2001:A11.

47. Liebeskind DS, Kidwell CS, Sayre JW et al. Evidence of publication bias in reporting acute stroke clinical trials. *Neurology.* 2006;67(6):973–79.

48. Mitka M. Critics bash HIV vaccine trial analysis. *JAMA.* 2003;289(12):1491.

49. VaxGen Inc. Press release: VaxGen announces results of its Phase III HIV vaccine trial in Thailand: Vaccine fails to meet endpoints. Issued November 12, 2003. Available at: http://www.secinfo.com/d13Wqv.26C5.d.htm#1st Page. Accessed in June 2007.

50. Lipton E. U.S. cancels order for 75 million doses of anthrax vaccine. *New York Times.* December 20, 2006.

51. Herper M. FDA Fix no. 1: Pay up. *Forbes.* January 12, 2005.

52. Institute of Medicine. The future of drug safety: Promoting and protecting the health of the public. Washington, DC: National Academies Press, 2006.

53. U.S. Government Accountability Office. Drug safety: Improvements needed in FDA's postmarket decision-making and oversight process. March 2006. Report no. GAO-06-402.

54. Carpenter D, Bowers J, Grimmer J et al. Deadline effect in regulatory drug review: a methodological and empirical analysis. Paper prepared for "Strengthening the FDA" workshop of the Project on Scientific Knowledge and Public Policy (SKAPP) at the George Washington University, Washington, DC. March 2007. Available at: http://www.defendingscience.org/newsroom/upload/Carpenter_FDA_Deadlines-2.pdf. Accessed in June 2007.

55. Psaty BM, Burke SP. Protecting the health of the public: Institute of Medicine recommendations on drug safety. *NEJM.* 2006;355(17):1753–55.

56. Gale EA. Lessons from the glitazones: A story of drug development. *Lancet.* 2001;357(9271):1870–75.

57. Pope C, Rauber P. *Strategic Ignorance: Why the Bush Administration Is Recklessly Destroying a Century of Environmental Progress.* San Francisco: Sierra Club Books, 2004.

58. Willman D. The new FDA: Case study: Rezulin. *Los Angeles Times.* December 20, 2000. Available at: http://www.pulitzer.org/year/2001/investigative-reporting/works/rezulin.html. Accessed in June 2007.

59. U.S. Food and Drug Administration, Center for Drug Evaluation and Research, Nonprescription Drugs Advisory Committee. Transcript: Meet-

ing on safety issues of phenylpropanolamine (PPA) in over-the-counter drug products. October 19, 2000. Available at: http://www.fda.gov/ohrms/ dockets/ac/00/transcripts/3647t1.doc. Accessed in June 2007.

60. Horwitz RI, Brass LM, Kernan WN et al. Phenylpropanolamine and risk of hemorrhagic stroke: Final report of the Hemorrhagic Stroke Project. May 10, 2000. Available at: http://www.defendingscience.org/courts/ upload/Yale-HSP-Final-FDA-Report-on-Phenylproanolamine-and-risk-of-hemorrhagic-stroke.pdf. Accessed in June 2007.

61. Kernan WN, Viscoli CM, Brass LM et al. Phenylpropanolamine and the risk of hemorrhagic stroke. *NEJM.* 2000;343(25):1826–32.

62. Kirton W (Bayer US). Email to Glass T, Hammes C, Kosio R, Dex T, Shook C, Schumm R. Subject: CHPA Yale study meeting, 1/21/99. 2000. Available at: http://www.latimes.com/media/acrobat/2004–03/11953872 .pdf. Accessed in June 2007.

63. Mundy A, Sack K. A dose of denial: How drug makers sought to keep popular cold and diet remedies on store shelves after their own study. *Los Angeles Times.* March 28, 2004.

64. Michaels D. Doubt is their product. *Sci Am.* 2005;292(6):96–101.

65. Giles J. Drug trials: Stacking the deck. *Nature Medicine.* 2006;440(7082): 270–72.

66. Stone MB, Jones ML. Clinical review: Relationship between antidepressant drugs and suicidality in adults. November 17, 2006. Available at: http:// www.fda.gov/OHRMS/DOCKETS/AC/06/briefing/2006-4272b1-01-FDA.pdf. Accessed in October 2007.

67. Levenson M, Holland C (Statistical reviewers, U.S. Food and Drug Administration, Center for Drug Evaluation and Research, Office of Translational Science, Office of Biostatistics). Statistical evaluation of suicidality in adults treated with antidepressants. November 17, 2006. Available at: http://www.fda.gov/OHRMS/DOCKETS/AC/06/briefing/2006-4272b1-01-FDA.pdf. Accessed in October 2007.

68. U.S. Food and Drug Administration. Public health advisory: Suicidality in children and adolescents being treated with antidepressant medications. Issued October 15, 2004. Available at: http://www.fda.gov/cder/drug/ antidepressants/SSRIPHA200410.htm. Accessed in June 2007.

69. Saldanha C. *Daubert* and suicide risk of antidepressants in children. *J Am Acad Psych Law.* 2005;33(1):123–25.

70. Josefson D. Jury finds drug 80% responsible for killings. *BMJ.* 2001;322 (7300):1446.

71. Cato J. U.S. Jury finds that antidepressant did not cause boy to kill his grandparents. *BMJ.* 2005;330(7489):438.

72. Chan A, Hróbjartsson A, Haahr MT et al. Empirical evidence for selective reporting of outcomes in randomized trials: comparison of protocols to published articles. *JAMA.* 2004;291(20):2457–65.

73. American Medical Association. Press release: AMA recommends that DHHS establish a registry for all U.S. clinical trials. Issued June 15, 2004.

74. DeAngelis CD, Drazen JM, Frizelle F et al. Is this clinical trial fully registered? A statement from the International Committee of Medical Journal Editors. *NEJM.* 2005;352(23):2436–38.

75. Drazen JM, Wood AJ. Trial registration report card. *NEJM.* 2005;353(26): 2809–11.

76. Zarin DA, Tse T, Ide NC. Trial registration at ClinicalTrials.gov between May and October 2005. *NEJM.* 2005;353(26):2779–87.

77. Chalmers I. From optimism to disillusion about commitment to transparency in the medico-industrial complex. *J R Soc Med.* 2006;99(7):337–41.

78. Rennie D. Thyroid storm. *JAMA.* 1997;277(15):1238–43.

79. Kahn JO, Cherng DW, Mayer K et al. Evaluation of HIV-1 immunogen, an immunologic modifier, administered to patients infected with HIV having 300 to 549 x 10(6)/L CD4 cell counts: A randomized controlled trial. *JAMA.* 2000;284(17):2193–2202.

80. Blumenthal D, Campbell EG, Anderson MS et al. Withholding research results in academic life science: Evidence from a national survey of faculty. *JAMA.* 1997;277(15):1224–28.

81. Davidoff F, DeAngelis CD, Drazen JM et al. Sponsorship, authorship, and accountability. *NEJM.* 2001;345(11):825–26; discussion 826–27.

82. Brownlee S. Doctors without borders: Why you can't trust medical journals anymore. *Washington Monthly.* April 2004.

83. Jones PB, Barnes TR, Davies L et al. Randomized controlled trial of the effect on quality of life of second- vs first-generation antipsychotic drugs in schizophrenia: Cost Utility of the Latest Antipsychotic Drugs in Schizophrenia Study (CUtLASS 1). *Arch Gen Psychiatry.* 2006;63(10): 1079–87.

84. Rosenheck RA. Outcomes, costs, and policy caution. A commentary on the Cost Utility of the Latest Antipsychotic Drugs in Schizophrenia Study (CUtLASS 1). *Arch Gen Psychiatry.* 2006;63(10):1074–76.

85. Lurie P. Selling new drugs using smoke and mirrors. *Worst Pills, Best Pills News.* March 2003:18–20.

86. Meier B. Results of drug trials can mystify doctors through omission. *New York Times.* July 21, 2004:C1.

87. Harris G. FDA official admits "lapses" on Vioxx. *New York Times.* March 2, 2005:A15.

CHAPTER 13

1. Annas GJ. Scientific evidence in the courtroom: The death of the *Frye* rule. *NEJM.* 1994;330(14):1018–21.

2. *Frye v. United States*, 293 F 1013 (December 3, 1923).

3. *Daubert v. Merrell Dow Pharmaceuticals, Inc.*, 113 S.Ct. 2786 (June 28, 1993).

4. *Fed. Rule Evid.* 702. Available at: http://www.law.cornell.edu/rules/fre/rules.htm#Rule702. Accessed in June 2007.

5. Edmond G, Mercer D. *Daubert* and the exclusionary ethos: The convergence of corporate and judicial attitudes toward the admissibility of expert evidence in tort litigation. *Law and Policy.* 2004;26(2):231–57.

6. Cranor C. *Toxic Torts: Science, Law, and the Possibility of Justice.* New York: Cambridge University Press, 2006.

7. *Daubert v. Merrell Dow Pharmaceuticals, Inc. (Daubert II)*, 43 F3d 1311 (1995).

8. *General Electric Co. v. Joiner*, 522 U.S. 136 (1997).

9. *Kumho Tire Co. v. Carmichael*, 526 U.S. 137 (1999).

10. Conley JM, Gaylord SW. Science in the state courts: *Daubert* and the problem of outcomes. *Judges' J.* 2005;44(5):6–15.

11. *Logerquist v. McVey*, 1 P.3d 113 (April 19, 2000).

12. Rothman KJ, Greenland S. Causation and causal inference in epidemiology. *Am J Public Health.* 2005;95(suppl 1):S144–S50.

13. Haack S. Trial and error: The Supreme Court's philosophy of science. *Am J Public Health.* 2005;95(suppl 1):S66–S73.

14. Ozonoff D. Epistemology in the courtroom: A little "knowledge" is a dangerous thing. *Am J Public Health.* 2005;95(suppl 1):S13–S15.

15. Kassirer JP, Cecil JS. Inconsistency in evidentiary standards for medical testimony: Disorder in the courts. *JAMA.* 2002;288(11):1382–87.

16. McGarity T. On the prospect of "*Daubert*izing" judicial review of risk assessment. *Law and Contemporary Problems.* 2003;66(155).

17. *Weisgram et al. v. Marley Co. et al.*, 528 U.S. 440 (February 22, 2000). Available at: http://www.law.cornell.edu/supct/html/99-161.ZS.html. Accessed in June 2007.

18. Ozonoff D. Legal causation and responsibility for causing harm. *Am J Public Health.* 2005;95(suppl 1):S35–S38.

19. Huber PW. *Galileo's Revenge: Junk Science in the Courtroom.* New York: Basic Books, 1993.

20. Vidmar N. Expert evidence, the adversary system, and the jury. *Am J Public Health.* 2005;95(suppl 1):S137–S43.

21. *Allison v. McGhan Medical Corporation*, 184 F3d 1300 (1999).

22. Lempert R. Civil juries and complex cases: Taking stock after twelve years. In: Litan RE, ed. *Verdict: Assessing the Civil Jury System.* Washington, DC: Brookings Institution, 1993:181–247.

23. Berger M. Statements made during interviews conducted with SKAPP staff, May 15–June 6, 2003.

24. *Castellow v. Chevron USA*, 97 F.Supp. 2d 780 (2000).

25. Court order no. 29: Addressing subject-matter jurisdiction, expert testimony, and sanctions. In re: silica products litigation; MDL docket no. 1553.

Signed by U.S. District Judge Jack JG of the Southern District of Texas, Corpus Christi Division. June 30, 2005. Available at: http://www.nytimes .com/packages/pdf/business/MDL-1553.pdf. Accessed in June 2007.

26. Glater JD. The tort wars, at a turning point. *New York Times.* October 9, 2005.

27. U.S. Environmental Protection Agency. Chemical hazard data availability study: What do we really know about the safety of high production volume chemicals? April 1998. Available at: http://www.epa.gov/chemrtk/pubs/ general/hazchem.pdf. Accessed in June 2007.

28. Gatowski SI, Dobbin SA, Richardson JT et al. Asking the gatekeepers: A national survey of judges on judging expert evidence in a post-*Daubert* world. *Law Hum Behav.* 2001;25(5):433–58.

29. *Nelson v. American Home Products Corp.,* 92 F.Supp. 2d 954 (March 24, 2000).

30. U.S. Food and Drug Administration. Press release: FDA moves to end use of bromocriptine for post-partum breast engorgement. Issued August 17, 1994. Available at: http://www.fda.gov/bbs/topics/ANSWERS/ANS00594 .html. Accessed in June 2007.

31. *Brasher v. Sandoz Pharmaceuticals,* 160 F.Supp. 2d 1291 (September 21, 2001).

32. Cecil JS. Ten years of judicial gatekeeping under *Daubert. Am J Public Health.* 2005;95(suppl 1):S74–S80. Available at:

33. Jasanoff S. Law's knowledge: science for justice in legal settings. *Am J Public Health* 2005;95(suppl 1):S49-S58.

34. Friedman LC, Daynard RA, Banthin CN. How tobacco-friendly science escapes scrutiny in the courtroom. *Am J Public Health.* 2005;95(suppl 1): S16–S20.

35. Berger MA. What has a decade of *Daubert* wrought? *Am J Public Health.* 2005;95(suppl 1):S59–S65.

36. RAND Institute. Changes in the standards for admitting expert evidence in federal civil cases since the *Daubert* decision. 2001. Available at: http://www .rand.org/pubs/monograph_reports/2005/MR1439.pdf. Accessed in June 2007.

37. Goldsmith WJ. Testimony before the Subcommittee on Workforce Protections of the Committee on Education and the Workforce of the U.S. House of Representatives. June 14, 2001.

38. U.S. Chamber of Commerce. Scientific information in federal rulemaking. 2002. Available at: http://www.uschamber.com/issues/index/regulatory/ scientific_rulemaking.htm. Accessed in June 2007.

39. Krimsky S. The weight of scientific evidence in policy and law. *Am J Public Health.* 2005;95(suppl 1):S129–S36.

40. McGarity TO. *Daubert* and the proper role for the courts in health, safety, and environmental regulation. *Am J Public Health.* 2005;95(suppl 1): S92–S98.

41. Neff RA, Goldman LR. Regulatory parallels to *Daubert:* Stakeholder influence, "sound science," and the delayed adoption of health-protective standards. *Am J Public Health.* 2005;95(suppl 1):S81–S91.

42. Wagner W. The perils of relying on interested parties to evaluate scientific quality. *Am J Public Health.* 2005;95(suppl 1):S99–S106.

CHAPTER 14

1. Omnibus Consolidated and Emergency Supplemental Appropriations Act, 1999 (also known as the Data Access Law/Act or Shelby Amendment). Public law no. 105–277, October 21, 1998.

2. Dockery DW, Pope CA, III, Zu Z et al. An association between air pollution and mortality in six U.S. cities. *NEJM.* 1993;329(24):1753–59.

3. Davis D. *When Smoke Ran Like Water: Tales of Environmental Deception and the Battle against Pollution.* New York: Basic Books, 2002.

4. U.S. Environmental Protection Agency. Press release: PR fact sheets to EPA proposes air standards for ozone. Issued November 27, 1996. Available at: http://yosemite.epa.gov/opa/admpress.nsf/8df5e230d6ef1224852570 1c005e0 d28/e55169512c4fea6b8525646000192bbb!OpenDocument. Accessed in June 2007.

5. Sound Science Project. May 1997. Philip Morris document no. 2081324784/ 4788. Available at: http://legacy.library.ucsf.edu/tid/xcx65c00. Accessed in June 2007.

6. Philip Morris. Force field analysis (draft). 1997. Philip Morris document no. 2081324814/4818. Available at: http://legacy.library.ucsf.edu/tid/ adx65c00. Accessed in June 2007.

7. Baba A, Cook DM, McGarity TO et al. Legislating "sound science": The role of the tobacco industry. *Am J Public Health.* 2005;95(suppl 1):S20–S27.

8. Russo E. Debating Shelby. *Scientist.* 2001 Apr 2;15(7):14.

9. Treasury and General Government Appropriations Act for Fiscal Year 2001: §515 (also known as the Data Quality Act or Information Quality Act). Public law no. 106–554, 2000.

10. Unofficial Transcript: Peer review standards for regulatory science and technical information (Workshop hosted by the National Research Council Policy and Global Affairs Division: Science, Technology, and Law Program.) November 18, 2003. Available at: http://www7.nationalacademies .org/stl/peer_review_transcript.pdf. Accessed in July 2007.

11. Geewax M. New law means more federal rules can be challenged. *Cox News Service.* September 30, 2002. Available at: http://thecre.com/news2003.html *(excerpts only).* Accessed in September 2006.

12. Rosenstock L. Protecting special interests in the name of "good science." *JAMA.* 2006;295(20):2407–10.

13. Hornstein DT. Accounting for science: The independence of public research in the new, subterranean administrative law. *Law and Contemporary Problems.* 2003;66(4):227–46.

14. Tozzi J (Center for Regulatory Effectiveness [CRE]) on behalf of the CRE, Kansas Corn Growers Association, Triazine Network. Request for correction of information contained in the Atrazine Environmental Risk Assessment. November 25, 2002. Available at: http://www.epa.gov/quality/informationguidelines/documents/2807.pdf. Accessed in June 2007.

15. Hayes TB, Collins A, Lee M et al. Hermaphroditic, demasculinized frogs after exposure to the herbicide atrazine at low ecologically relevant doses. *PNAS.* 2002;99(8):5476–80.

16. U.S. Environmental Protection Agency, Office of Prevention, Pesticides and Toxic Substances. Response to comments (OPP 02– 0026– 0198) by the Center for Regulatory Effectiveness (CRE) on the Atrazine Environmental Fate and Effects Risk Assessment (docket control no. OPP-34237C), November 4, 2002. Available at: http://www.epa.gov/quality/information guidelines/documents/2807Response_03_27_03.pdf, pp. 17–21. Accessed in June 2007.

17. National Assessment Synthesis Team, U.S. Global Change Research Program. Climate change impacts on the United States: The potential consequences of climate variability and change. 2000. Available at: http://www.usgcrp.gov/usgcrp/nacc/. Accessed in June 2007.

18. Horner CC (senior fellow, Competitive Enterprise Institute). Letter to Whitman CT (administrator, U.S. Environmental Protection Agency). Re: Petition under Federal Data Quality Act to Prohibit Further Dissemination of "Climate Action Report 2002." June 4, 2002. Available at: http://www.cei.org/gencon/027,03040.cfm. Accessed in July 2007.

19. National Research Council. Climate change science: An analysis of some key questions. Washington, DC: National Academy Press, 2001.

20. Competitive Enterprise Institute. Press release: White House acknowledges climate report was not subjected to sound science law; CEI drops lawsuit against Bush Administration. Issued November 6, 2003. Available at: http://www.cei.org/gencon/003,03740.cfm. Accessed in June 2007.

21. Privitera D (Morgan Lewis, counselors at law). Letter to Office of Information Quality Guidelines; U.S. Environmental Protection Agency. Re: Request for correction of information. August 19, 2003. Available at: http://www.epa.gov/quality/informationguidelines/documents/12467.pdf. Accessed in June 2007.

22. U.S. Environmental Protection Agency. Guidance for preventing asbestos disease among auto mechanics. June 1986. Publication no. EPA-560-OPTS-86– 002. Available at: http://www.defendingscience.org/public_health_regulations/upload/EPA-Gold-Book-1986.pdf. Accessed in July 2007.

23. Hazen SB (principal deputy assistant administrator, Office of Prevention, Pesticides and Toxic Substances, U.S. Environmental Protection Agency). Letter to Privitera D (Morgan Lewis, LLP). Re: Response to request for correction (FRC) regarding the United States (U.S.) Environmental Protection Agency's (EPA's) *Guidance for Preventing Asbestos Disease among Auto Mechanics* (the Gold Book) pursuant to the U.S. EPA's Information Quality Guidelines (RFC no. 12467). November 24, 2003. Available at: http://www.epa.gov/quality/informationguidelines/documents/12467 response-morgan-lewis.pdf. Accessed in June 2007.

24. U.S. Environmental Protection Agency. Current Best Practices for Preventing Asbestos Exposure Among Brake and Clutch Repair Workers. March 2007. Publication no. EPA-747-F-04-004.

25. Michaels D, Monforton C. How litigation shapes the scientific literature: asbestos and disease among automobile mechanics. *J Law Policy*. 2007;15(3): 1137–1169.

26. Goodman M, Morgan RW, Ray R et al. Cancer in asbestos-exposed occupational cohorts: A meta-analysis. *Cancer Causes Control*. 1999;10(5):453–65.

27. Paustenbach DJ, Richter RO, Finley BL et al. An evaluation of the historical exposures of mechanics to asbestos in brake dust. *Appl Occup Environ Hyg*. 2003;18(10):786–804.

28. Paustenbach DJ, Finley BL, Lu ET et al. Environmental and occupational health hazards associated with the presence of asbestos in brake linings and pads (1900 to present): A "state-of-the-art" review. *J Toxicol Environ Health B Crit Rev*. 2004;7(1):25–80.

29. Goodman M, Teta MJ, Hessel PA et al. Mesothelioma and lung cancer among motor vehicle mechanics: A meta-analysis. *Ann Occup Hyg*. 2004;48 (4):309–26.

30. Hessel PA, Teta MJ, Goodman M et al. Mesothelioma among brake mechanics: An expanded analysis of a case control study. *Risk Analysis*. 2004; 24(3):547–52.

31. Paustenbach DJ, Finley BL, Sheehan PJ et al. Re: Evaluation of the size and type of free particulates collected from unused asbestos-containing brake components as related to potential for respirability. *Am J Ind Med*. 2006;49(1):60–61; author reply 62–64.

32. Egilman DS, Bohme SR. Author reply to Paustenbach DJ. Scientific method questioned. *Int J Occup Environ Health* 2006;12(3):290–92. *Int J Occup Environ Health*. 2006;12(3):292–93.

33. Castleman B. Letter to Docket EPA-HQ-OPPT-2006–0398: Release of updated guidance for preventing asbestos exposure among brake and clutch repair workers. Re: EPA revised Gold Book. October 23, 2006. Document no. EPA-HQ-OPPT-2006–0398–0011.

34. Available at: http://www.defendingscience.org/upload/Exponent_invoices .pdf. Accessed in December 2007.

35. Kelsh MA, Craven VA (principal scientist and managing scientist, respectively, Exponent Health Sciences, Inc.). Letter to Docket EPA-HQ-OPPT-2006–0398: Release of updated guidance for preventing asbestos exposure among brake and clutch repair workers. October 20, 2006. Document no. EPA-HQ-OPPT-2006–0398–0007.1.

36. Kovacs WL, Hanneman RL (Vice President, Environment, Technology, and Regulatory Affairs, U.S. Chamber of Commerce, and president, the Salt Institute, respectively). Letter to Office of Communications, National Heart, Lung, and Blood Institute. May 14, 2003. Available at: http://aspe.hhs.gov/infoquality/request&response/8a.pdf. Accessed in June 2007.

37. Sacks FM, Svetkey LP, Vollmer WM et al. Effects on blood pressure of reduced dietary sodium and the Dietary Approaches to Stop Hypertension (DASH) diet. DASH–Sodium Collaborative Research Group. *NEJM.* 2001;344(1):3–10.

38. Roth CA (associate director for Scientific Program Operation, National Heart, Lung, and Blood Institute). Letter to Kovaks [*sic*] WL, Hanneman RL (Vice President, Environment, Technology, and Regulatory Affairs, Chamber of Commerce; and President, the Salt Institute, respectively). August 19, 2003. Available at: http://www.ombwatch.org/info/dataquality/HHS_SaltResponse.pdf. Accessed in June 2007.

39. Kovacs WL, Hanneman RL (vice president, Environment, Technology, and Regulatory Affairs, U.S. Chamber of Commerce; and President, the Salt Institute, respectively) Letter to associate director for Communications (National Institutes of Health). Re: U.S. Chamber/Salt Institute Information Quality Appeal. September 22, 2003. Available at: http://aspe.hhs.gov/infoquality/request&response/8c.pdf. Accessed in June 2007.

40. Alving B (Acting Director, National Heart, Blood, and Lung Institute). Letter to Kovaks [*sic*] WL, Hanneman RL (Vice President, Environment, Technology, and Regulatory Affairs, U.S. Chamber of Commerce; and president, the Salt Institute, respectively). Re: Request for reconsideration submitted September 22, 2003. February 11, 2004. Available at: http://aspe.hhs.gov/infoquality/request&response/8d.shtml. Accessed in June 2007.

41. *Salt Institute and U.S. Chamber of Commerce v. Tommy G. Thompson, Secretary, Health and Human Services,* case no. 04-CV-359 (complaint filed March 31, 2004).

42. *Salt Institute and U.S. Chamber of Commerce v. Tommy G. Thompson, Secretary, Health and Human Services,* civil action no. 04–359 (GBL) (dismissed November 15, 2004). Available at: http://www.ombwatch.org/info/dataquality/HHS_SaltCourtDecision.pdf. Accessed in June 2007.

43. Calabrese DB (vice president, Government Relations, Association of Home Appliance Manufacturers). Letter to Stevenson TA (secretary, U.S. Consumer Product Safety Commission). Re: Information Quality guidelines:

Final report on electric clothes dryers and lint ignition characteristics, May 2003. September 12, 2003. Available at: http://www.cpsc.gov/library/correction/electric.pdf. Accessed in June 2007.

44. Elder J (assistant executive director, Office of Hazard Identification and Reduction, U.S. Consumer Product Safety Commission). Letter to Calabrese DB (vice president, Government Relations, Association of Home Appliance Manufacturers). Re: Information Quality guidelines: Final report on electric clothes dryers and lint ignition characteristics, May 2003. November 21, 2003. Available at: http://www.cpsc.gov/library/correction/electric.pdf. Accessed in July 2007.

45. Cook JA (technical director, Chemical Products Corporation). Letter to Quality Guidelines Staff, U.S. Environmental Protection Agency. Subject: Request for correction of the IRIS barium and compounds substance file—Information disseminated by EPA that does not comply with EPA or OMB Information Quality Guidelines. October 29, 2002. Available at: http://www.epa.gov/quality/informationguidelines/documents/2293.pdf. Accessed in June 2007.

46. Gilman P (assistant administrator, Office of Research and Development, U.S. Environmental Protection Agency). Letter to Cook JA (technical director, Chemical Products Corporation). Re: Request for Correction of the IRIS Barium and Compounds Substance File Pursuant to EPA and OMB Information Quality Guidelines (IQG #2293). January 30, 2003. Available at: http://www.epa.gov/quality/informationguidelines/documents/2293Response.pdf. Accessed in June 2007.

47. Gilman P (assistant administrator, Office of Research and Development, U.S. Environmental Protection Agency). Letter to Cook JA (technical director, Chemical Products Corporation). Re: request for correction of the IRIS barium and compounds substance file pursuant to EPA and OMB information quality guidelines (IQG no. 2293). December 11, 2003.

48. Office of Management and Budget. Peer review and information quality proposed bulletin and request for comment. August 29, 2003.

49. U.S. Environmental Protection Agency. EPA Science Advisory Board. 2005. Available at: http://www.epa.gov/sab/. Accessed in June 2007.

50. Expert panel on the role of science at the EPA. Report to Reilly WK, EPA Administrator. Safeguarding the future: Credible science, credible decisions. 1992. Report no. EPA/600/9–91/050.

51. EPA Science Policy Council. Science Policy Council handbook: Peer review. January 1998. Document no. EPA 100-B-98-001.

52. EPA Science Policy Council. Science Policy Council handbook: Peer review. 2^d ed. December 2000. Document no. EPA-100-B-00-001.

53. Smith R. Peer review: Reform or revolution? *BMJ.* 1997;315(7111):759–60.

54. Lock S. *A Difficult Balance: Editorial Peer Review in Medicine.* London: Nuffield Provincial Hospitals Trust, 1985.

55. Gans JS, Shepherd GB. How are the mighty fallen: Rejected classic articles by leading economists. *J Econ Perspect.* 1994;8(1):165–79.

56. Shapiro S, Guston D. Comments on the Office of Management and Budget's Proposed Bulletin on Peer Review and Information Quality. December 12, 2003. Available at: http://www.whitehouse.gov/omb/inforeg/2003iq/87.pdf. Accessed in June 2007.

57. Jasanoff S. Comments on Office of Management and Budget Proposed Bulletin on Peer Review and Information Quality, December 16, 2003. Available at: http://www.whitehouse.gov/omb/inforeg/2003iq/159.pdf. Accessed in June 2007.

58. Taylor MR. Statement before the Committee on Peer Review Standards for Regulatory Science and Technical Information of the Science, Technology, and Law Program of the National Academies. November 18, 2003. Available at: http://www7.nationalacademies.org/stl/Taylor_Presentation _pdf.pdf. Accessed in June 2007.

59. American Association for the Advancement of Science (AAAS). AAAS Resolution: On the OMB Proposed Peer Review Bulletin. Approved by AAAS Council on March 9, 2004. Available at: http://archives.aaas.org/docs/resolutions.php?doc_id=434. Accessed in June 2007.

60. American Public Health Association. Interim policy statement late-breaker 03–1: "Threats to public health science." Adopted November 18, 2003.

61. Cohen JJ, Wells RD (president, American Association of Medical Colleges, and president, Federation of American Societies for Experimental Biology, respectively). Letter to Schwab M (Office of Information and Regulatory Affairs, Office of Management and Budget). Re: Proposed Bulletin on Peer Review and Information Quality, 68 FR 54023–29. December 4, 2003. Available at: http://www.whitehouse.gov/omb/inforeg/2003iq/23.pdf. Accessed in June 2007.

62. Phillips K (president, Council on Governmental Relations [COGR]). Letter to Schwab M (Office of Information and Regulatory Affairs, Office of Management and Budget). Re: Proposed Bulletin on Peer Review and Information Quality, 68 FR 54023–29. December 15, 2003. Available at: http://www.whitehouse.gov/omb/inforeg/2003iq/78.pdf. Accessed in June 2007.

63. Alberts B (president, National Academies of Science, and chair, National Research Council). Letter to Graham J (administrator, Office of Information and Regulatory Affairs, Office of Management and Budget). December 15, 2003. Available at: http://www.whitehouse.gov/omb/inforeg/2003iq/115.pdf. Accessed in June 2007.

64. King E (assistant general counsel, Pharmaceutical Research and Manufacturers of America). Letter to Schwab M (Office of Information and Regulatory Affairs, OMB). Re: Proposed Bulletin on Peer Review and Information Quality. *Fed. Reg.* September 15, 2003;68:54023. December 15, 2003.

Available at: http://www.whitehouse.gov/omb/inforeg/2003iq/118.pdf. Accessed in June 2007.

65. Kennedy D. Disclosure and disinterest. *Science.* 2004;303(5654):15.

66. Office of Management and Budget. Final Information Quality Bulletin for Peer Review. December 16, 2004.

67. OMB Watch. OMB Watch analysis on Final Peer Review Bulletin. 2005. Available at: http://www.ombwatch.org/article/articleview/2594/1/232? TopicID=3. Accessed in June 2007.

68. Houck O. Tales from a troubled marriage: Science and law in environmental policy. *Science.* 2003;302(5652):1926–29.

CHAPTER FIFTEEN

1. Centers for Disease Control and Prevention (CDC). Preventing Lead Poisoning in Young Children. Statement issued October 1991. Available at: http://www.cdc.gov/nceh/lead/publications/books/plpyc/contents.htm. Accessed in July 2007.

2. Blood lead levels—United States, 1999–2002. *Morbidity and Mortality Weekly Report.* 2005;54(20):513–516.

3. Ferber D. Overhaul of CDC panel revives lead safety debate. *Science.* 2002; 298(5594):732.

4. Agency for Toxic Substances and Disease Registry. Public Health Assessment for Omaha Lead Refinery, Omaha, Douglas County, Nebraska; EPA facility ID: NESFN0703481. June 7, 2004. Available at: http://www .atsdr.cdc.gov/hac/PHA/omahalead/omahalead.pdf. Accessed in June 2007.

5. Washington State Department of Ecology. Everett smelter site (Everett, Washington) integrated final cleanup action plan and final environmental impact statement for the upland area. Vol. 2, appendix B: Responsiveness survey. November 19, 1999. Available at: http://ecystage.ecy.wa.gov/programs/ tcp/sites/asarco/prospective_purchaser/Exhibit%20C/VOL%20II.PDF. Accessed in June 2007.

6. Staff of Rep. Markey EJ (D-MA-7). Turning lead into gold: How the Bush administration is poisoning the Lead Advisory Committee at the CDC [report]. October 8, 2002.

7. Weiss R. HHS seeks science advice to match Bush views. *Washington Post.* September 17, 2002:A1.

8. Tumulty K. Jesus and the FDA. *Time.* October 5, 2002.

9. On health and medicine: When politics trumps science. *San Francisco Chronicle.* January 5, 2003.

10. Couzin J. Plan B: A collision of science and politics. *Science.* 2005;310 (5745):38–39.

11. Michaels D, Bingham E, Boden L et al. Advice without dissent. *Science.* 2002;298(5594):703.

12. Howard III WE. Advice without dissent at the DOD. *Science.* 2002;298 (5597):1334–35.

13. Loomis D. Unpopular opinions need not apply. *Science.* 2002;298(5597): 1335–36.

14. U.S. General Accounting Office. Federal advisory committees: Additional guidance could help agencies better ensure independence and balance. Washington, DC; April 2004. Report no. GAO-04-328.

15. American Association for the Advancement of Science (AAAS). AAAS Resolution Regarding Membership On Federal Advisory Committees. Approved March 3, 2003. Available at: http://www.aaas.org/news/releases/ 2003/0305fair2.shtml. Accessed in June 2007.

16. American Public Health Association. Policy resolution 2003–6: Ensuring the scientific credibility of government public health advisory committees. Adopted by the Governing Council November 18, 2003.

17. National Academy of Engineering, Institute of Medicine. Science and technology in the national interest: Ensuring the best presidential and advisory committee appointments. Washington, DC: National Academies Press, 2005.

18. Kennedy D. An epidemic of politics. *Science.* 2003;299(5607):625.

19. Kennedy D. "Well, they were doing it, too." *Science.* 2003;302(5642):17.

20. Federal Advisory Committee Act. Public law no. 92–463, 1972.

21. Steinbrook R. Science, politics, and federal advisory committees. *NEJM.* 2004;350(14):1454–60.

22. Blackburn E. Bioethics and the political distortion of biomedical science. *NEJM.* 2004;350(14):1379–80.

23. Kass L. We don't play politics with science. *Washington Post.* March 3, 2004:A27.

24. Brumfiel G. Energy secretary ditches science advisers. *Nature.* 2006;440:725.

25. Gray G, Wehrum W (assistant administrator, EPA Office of Research and Development, and acting assistant administrator, EPA Office of Air and Radiation, respectively). Letter to Peacock M (deputy administrator, EPA). Re: Review of process for setting national ambient air quality standards. April 3, 2006. Available at: http://www.epa.gov/ttn/naaqs/naaqs_process_ report_march2006_cover.pdf. Accessed in June 2007.

26. Gelbspan R. Snowed. *Mother Jones.* May/June 2005.

27. Luntz F. Memo: The environment: A cleaner, safer, healthier America; ca. 2003. Available at: http://www.ewg.org:16080/briefings/luntzmemo. Accessed in June 2007.

28. Mooney C. Some like it hot. *Mother Jones.* May/June 2005.

29. ExxonMobil. Global climate science communications: Action plan. April 3, 1998. Available at: http://www.environmentaldefense.org/documents/3860 _GlobalClimateSciencePlanMemo.pdf. Accessed in June 2007.

30. Randol R (ExxonMobil, Washington office). Facsimile to Howard J (Council on Environmental Quality). Re: Bush team for IPCC negotiations. February 6, 2001. Available at: http://www.nrdc.org/media/docs/020403 .pdf. Accessed in June 2007.

31. Intergovernmental Panel on Climate Change. Climate change 2001: Third assessment report. 2001.

32. Bridgeland JM, Edson G (deputy assistant to the president for Domestic Policy and director, Domestic Policy Council; deputy assistant to the president for International Economic Affairs, respectively). Letter to Alberts B (National Academy of Sciences). May 11, 2001. In National Academy of Sciences, *Climate Change Science: An Analysis of Some Key Questions.* Washington, DC: National Academies Press. 2001:27.

33. National Research Council. Climate change science: An analysis of some key questions. Washington, DC: National Academy Press, 2001.

34. Letter from President Bush GW to Sens. Hagel, Helms, Craig, and Roberts. March 13, 2001. http://www.whitehouse.gov/news/releases/2001/03/ 20010314.html. Accessed in June 2007.

35. Gelbspan R. *Boiling Point: How Politicians, Big Oil and Coal, Journalists, and Activists Have Fueled the Climate Crisis—and What We Can Do to Avert Disaster.* New York: Basic Books, 2004.

36. Union of Concerned Scientists (UCS). Scientific integrity in policymaking: an investigation into the Bush administration's misuse of science. March 2004. Available at: http://www.ucsusa.org/scientific_integrity/interference/ reports-scientific-integrity-in-policy-making.html. Accessed in July 2007.

37. Stephenson JB (Director, Natural Resources and the Environment, U.S. General Accounting Office). Testimony before the Committee on Commerce, Science, and Transportation, U.S. Senate. Climate change: Preliminary observations on the administration's February 2002 climate initiative. October 1, 2003. Report no. GAO-04-131T.

38. Revkin AC. Climate expert says NASA tried to silence him. *New York Times.* January 29, 2006.

39. Revkin AC. NASA chief backs agency openness. *New York Times.* February 4, 2006.

40. Revkin AC. Call for openness at NASA adds to reports of pressure. *New York Times.* February 16, 2006.

41. Revkin AC. A young Bush appointee resigns his post at NASA. *New York Times.* February 8, 2006.

42. Regalado A, Carlton J. Politics and economics: Agency retreats from discounting global warming; hurricane dispute becomes flashpoint as scientists decry White House policies. *Wall Street Journal.* February 16, 2006:A4.

43. National Aeronautics and Space Administration (NASA). Statement on scientific openness. February 4, 2006. Available at: http://www.nasa.gov/ about/highlights/griffin_science.html. Accessed in June 2007.

44. National Oceanic and Atmospheric Administration (NOAA). Message from the under secretary: Encouragement of scientific debate and transparency within NOAA. February 14, 2006. Available at: http://www.peer.org/docs/noaa/06_15_2_sci_open.pdf. Accessed in June 2007.

45. Revkin AC. Bush aide softened greenhouse gas links to global warming. *New York Times.* June 8, 2005:A1.

46. Revkin AC. Former Bush aide who edited reports is hired by Exxon. *New York Times.* June 15, 2005.

47. White House Office of the Press Secretary. President Bush meets with supporters of U.S. military in Iraq and Afghanistan [transcript]. June 26, 2006. Available at: http://www.whitehouse.gov/news/releases/2006/06/20060626–2.html. Accessed in June 2007.

48. Oral Arguments for *Massachusetts et al. v. Environmental Protection Agency et al.* [Supreme Court transcript]. November 29, 2006. Available at: http://www.supremecourtus.gov/oral_arguments/argument_transcripts/05–1120.pdf. Accessed in June 2007.

49. Mufson S, Eilperin J. Energy firms come to terms with climate change. *Washington Post.* November 25, 2006:A1.

50. World Health Organization. Guidelines for drinking-water quality. 3^d ed. Vol. 1: Recommendations. Geneva, Switzerland; 2004.

51. National Research Council. Arsenic in drinking water: 2001 update. Washington, DC: National Academy Press, 2001.

52. Walsh E. Arsenic drinking water standard issued; after seven-month scientific review, EPA backs Clinton-established levels. *Washington Post.* June 8, 2001; section A:A31.

53. Mooney C. *The Republican War on Science.* New York: Basic Books; 2005.

54. U.S. Government Accountability Office. Clean Air Act: Observations on EPA's cost-benefit analysis of its mercury control options. February 2005. Report no. GAO-05–252.

55. Eilperin J. Report accuses EPA of slanting analysis; Hill researchers say agency fixed pollution study to favor Bush's "Clear Skies." *Washington Post.* December 3, 2005:A8.

56. Miller AC, Hamburger T. EPA relied on industry for plywood plant pollution rule. *Los Angeles Times.* May 21, 2004.

57. Hauptmann M, Lubin JH, Stewart PA et al. Mortality from lymphohematopoietic malignancies among workers in formaldehyde industries. *J Natl Cancer Inst.* 2003;95(21):1615–23.

58. Pinkerton LE, Hein MJ, Stayner LT. Mortality among a cohort of garment workers exposed to formaldehyde: An update. *Occup Environ Med.* 2004; 61(3):193–200.

59. International Agency for Research on Cancer. IARC Monographs on the Evaluation of Carcinogenic Risks to Humans, Vol. 88: Formaldehyde, 2-Butoxyethanol, and 1-tert-Butoxypropan-2-ol. December 2006.

60. Trombulak SC, Wilcove DS, Male TD. Science as a smoke screen. *Science.* 2006;312(5776):973.

61. Michaels D. Statement before the House of Representatives Subcommittee on Energy and Mineral Resources' oversight hearing: The impact of science on public policy. February 4, 2004. Available at: http://www.defendingscience .org/public_health_regulations/upload/Michaels-Testimony-Oversight-Hearing-The-Impact-of-Science-on-Public-Policy-The-House-of-Representatives-Subcommittee-on-Energy-and-Mineral-Resources-2004.pdf. Accessed in June 2007.

62. H.R. 1662. Sound Science for Endangered Species Act Planning Act of 2003. Introduced April 8, 2003, by Rep. Walden G (R-OR-2).

63. H.R. 3824. Threatened and Endangered Species Recovery Act of 2005. Introduced September 19, 2005, by Rep. Pombo RW (R-CA-11).

64. Cart J. Land study on grazing denounced: Two retired specialists say Interior excised their warnings on the effects on wildlife and water. *Los Angeles Times.* June 18, 2005.

65. U.S. Food and Drug Administration. Press release: FDA announces framework for moving emergency contraception medication to over-the-counter status. Issued July 31, 2006. Available at: http://www.fda.gov/bbs/topics/ NEWS/2006/NEW01421.html. Accessed in June 2007.

66. Trussell J, Hatcher RA, Cates Jr. W et al. Contraceptive failure in the United States: An update. *Studies in Family Planning.* 1990;21(1):51–54.

67. Jones EF, Forrest JD. Contraceptive failure rates based on the 1988 NSFG. *Family Planning Perspectives.* 1992;24(1):12–19.

68. U.S. House Committee on Governmental Reform, minority staff. The content of federally funded abstinence-only education programs (report prepared for Rep. Waxman HA). 2004. Available at: http://www.democrats .reform.house.gov/Documents/20041201102153–50247.pdf. Accessed in June 2007.

69. Stein R. Health experts criticize changes in STD panel. *Washington Post.* May 9, 2006:A3.

70. American Medical Association. Resolution 443: FDA rejection of over-the-counter status for emergency contraception pills. June 2004. Available at: http://www.ama-assn.org/ama1/pub/upload/mm/15/res_hod443_a04.doc. Accessed in June 2007.

71. Malec K. The abortion–breast cancer link: How politics trumped science and informed consent. *J Am Physicians and Surgeons.* 2003;8(2):41–45.

72. U.S. House Committee on Governmental Reform, minority staff. False and misleading information provided by federally funded pregnancy resource centers (report prepared for Rep. Waxman HA). July 2006. Available at: http://www.democrats.reform.house.gov/Documents/20060717101140–30092.pdf. Accessed in July 2007.

73. Keiger D. Political science. *Johns Hopkins Magazine.* 2004;56(5).

74. U.S. General Accounting Office. Needle exchange programs: Research suggests promise as an AIDS prevention strategy. March 1993. Report no. GAO/HRD-93-60.

75. Lurie P, Reingold AL, Bowser B et al. The public health impact of needle exchange programs in the United States and abroad: Summary, conclusions, and recommendations. Prepared by the School of Public Health, University of California–Berkeley, and the Institute for Health Policy Studies, University of California–San Francisco, for the Centers for Disease Control (CDC). October 1993. Available at: http://www.caps.ucsf.edu/pubs/reports/pdf/NEPReportSummary1993.pdf. Accessed in June 2007.

76. Experts blast Shalala on needle exchange remarks. *AIDS Alert.* 1996;11(3): 33–34.

77. U.S. Department of Health and Human Services. Press release: Research shows needle exchange programs reduce HIV infections without increasing drug use. Issued April 20, 1998. Available at: http://www.hhs.gov/news/press/1998pres/980420a.html. Accessed in June 2007.

78. Pear R. Inquiry confirms top Medicare official threatened actuary over cost of drug benefits. *New York Times.* July 7, 2004.

79. Pear R. New White House estimate lifts drug benefit cost to $720 billion. *New York Times.* February 9, 2005.

80. Jacoby M. EU chemicals proposal prompts global mobilization led by U.S. *Wall Street Journal.* June 27, 2006:A6.

81. SourceWatch. C. Boyden Gray. 2006. Available at: http://www.sourcewatch.org/index.php?title=C._Boyden_Gray. Accessed in June 2007.

82. World Health Organization. Diet, nutrition, and the prevention of chronic diseases: Report of a joint WHO/FAO expert consultation. Geneva, Switzerland, 2003.

83. Steiger WR (special assistant to the Secretary for International Affairs, U.S. Department of Health and Human Services). Letter to Lee JW (director general, WHO). January 5, 2004. Available at: http://www.commercialalert.org/bushadmincomment.pdf. Accessed in June 2007.

84. Dyer O. U.S. government rejects WHO's attempts to improve diet. *BMJ.* 2004;328(7433):185.

85. Dyer O. United States wins more time to lobby against WHO diet plan. *BMJ.* 2004;328(7434):245.

86. Avorn J (professor of medicine, Harvard Medical School, and chief, Division of Pharmacoepidemiology and Pharmacoeconomics, Brigham and Women's Hospital). Letter to Rep. Waxman H (D-CA-30). May 25, 2006. Available at: http://www.democrats.reform.house.gov/Documents/20060626111957–56484.pdf. Accessed in June 2007.

87. U.S. House Committee on Governmental Reform, minority staff. Prescription for harm: The decline in FDA enforcement activity (report prepared for Rep. Waxman HA). June 2006. Available at: http://www.democrats

.reform.house.gov/Documents/20060627101434-98349.pdf. Accessed in June 2007.

88. Goozner M. FDA seeking early retirements. GoozNews [blog]. June 23, 2006. Available at: http://www.gooznews.com/archives/000432.html. Accessed in June 2007.

89. Union of Concerned Scientists, Public Employees for Environmental Responsibility. U.S. Fish and Wildlife Service Survey Summary. 2005. Available at: http://www.ucsusa.org/scientific_integrity/interference/us-fish-wildlife-service-survey.html. Accessed in June 2007.

90. Union of Concerned Scientists. Summary of National Oceanic & Atmospheric Administration Fisheries Service Scientist Survey. 2005. Available at: http://www.ucsusa.org/scientific_integrity/interference/survey-political-interference-at-noaa-fisheries.html. Accessed in June 2007.

91. Emergency Planning and Community Right-to-Know Act. Public law no. 99-499, 1986.

92. Graham M. Regulation by shaming. *Atlantic Monthly.* 2000;285(4):36-40.

93. Alert: EPA proposes rollback on toxic pollution reporting. *OMB Watch.* 2005;6(20). Available at: http://www.ombwatch.org/article/articleview/3117/1/396. Accessed in June 2007.

94. U.S. Environmental Protection Agency. Toxics Release Inventory (TRI) Program. TRI chemical list changes (1987-2005). Available at: http://www.epa.gov/triinter/chemical/ChemListChanges05.pdf. Accessed in June 2007.

95. Society of the Plastics Industry, Inc. Comments on the Toxics Release Inventory burden reduction proposed rule. *Fed. Reg.* October 4, 2005; 70:57822. January 12, 2006. Submitted to Docket EPA-HQ-TRI-2005-0073. Document no. EPA-HQ-TRI-2005-0073-1958.1.

96. National Association of Manufacturers. Comments on Toxics Release Inventory burden reduction: Proposed rule. January 10, 2005. Docket no. EPA-HQ-TRI-2005-0073. Document no. EPA-HQ-TRI-2005-0073-3022.

97. Edison Electric Institute. Comments on "Toxics Release Inventory burden reduction proposed rule." January 13, 2006. Docket no. EPA-HQ-TRI-2005-0073. Document no. EPA-HQ-TRI-2005-0073-2720.1.

98. Synthetic Organic Chemical Manufacturers Association (SOCMA). Comments on the Toxics Release Inventory burden reduction proposed rule (10/04/05, 70 FR 57822). January 13, 2005. Docket no. EPA-HQ-TRI-2005-0073.

99. U.S. Environmental Protection Agency. Toxics Release Inventory burden reduction final rule. *Fed. Reg.* 2006;71(246):76932-45.

100. Downey K. U.S. drops report on mass layoffs. *Washington Post.* January 2, 2003:D11.

101. Schemo DJ. Nation's charter schools lagging behind, U.S. test scores reveal. *New York Times.* August 17, 2004.

102. Schemo DJ. U.S. cutting back on details in data about charter schools. *New York Times.* August 29, 2004.

103. Krugman P. The great wealth transfer. *Rolling Stone.* November 30, 2006.

104. Glasser SB. Annual terror report won't include numbers. *Washington Post.* April 19, 2005:A17.

105. Rood J. Bush admin won't release Iraq attack numbers. TPM Muckraker .com [blog]. Available at: http://www.tpmmuckraker.com/archives/002169 .php. Accessed in July 2007.

106. Levey NN, Zavis A. U.S. drops Baghdad electricity reports. *Los Angeles Times.* July 27, 2007.

107. Mervis J. Climate sensors dropped from U.S. weather satellite package. *Science.* 2006;312(5780):1580.

108. Mervis J. NOAA loses funding to gather long-term climate data. *Science.* 2005;307(5707):188.

CHAPTER SIXTEEN

1. U.S. Department of Energy; Office of Environmental Management. Closing the circle on the splitting of the atom: The environmental legacy of nuclear weapons production in the United States and what the Department of Energy is doing about it. January 1995. Report no. DOE/EM-0266.

2. Groves LM. *Now It Can Be Told: The Story of the Manhattan Project.* New York: Da Capo, 1962.

3. Smyth HD. *Atomic Energy for Military Purposes: The Official Report on the Development of the Atomic Bomb under the Auspices of the United States Government, 1940–1945.* Princeton, NJ: Princeton University Press, 1945.

4. Robinson GO. *The Oak Ridge Story: The Saga of a People Who Share in History.* Kingsport, TN: Southern Publishers, 1950.

5. O'Neill K. Building the bomb. In: Schwartz SI, ed. *Atomic Audit: The Costs and Consequences of U.S. Nuclear Weapons since 1940.* Washington, DC: Brookings Institution Press, 1998:33–104.

6. Dean G. *Report on the Atom: What You Should Know about the Atomic Energy Program of the United States.* New York: Knopf, 1953.

7. Makhijani A, Schwartz SI, Weida WJ. Nuclear waste management and environmental remediation. In: Schwartz SI, ed. *Atomic Audit: The Costs and Consequences of U.S. Nuclear Weapons since 1940.* Washington, DC: Brookings Institution Press, 1998:353–94.

8. Norris RS, Kosiak SM, Schwartz SI. Deploying the bomb. In: Schwartz SI, ed. *Atomic Audit: The Costs and Consequences of U.S. Nuclear Weapons since 1940.* Washington, DC: Brookings Institution Press, 1998:105–96.

9. U.S. Department of Energy, Highly Enriched Uranium Working Group. Environmental, safety, and health vulnerabilities associated with the depart-

ment's storage of highly enriched uranium; December 1996. Report no. DOE/EH-0525.

10. U.S. Department of Energy, Plutonium Working Group. Environmental, safety, and health vulnerabilities associated with the department's plutonium storage; November 1994. Report no. DOE/EH-0415.

11. Hacker BC. *The Dragon's Tail: Radiation Safety in the Manhattan Project, 1942–1946.* Los Angeles: University of California Press, 1987.

12. Franklin JC (Manager, Oak Ridge Operations) to Wilson CL (General Manager, Washington). Subject: Medical Policy. September 26, 1947. Available at: http://www.defendingscience.org/upload/Franklin_1947.pdf. Accessed in December 2007.

13. ChemRisk, Inc. Task 2 Report- Mercury Releases from Lithium Enrichment at the Oak Ridge Y-12 Plant- A Reconstruction of Historical Releases and Off-Site Doses and Health Risks. Submitted to the Tennessee Department of Health. July 1999.

14. National Research Council. Toxicological effects of methylmercury. Washington, DC: National Academy Press, 2000.

15. Magnuson E. They lied to us: Unsafe, aging U.S. weapons plants are stirring fear and disillusion. *Time.* October 31, 1988:60–65.

16. U.S. Department of Energy, Office of Environmental Management, Depleted Uranium Hexafluoride Management Program. Overview of Depleted Uranium Hexafluoride Management Program. Fall 2001.

17. Anigstein R, Thurber WC, Mauro JJ et al. (S. Cohen and Associates, under contract no. 1W-2603-LTNX with U.S. Environmental Protection Agency, Office of Radiation and Indoor Air). Technical support document: Potential recycling of scrap metal from nuclear facilities. Part 1: Radiological assessment of exposed individuals. Vol. 1, 2001. Chapter 4: Quantities and characteristics of potential sources of scrap metal from DOE facilities and commercial nuclear power plants. Available at: http://www.epa.gov/radiation/docs/cleanmetals/tsd/scrap_tsd_041802_ch4.pdf. Accessed in June 2007.

18. U.S. Department of Energy Top-to-Bottom Review Team. Review of the Environmental Management Program. February 4, 2002.

19. Memorandum from Wilson CE (chief, Insurance Branch, AEC) to Vallado AC (deputy declassification officer, Declassification Branch, AEC). Re: Review of document by Knowlton. December 20, 1948. Available at http://www.defendingscience.org/upload/Wilson_1948.pdf. Accessed in December 2007.

20. Michaels D. In memorium: Thomas F. Mancuso, MD, MPH (1912–2004). *Am J Ind Med.* 2005;47(1):1–3.

21. Mancuso TF, Stewart AM, Kneale GW. Radiation exposures of Hanford workers dying from cancer and other causes. *Health Physics.* 1977;33:369–85.

22. Kneale GW, Mancuso TF, Stewart AM. Hanford radiation study 3: A cohort study of the cancer risks from radiation to workers at Hanford (1944–1977 deaths) by the method of regression models in life-table. *Br J Ind Med.* 1981;38:156–66.

23. Kneale GW, Mancuso TF, Stewart AM. Identification of occupational mortality risks for Hanford workers. *Br J Ind Med.* 1984;41:6–8.

24. Kneale GW, Mancuso TF, Stewart AM. Job-related mortality risks of Hanford workers and their relation to cancer effects of measured doses of external radiation. *Br J Ind Med.* 1984;41:9–14.

25. President's Advisory Committee on Human Radiation Experiments. Chapter 10: Atomic veterans: Human experimentation in connection with atomic bomb tests. *The Human Radiation Experiments: The Final Report of the President's Advisory Committee.* New York: Oxford University Press, 1996.

26. Radiation-exposed Veterans Compensation Act. Public law no. 100–321, May 20, 1988.

27. Orphan Drug Act. Public law no. 97–414, January 4, 1983.

28. Report of the National Institutes of Health ad hoc Working Group to Develop Radioepidemiology Tables. 1985.

29. Eisenbud M. *An Environmental Odyssey: People, Pollution, and Politics in the Life of a Practical Scientist.* Seattle, WA: University of Washington Press, 1990.

30. Ball H. *Justice Downwind: America's Atomic Testing Program in the 1950s.* New York: Oxford University Press, 1986.

31. Udall SL. *The Myths of August.* New York: Pantheon, 1994.

32. Radiation Exposure Compensation Act (RECA). Public law no. 101–426, October 15, 1990.

33. Parascandola M. Uncertain science and a failure of trust: The NIH radioepidemiologic tables and compensation for radiation-induced cancer. *Isis.* 2002;93:559–84.

34. Janofsky M. 111 uranium miners left waiting as payments for exposure lapse. *New York Times.* March 27, 2001:A1.

35. Michaels D (assistant secretary for Environment Safety and Health, Department of Energy). Memorandum to Minsk R (National Economic Council). Subject: Work products from interagency working groups. March 31, 2000.

36. Warrick J. Paducah workers sue firms; class action cites radiation exposure, seeks $10 billion. *Washington Post.* September 4, 1999:A1.

37. Warrick J. Administration sides with workers in uranium factory suit. *Washington Post.* May 31, 2003:A2.

38. U.S. Department of Energy, Office of Environment, Safety, and Health. Phase 2 independent investigation of the Paducah gaseous diffusion plant: Environment, safety, and health practices, 1952–1990. February 2000.

39. Memorandum to the files of Dunham CL (director, Division of Biology and Medicine, AEC) and Bruner HD (chief, Medical Research Branch,

Division of Biology and Medicine, AEC). Subject: Neptunium^{237} contamination problem, Paducah, Kentucky, February 4, 1960; filed March 11, 1960. Available at: http://www.defendingscience.org/upload/Paducah_1960.pdf. Accessed in December 2007.

40. U.S. Department of Energy, Office of Environment Safety and Health. Independent investigation of the Portsmouth gaseous diffusion plant. Vol. 1: Past environment, safety, and health practices. May 2000.

41. U.S. Department of Energy, Office of Environment, Safety, and Health. Independent investigation of the East Tennessee Technology Park. Vol. 1: Past environment, safety, and health practices. October 2000.

42. Transcript: U.S. Department of Energy public meeting with assistant secretary of Energy, Dr. David Michaels, for employees of the Portsmouth gaseous diffusion plant. Comfort Inn, Piketon, OH. October 31, 1999.

43. Transcript: U.S. Department of Energy public hearing—injured [Los Alamos National Laboratory] workers. Northern New Mexico Community College, Espanola, NM. March 18, 2000.

44. Transcript: U.S. Department of Energy public meeting: Workers' Compensation initiative [for Pantex Plant employees]. Civic Center Grand Plaza, Amarillo, TX. June 29, 2000.

45. Energy Employees Occupational Illness Compensation Program Act (EEOICPA). Public law no. 106–398, October 30, 2000.

46. Government Accountability Office. Department of Energy, Office of Worker Advocacy: Deficient controls led to millions of dollars in improper and questionable payments to contractors. May 2006. Report no. GAO-06-547.

47. Office of Sen. Grassley C (R-IA). Press release: Grassley urges Senate conferees to support changes to Energy Employee Occupational Illness Compensation Program. Issued September 14, 2004. Available at: http://grassley.senate.gov/index.cfm?FuseAction=PressReleases.Detail&PressRelease_id=147&Month=9&Year=2004. Accessed in July 2007.

48. Ronald W. Reagan National Defense Authorization Act for Fiscal Year 2005: Part 4, Division C, Subtitle E: Energy Employees Occupational Illness Compensation Program. Public law no. 108–375, October 28, 2004.

CHAPTER SEVENTEEN

1. Mintz M. *At Any Cost: Corporate Greed, Women, and the Dalkon Shield.* New York: Pantheon, 1985.

2. Hicks K. *Surviving the Dalkon Shield IUD: Women v. the Pharmaceutical Industry.* New York: Teachers College Press, 1994.

3. Mundy A. *Dispensing with the Truth: The Victims, the Drug Companies, and the Dramatic Story behind the Battle over Fen-Phen.* New York: St. Martin's Press, 2001.

4. Marshall E. Buried data can be hazardous to a company's health. *Science.* 2004;304:1576–77.
5. Nissen SE, Wolski K. Effect of rosiglitazone on the risk of myocardial infarction and death from cardiovascular causes. *NEJM* 2007;356: 2457–71.
6. Psaty BM, Furberg CD. Rosiglitazone and cardiovascular risk. *NEJM* 2007;356:2522–4.
7. Vernick JS, Mair JS, Teret SP et al. Role of litigation in preventing product-related injuries. *Epidemiol Rev.* 2003;25(1):90–98.
8. Transportation Recall Enhancement, Accountability, and Documentation (TREAD) Act. Public law no. 106–414, November 1, 2000.
9. Public Citizen, Safetyforum.com. The real root cause of the Ford-Firestone tragedy: Why the public is still at risk. April 2001. Available at: http://www.citizen.org/documents/rootcause.pdf. Accessed in June 2007.
10. Conrad JW Jr. Open secrets: The widespread availability of information about the health and environmental effects of chemicals. *Law and Contemporary Problems.* 2006;69(3):141–65.
11. Givelber DJ, Robbins A. Public health vs. court-sponsored secrecy. *Law and Contemporary Problems.* 2006;69(3):131–39.
12. Felcher EM. *It's No Accident: How Corporations Sell Dangerous Baby Products.* Monroe, ME, and Philadelphia, PA: Common Courage Press, 2001.
13. Anderson JS. Hidden from the public by order of the court: The case against government-enforced secrecy. *SC Law Rev.* 2004;55:711–59.
14. Casey M. OSHA: Discounted lives. *Kansas City Star.* December 11, 2005:A1.
15. Barab J. *Kansas City Star* clobbers OSHA. Confined Space Blog. December 12, 2005. Available at: http://spewingforth.blogspot.com/2005/12/kansas-city-star-clobbers-osha.html. Accessed in June 2007.
16. Barab J. What's more effective? OSHA penalties or suing the bastards? Confined Space Blog. February 2, 2006. Available at: http://spewingforth.blogspot.com/2006/02/whats-more-effective-osha-penalties-or.html. Accessed in June 2007.
17. Vladeck DC. Federal preemptions of state tort law: The problem of medical drugs and devices: Preemption and regulatory failure. *Pepp L Rev.* 2005; 33:95–131.
18. Levin M, Miller AC. Industries get quiet protection from lawsuits. *Los Angeles Times.* February 19, 2006.
19. Sharkey CM. Preemption by preamble: Federal agencies and the federalization of tort reform. *DePaul Law Review.* 2007;56.
20. Associated Press. Vioxx judge finds FDA approval of drug label doesn't avert claims. *Wall Street Journal* (online). July 3, 2007.
21. Tesoriero HW. Merck's Vioxx troubles may ebb with ruling poised to aid defense. *Wall Street Journal.* April 13, 2007:A3.

CHAPTER EIGHTEEN

1. Dyckman LJ (Director, Food and Agriculture Issues, Resources, Community, and Economic Development Division, U.S. General Accounting Office). Testimony before the Subcommittee on Oversight of Government Management, Restructuring, and the District of Columbia; Committee on Governmental Affairs, U.S. Senate. Food Safety: U.S. needs a single agency to administer a unified, risk-based inspection system. August 4, 1999. Report no. GAO/T-RCED-99-256.

2. Americans growing less confident in FDA's job on safety, poll shows. *Wall Street Journal* (online). May 24, 2006.

3. World Health Organization. Fact sheet no. 187: Air pollution. September 2000. Available at: http://www.who.int//inf-fs/en/fact187.html. Accessed in July 2007.

4. Merton RK. Priorities in scientific discovery: A chapter in the sociology of science. *Amer Soc Rev.* 1957;22(6):635–59.

5. American Competitiveness and Corporate Accountability Act (also known as the Sarbanes-Oxley Act). Public law no. 107–204, 2002.

6. Union of Concerned Scientists. Restoring scientific integrity in policymaking [letter]. 2006. Available at: http://www.ucsusa.org/scientific_integrity/interference/scientists-signon-statement.html. Accessed in June 2007.

7. Davidoff F, DeAngelis CD, Drazen JM et al. Sponsorship, authorship, and accountability. *JAMA.* 2002;286(10):1232–34.

8. Michaels D, Wagner W. Disclosure in regulatory science. *Science.* 2003;302(5653):2073.

9. S. 2812. Proposed amendments to the Federal Food, Drug, and Cosmetic Act. Introduced November 4, 1971, by Sen. Nelson G (D-WI).

10. Krimsky S. *Science in the Private Interest: Has the Lure of Profits Corrupted Biomedical Research?* Lanham, MD: Rowman and Littlefield, 2003.

11. Guerrero PF (director; Environmental Protection Issues; Resources, Community, and Economic Development Division; U.S. General Accounting Office). Testimony before the Subcommittee on Toxic Substances, Research, and Development; Committee on Environment and Public Works, U.S. Senate. Toxic Substances Control Act: EPA's limited progress in regulating toxic chemicals. May 17, 1994. Report no. GAO/T-RCED-94-212.

12. Stephenson JB (Director, Natural Resources and Environment, U.S. Government Accountability Office). Testimony before the Committee on the Environment and Public Works, U.S. Senate). Chemical regulation: Options are needed to improve the effectiveness of EPA's Chemical Review Program. August 2, 2006. Report no. GAO-06-1032T.

13. Environmental Defense Fund. Toxic ignorance: The continuing absence of basic health testing for top-selling chemicals in the United States.

1997. Available at: http://www.environmentaldefense.org/documents/243 _toxicignorance.pdf. Accessed in July 2007.

14. U.S. Environmental Protection Agency. Chemical hazard data availability study: What do we really know about the safety of high production volume chemicals? April 1998.

15. U.S. Environmental Protection Agency. 267 unsponsored chemicals. November 30, 2006. Available at: http://www.epa.gov/chemrtk/pubs/general/ hpvunspn.pdf. Accessed in July 2007.

16. European Commission. The new EU chemicals regulation: REACH (Registration, Evaluation, and Authorisation of Chemicals). 2006. Available at: http://ec.europa.eu/enterprise/reach/overview_en.htm. Accessed in June 2007.

17. Toxic Substances Control Act. Public law no. 94–469. 1976.

18. Office of the Special Inspector General for Iraq Reconstruction. Interim audit report on inappropriate use of proprietary data markings by the Logistics Civil Augmentation Program (LOGCAP) contractor. October 26, 2006. Report no. SIGIR-06-035.

19. Jasanoff S. Transparency in public science: Purposes, reasons, limits. *Law and Contemporary Problems.* 2006;69(3):21–45.

20. Wagner W, Michaels D. Equal treatment for regulatory science: Extending the controls governing the quality of public research to private research. *Am J Law Med.* 2004;30:119–54.

21. Krewski D, Burnett RT, Goldberg M et al. Reanalysis of the Harvard Six Cities Study. Part 1: Validation and replication. *Inhal Toxicol.* 2005;17 (7–8):335–42.

22. Neutra RR, Cohen A, Fletcher T et al. Toward guidelines for the ethical reanalysis and reinterpretation of another's research. *Epidemiology.* 2006; 17(3):335–38.

23. U.S. Small Business Administration, Office of Advocacy. Small Business Regulatory Enforcement Fairness Act of 1996 (overview). 2002.

24. Committee on Ensuring the Best Presidential and Federal Advisory Committee Science and Technology Appointments, National Academy of Sciences, National Academy of Engineering, Institute of Medicine. Science and technology in the national interest: Ensuring the best presidential and federal advisory committee science and technology appointments. Washington, DC: National Academies Press, 2005.

25. Departments of Labor, Health and Human Services, and Education, and Related Agencies Appropriations Act, 2006, §5519. Public law no. 109–149, December 30, 2005.

26. Steinbrook R. Financial conflicts of interest and the Food and Drug Administration's advisory committees. *NEJM.* 2005;353(2):116.

27. U.S. Food and Drug Administration. Draft guidance for the public, FDA advisory committee members, and FDA staff on procedures for

determining conflict of interest and eligibility for participation in FDA advisory committees; Availability. [Notice]. *Fed. Reg.* 2007;72(56): 13805.

28. Marchione M. Groups question doctors' ties to drug firms: Federal cholesterol guidelines promoted by physicians paid by private companies prompt conflict concerns. *Associated Press.* October 17, 2004. Available at: http:// www.commondreams.org/headlines04/1017-08.htm. Accessed in July 2007.

29. International Agency for Research on Cancer. IARC Monographs on the Evaluation of Carcinogenic Risks to Humans: Preamble. January 2006.

30. Brandeis LD. *Other People's Money and How the Banks Use It.* New York: Stokes, 1914.

31. Graham M. Regulation by shaming. *Atlantic Monthly.* 2000;285(4):36–40.

32. U.S. Department of Energy. Press release: Los Alamos National Lab cited for nuclear safety violations. Issued September 8, 1999.

33. OSHA. Air contaminants: Final rule. *Fed. Reg.* 1993;58:35338–51.

34. Barab J. Wild animals? Lock the cage—even if there's no OSHA standard. Confined Space Blog. January 18, 2006. Available at: http://spewingforth .blogspot.com/2005/01/wild-animals-lock-cage-even-if-theres.html. Accessed in June 2007.

35. Worker critical after bear attacks. *Chicago Sun Times.* September 13, 2004.

36. AFL-CIO. *Death on the Job: The Toll of Neglect. A National and State-by-State Profile of Worker Safety and Health in the United States.* 16th ed. April 2007. Available at: http://www.aflcio.org/issues/safety/memorial/upload/ doj_2007.pdf. Accessed in July 2007.

37. Food Quality Protection Act. Public law no. 104–170. August 3, 1996.

38. Wigle DT, Lanphear BP. Human health risks from low-level environmental exposures: No apparent safety thresholds. *PLoS Med.* 2005;2(12): 1232–34.

39. Lanphear BP, Hornung R, Khoury J et al. Low-level environmental lead exposure and children's intellectual function: An international pooled analysis. *Environ Health Perspect.* 2005;113(7):894–99.

40. World Health Organization–Europe. Health aspects of air pollution: Results from the WHO project "Systemic Review of Health Aspects of Air Pollution in Europe." June 2004. Available at: http://www.euro.who.int/ document/E83080.pdf. Accessed in June 2007.

41. National Research Council. Health risks from exposure to low levels of ionizing radiation: BEIR VII Phase 2 (2006). Washington, DC: National Academies Press, 2006.

42. U.S. Department of Energy. DOE occupational radiation exposure: 2001 report. Report no. DOE/EH-0660.

43. Takahashi W, Wong L, Rogers BJ et al. Depression of sperm counts among agricultural workers exposed to dibromochloropropane and ethylene dibromide. *Bull Environ Contam Toxicol.* 1981;27(4):551–58.

44. Epidemiologic notes and reports: Human lead absorption—Texas. *Morbidity and Mortality Weekly Report.* 1997;46(37):871–77.

45. Associated Press. BP's Texas City refinery nation's top polluter. May 7, 2006.

46. Barstow D, Bergman L. At a Texas foundry, an indifference to life. *New York Times.* January 8, 2003.

47. Barstow D, Bergman L. Family's profits, wrung from blood and sweat. *New York Times.* January 9, 2003.

48. Barstow D, Bergman L. Deaths on the job, slaps on the wrist. *New York Times.* January 10, 2003.

49. U.S. Department of Justice. Press release: McWane, Inc., and company executive plead guilty and McWane sentenced for environmental crimes. Issued February 8, 2006. Available at: http://www.usdoj.gov/opa/pr/2006/February/06_enrd_065.html. Accessed in June 2007.

50. California Office of Environmental Health Hazard Assessment. Proposition 65: Safe Drinking Water and Toxic Enforcement Act of 1986. Available at: http://www.oehha.ca.gov/prop65/law/P65law72003.html. Accessed in July 2007.

51. Mendelson N. Bullies along the Potomac. *New York Times.* July 5, 2006.

52. H.R. 4167. National Uniformity for Food Act. Introduced October 27, 2005, by Rep. Rogers MJ (R-MI-8).

53. Wilson MP. Green chemistry in California: A framework for leadership in chemicals policy and innovation. California Policy Research Center at the University of California for the California Senate Environmental Quality Committee and the California Assembly Committee on Environmental Safety and Toxic Materials; 2006. Available at: http://coeh.berkeley.edu/news/06_wilson_policy.htm. Accessed in June 2007.

Index

abortion, 206
abstinence, 205
accountability, 252–53
accounting, 243, 244
acroosteolysis, 35, 36
ACS. *See* American Cancer Society
Action on Smoking and Health, 83
addiction, 3, 10, 90
Administrative Procedures Act, 254
advertising, 5, 10, 90, 208
advisory committees, 193–95, 196
AEC. *See* Atomic Energy Commission
AFL-CIO, 83
A.H. Robbins (co.), 233
AIDS. *See* HIV/AIDS
AidsVax, 151
air pollution, 31, 43, 46, 50, 56–57, 62,
    85, 176–77, 242, 252, 261
ALARA (as low as reasonably achievable),
    260–61
Alberts, Bruce, 188
Aleve. *See* naproxen
Allied Chemical and Dye Corporation,
    21, 27, 28, 92–94, 100

alternative compensation programs, 237–38
Amarillo (Tex.), 227–28
American Association for the Advancement
    of Science, 188, 195
American Association of Medical
    Colleges, 188
American Beverage Association, 48
American Cancer Society (ACS), 6, 7, 87
American Chemistry Council, 189
American Competitiveness and Corporate
    Accountability Act. *See* Sarbanes-
    Oxley
American Conference of Governmental
    Industrial Hygienists, 15
American Home Products, 171
American Journal of Disease in Children, 39
American Medical Association, 6, 89,
    158, 206
American National Standards Institute, 97
American Petroleum Institute (API), 41,
    48, 70, 74–77, 201
American Public Health Association,
    188, 195
American Trucking Association, 120

357

junk science, xi–xii, 57–58, 122, 164, 179, 197, 202
juries, 161, 166–68, 172

Kaiser Permanente, 154
Kass, Leon, 196
Kassirer, Jerome, 166, 171
Kennedy, Donald, 189, 193, 195
Kennedy, John F., 29
Kennedy, Ted, 228
Kessler, David, 156
Keusch, Gerald, 196
Key, Marcus, 36
Koop, C. Everett, 10, 89
Kornegay, Horace, 79
Kovacs, William, 180
Krimsky, Sheldon, 247
Kumbo Tire Co. v. Carmichael, 164, 169
Kweder, Sandra, 160
Kyoto Accords, 199

labor unions, 32
Lanphear, Bruce, 192
Lanza, Anthony, 13–14
Lasker, Mary, 7
lawsuits, 233–34, 236–37
lead, 31, 35, 261
Lead-based Paint Poisoning Prevention Act, 39
lead-based paints, 38–40
leaded gasoline, 23–24, 40–44
Lead Industries Associaton, 39
lead poisoning, xi, 38–44, 192–93
Lempert, Richard O., 168
leukemia, 62–63, 66–67, 70–73, 75, 77, 203, 218, 219
Levy, Paul, 50
lie detector test, 162
life insurance, 13
lifespan, 4, 7
Lilley, Floy, 58
liquor, 51
lithium, 215
litigation avoidance, 234
Little, Clarence Cook, 7
liver, 34–35, 66, 155, 160
Lockheed Martin, 48, 56, 224, 225

London Principles, 88
Loomis, Dana, 194
López, Pete, 227
Lorain (Ohio), 125, 134, 135
Los Alamos (N.M.), 213, 217, 226–27, 257–58
Love Canal, 30, 51
lung cancer
  and asbestos, 16, 17, 50, 61, 62, 66, 82, 177, 232, 242
  and beryllium, 128, 130, 132, 139, 141
  and carbon black, 55
  and chromium, 54, 98–100, 102, 104–7, 253
  and exposure to PCBs, 163, 166
  and radon, 220
  and smoking, 4, 5, 9, 50, 66, 80, 82, 87, 177, 232
  and uranium, 221
lung disease, 110–19, 221, 247
Luntz, Frank, xi, 197–98, 201
Lurie, Peter, 102, 159, 207

Machle, Willard, 125, 127
MacMahon, Brian, 130, 132, 141
malaria, 20, 202
Maltoni, Cesare, 35, 36
mammals, 67
Mancuso, Thomas, 27, 36, 98, 100, 104, 128, 129, 217–18
Manhattan Institute, 164
Manhattan Project, 124–25, 213
manufactured uncertainty, x, 124, 137, 140
Manufacturing Chemists Association, 93
Marathon Oil, 77
Markowitz, Gerald, 35, 38, 39
Marshall, Ray, 130
Marshall Islands, 218
Martin Marietta (co.), 224
Massachusetts, 126
mattress flammability, 239
mauve, 20
Maxcy, Margaret, 58
Mazzocchi, Tony, 113
McGarity, Tom, 169, 183

New Mexico, 219
Nexium, 159–60
Niagara Falls (N.Y.), 30, 92, 93–94
nicotine, 3, 10, 90
9/11 terrorist attack, 238
NIOSH. *See* National Institute for
    Occupational Safety and Health
Nissen, Steven, 233
nitrogen dioxide, 31
Nixon, Richard, 30, 31, 33, 39, 43
NOAA. *See* National Oceanic and
    Atmospheric Administration
nonexclusive compensation scheme, 237–38
nonsteroidal anti-inflammatory drugs
    (NSAIDs), 143, 145, 146, 149
North Dakota Lignite Research Council,
    50
Novartis, 27
NSAIDs. *See* nonsteroidal anti-
    inflammatory drugs
Nuclear Regulatory Commission, 228–29
nuclear weapons, 125, 140, 196, 212, 214,
    215, 220, 257–58, 259
nuclear weapons workers, x, xii, 122, 125,
    212, 214, 217–31, 236, 237, 261

Oak Ridge (Tenn.), 213, 214, 215, 223–26
obesity, 48, 56, 208, 209
Occidental Chemical, 31–32
Occupational Safety and Health
    Administration (OSHA)
    and benzene exposure standards, 71,
        73–76
    beryllium standard, 126, 131, 138–39,
        140
    and chromium standards, 97–110, 253
    creation of, 30, 258
    ergonomics standard, 121, 123, 195
    move to regulate benzidine, 91, 94
    and "popcorn lung," 110–19, 234
    possible conflict of interest in studies,
        246
    regulation of corporations, 232
    risk assessments, 69, 99
    and smoking, 3, 50, 80, 83–85, 90
    standards, 31–32, 70, 97–100, 120–23,
        174, 234, 242, 254, 258

and state governments, 263
    surrender to special interests, 202
    vinyl chloride exposure levels, 36, 37, 45
    weakness of chemical hazard regulation,
        241
Occupational Tumors and Allied Diseases
    (Hueper), 24
Office of Management and Budget
    (OMB), ix, 178, 180, 183–90, 225
Oil, Chemical, and Atomic Workers
    Union, 43, 91, 99, 222
oil industry, 72, 73, 77, 78, 201–2, 262
oil refineries, 72, 73, 77
OMB. *See* Office of Management and
    Budget
omeprazole, 159–60
Ong, Elisa, 58
optic neuropathy, 171
ortho-toluidine (OT), 92–94, 96
Orville Redenbacher popcorn, 118
Orwell, George, xi
OSHA. *See* Occupational Safety and
    Health Administration
OT. *See* orthotoluidine
Oxford University, 148
Oxley, Michael, 244
ozone, 31, 45

Pachauri, Rajendra, 199
Pacific Gas and Electric, 52
Paducah (Ky.), 213, 216, 225–26
pain, 146
paint, 38–40
Pantex (co.), 227
Parkinson's disease, 49
Parlodel, 171–72
Parmet, Allan, 110, 114
particulate matter, 31, 57
patents, 243
Patterson, Clair, 41, 42
Paustenbach, Dennis, 51, 52, 74–75, 76,
    100, 103, 138, 193
Paxil, 233
PCBs (polychlorinated biphenyls), 30, 52,
    163, 166, 248
peer review, 53–55, 57, 181, 183–90, 199
Pennsylvania, 221

Switzerland, 21, 22, 28
Syngenta (co.), 49
synthetic rubber. *See* rubber hydrochloride

TASSC. *See* The Advancement of Sound
    Science Coalition
tax cuts, 211
"taxicab standard," 125–27, 129
Taylor, Michael, 188
Teller, Edward, 212
terrorism, 211
tetraethyl lead. *See* ethyl
Thacker, Paul, 49
The Advancement of Sound Science
    Coalition (TASSC), 58, 85
think tanks, 55–56
Thompson, Tommy, 194, 195, 196, 209
Thoreau, Henry David, 29
Thurmond, Strom, 228
Time magazine, 30, 215
Times Beach (Mo.), 51
tire defects, 233–34
Titanic, 239
titanium, 39
tobacco industry, 38, 50
    advertising, 5, 10, 90
    civil litigation in, 30
    and Data Quality Act, 178–79, 190, 191
    defense of secondhand smoke, 79–90,
        133, 177
    denials of health hazards, 4
    doubt as strategy of, x, 3–11
    and expert witnesses, 173
    and health, 6–10
    and press, 5
    science of, 79–82, 84, 86, 90
    sequestering of data, 242
Tobacco Industry Research Committee,
    6, 7, 10, 127
Torkelson, Theodore, 32, 34
tort reform, 164, 235
toxic chemicals, 32–33, 46, 208, 210, 214,
    242, 247–50, 258, 264
toxicity, 249–51, 261–63, 264
toxicology studies, 67
Toxic Substances Control Act (TSCA),
    30, 247–51

toxic tort cases, 163, 164, 236
Tozzi, Jim, 58, 88, 179, 180
trade secrets, 250
Traditional Values Coalition, 206
Treasury Department, 211
Trenberth, Kevin, 211
Trichopoulos, Dimitrios, 135, 141
Trigg, Bruce, 205–6
Trudeau Sanatorium, 14
TSCA. *See* Toxic Substances Control Act
Tsuji, Joyce, 192

Udall, Stewart, 220
Udall, Tom, 220
Union Carbide, 210, 224, 225
Union of Concerned Scientists, 210, 244
United Food and Commercial Workers, 115
United Parcel Service, 120, 122
University of California, 86, 207, 227, 258
University of Michigan, 35
Upjohn Company, 94
uranium, 213, 214, 216, 219–21, 225–26,
    230–31
uranium hexafluoride, 216
U.S. Chamber of Commerce, 174, 182, 189
Utah, 220, 226

vaccines, 237
Vanity Fair, 4
VaxGen (co.), 151
vehicle rollovers, 239
Veneman, Ann, 188
ventricular arrhythmia, 171
Viagra, 145
Vidmar, Neil, 168
vinyl chloride, 34–37, 45, 66, 175
Viola, Pierluigi, 35
Vioxx, 146–49, 153–55, 157, 160, 240,
    255–56
Vladeck, David, 239
Voinovich, George, 226

Wagner, Wendy, 246
Walden (Thoreau), 29
Wall Street Journal, 52, 130
Warner-Lambert, 155
Warren, Christian, 42